UNITED STATES SENATE

ELECTION, EXPULSION AND CENSURE CASES

1793–1990

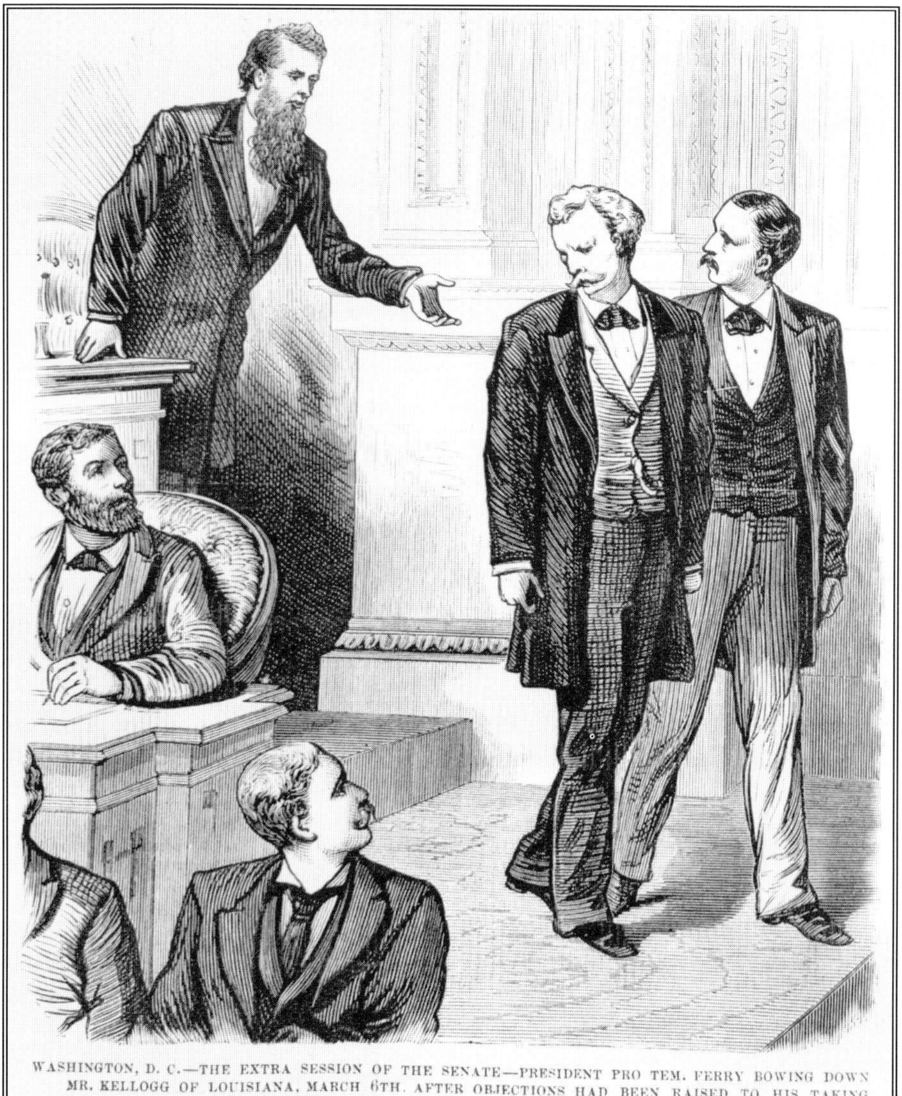

WASHINGTON, D. C.—THE EXTRA SESSION OF THE SENATE—PRESIDENT PRO TEM. FERRY BOWING DOWN MR. KELLOGG OF LOUISIANA, MARCH 6TH. AFTER OBJECTIONS HAD BEEN RAISED TO HIS TAKING THE OATH OF OFFICE. — FROM SKETCHES BY OUR SPECIAL ARTISTS, ALBERT BERGHAUS AND HARRY OGDEN.

A SENATOR BEING DENIED THE OATH OF OFFICE WHILE HIS CREDENTIALS ARE SENT TO COMMITTEE *(See Case 63). From Frank Leslie's Illustrated Newspaper, March 24, 1877. U.S. Senate Collection*

United States Senate
Election, Expulsion and Censure Cases
1793–1990

by
Anne M. Butler and Wendy Wolff
U.S. Senate Historical Office

Prepared under the direction of
Sheila P. Burke
Secretary of the Senate

Washington: Government Printing Office

103d Cong., 1st sess.
S. Con. Res. 6
U.S. Senate

Senate Document 103–33
U.S. Government Printing Office
Washington: 1995

Supt. of Docs. No.: 052–071–01127–7

Library of Congress Cataloging-in-Publication Data

Butler, Anne M., 1938–
Senate election, expulsion, and censure cases from 1793 to 1990 / by Anne M. Butler and Wendy Wolff ; prepared under the direction of Sheila P. Burke.
p. cm.
Rev. ed. of: Senate election, expulsion, and censure cases from 1793 to 1972. 1972.
Includes bibliographical references and index.
1. United States. Congress. Senate—Contested elections—Digests.
2. United States. Congress. Senate—Expulsion—Digests. 3. United States. Congress. Senate—Censures—Digests. I. Wolff, Wendy. II. Burke, Sheila P. III. Senate election, expulsion, and censure cases from 1793 to 1972.
IV. Title.
KF4976.A2 1995 95–35521
328.73'073—dc20 CIP

For sale by U.S. Government Printing Office
Superintendent of Documents, Mail Stop: SSOP, Washington, DC 20402–9328

Contents

and scholarly articles about the senators involved, as well as broader studies of the era in question. For those who wish to review the Senate documents for a case, citations are again included to committee reports and to the *Congressional Globe* or *Congressional Record* accounts of the relevant debates.

Some of the cases that appeared in the earlier publications have been dropped from the present volume. Election cases are included if either the full Senate or a Senate committee took some action on the matter. The criteria for including disciplinary cases prior to 1964 are the same. Starting in 1964, when the Select Committee on Standards and Conduct was established (followed in 1977 by its successor the Select Committee on Ethics), disciplinary cases are included only if one of these committees filed a report recommending that the Senate act or if the full Senate took some action. Because the case numbers used in this volume thus differ from those used in the 1962 and 1972 books, a cross reference is included in Appendix D showing both the old and new case numbers.

In 1982 the secretary of the Senate assigned the Senate Historical Office responsibility for updating this volume. Over the following two years, Anne M. Butler, now a member of the department of history at Utah State University, thoroughly researched more than 160 of the original cases. She examined hundreds of primary source documents to capture the historical context and political complexity of each case. Her narrative description comprises the major portion of this compilation.

In 1985, the Historical Office took on several major publication projects associated with the Senate's forthcoming two-hundredth anniversary commemoration. These obligations caused this project to be set aside until the early 1990s. Work resumed under the editorial direction of Wendy Wolff, who reviewed and updated each case where necessary, prepared the introduction, devised an organizational structure to permit quick identification of comparable cases, and edited the entire volume. Essential assistance was also provided by current and former Historical Office staff Richard A. Baker, Kathryne Bomberger, Diane Boyle, Ellen T. McDougall, Jo Anne McCormick Quatannens, Donald A. Ritchie, Matthew Schwartz, and Elizabeth Strannigan.

Sheila P. Burke
Secretary of the Senate

Introduction

The United States Constitution gives each house of Congress the power to be the judge of the "elections, returns, and qualifications of its own members" and to "punish its members for disorderly behavior" (Article I, section 5). Over its more than two-hundred-year history, the Senate has jealously guarded this prerogative. The body has therefore developed its own procedures for judging the qualifications of its members in contested elections and for taking disciplinary action against members through such measures as formal censure or actual expulsion from the Senate. By far the largest number of the 141 cases in this book deal with election contests; only about 41 of them relate to the Senate's disciplinary power.

I. Elections

Senators serve for six-year terms. The Constitution in Article I, section 3, states that the Senate should be divided as equally as possible into three classes, so that one-third of the Senate will be chosen every two years. Until 1913, senators were elected by the legislatures of their respective states; since the Seventeenth Amendment became part of the Constitution, senators have been elected by direct popular vote. Under both the new and the old system, the Constitution permits state governors to make temporary appointments to fill Senate vacancies. Election disputes reviewed by the Senate have fallen into several general categories, including the form of the credentials presented and the conduct of the election. During the sectional conflicts prior to the Civil War, and in the war's aftermath as the former Confederate states sought to return to the Union and send senators to Washington, questions often arose regarding the legality of the legislature carrying out the election. Later in the nineteenth century and into the early twentieth century, corrupt use of money in elections became an issue, and the resulting public furor contributed to the eventual adoption of the Seventeenth Amendment. Since that time, campaign expenditures, demands for recounts in close elections, and complaints of election irregularities or outright fraud have constituted the dominant issues.

Election Laws

The laws governing Senate elections have evolved slowly over time. The Constitution simply states that "The Times, Places and Manner of holding Elections for Senators and Representatives, shall be prescribed in each State by the Legislature thereof; but the Congress may at any time by Law make or alter such Regulations" (Article I, section 4). For almost eighty years, the Senate left the supervision of senatorial elections entirely in the hands of the state legislatures. After frequent and flagrant abuses, however, Congress decided to exercise its constitutional prerogative to impose some order on the process.

1866 Act

In the years just before and during the Civil War, the Democratic and Republican parties within state legislatures matured to the point that they could hold their members to party discipline, leaving less room for compromise. As a result, a party caucus was often able to prevent an election from being completed until the caucus members could agree on a candidate to support. One frequent stalling tactic was for the upper chamber of a legislature to block a U.S. Senate election by refusing to send a quorum of its members to a joint assembly of the two houses. To prevent this abuse, Congress in 1866 passed an act governing election of senators that established rules for a joint assembly in which the two houses of a legislature lost their individual character and merged into a unique body to elect a U.S. senator.[1] By stipulating that the joint assembly took jurisdiction over an election only after one house had failed to elect, the Senate ended the right of the two houses to act separately when stalemated and instead encouraged them to complete the election through the joint assembly. Because the terms of state legislatures varied and there had been cases of a later legislature seeking to override a senatorial election carried out by its predecessor, the law stipulated specifically that the election be carried out by "the legislature of each state which is chosen next preceding the expiration of the time for which any senator was elected to represent such state in Congress." The election was to begin on "the second Tuesday after the meeting and organization" of that legislature. The act then outlined the manner in which the legislature was to conduct the election. Provision was also made for filling vacancies by a similar election.

Reconstruction Acts (1867–1868)

At the close of the Civil War, the Union needed to develop a process for readmitting the former Confederate states. The initial phase of Reconstruction under presidents Abraham Lincoln and Andrew Johnson sought to return the seceding states to the Union as quickly as possible. During this period, from 1865 to 1867, states were required simply to ratify the Thirteenth Amendment abolishing slavery and to swear allegiance to the Union. It soon became apparent, however, that former Confederates were being elected to state and local office in governments that did little to protect the rights of the recently freed slaves. In fact, many states adopted black codes that forbade

[1] An Act to regulate the Times and Manner of holding Elections for Senators in Congress, 14 Stat. 243, Ch. 245 (1866).

African American citizens to vote or hold office, and incidents of violence against both blacks and white unionists proliferated throughout the South. As a result, some states, which in 1866 had adopted new constitutions that repudiated secession but failed to provide adequate rights and safeguards for the freedmen, found that the House and Senate refused to admit the representatives and senators they sent to Washington.

Increasingly, Republicans in Congress began to assert themselves on Reconstruction issues. In December 1865, Congress established the Joint Committee of Thirteen on Reconstruction, and in the 1866 elections, Radical Republicans gained sufficient strength in both houses to override presidential vetoes on such legislation as renewal of the Freedmen's Bureau. Then, in 1867 and 1868, over President Johnson's veto, Congress passed a series of Reconstruction acts, setting forth new, more stringent requirements to be met before states could be accepted back into the Union. These criteria included ratification of the Fourteenth Amendment, which ensured citizenship for blacks. The amendment also disqualified from holding state or federal office those former Confederates who had held government posts before the war and thus had violated their oath to uphold the Constitution. States were again placed under military control and required to adopt new constitutions allowing black citizens to vote. Once a state had satisfactorily complied with these requirements and had also ratified the Fifteenth Amendment guaranteeing black suffrage, Congress would pass a law specifically returning the state to representation in the House and Senate. In 1866, Tennessee became the first state readmitted under this procedure, followed in June 1868 by Alabama, Arkansas, Florida, Louisiana, North Carolina, and South Carolina. Georgia, Mississippi, Texas, and Virginia returned to the Union in 1870.

Campaign Finance Laws (1883–1911)

The laws governing the financing of federal election campaigns have evolved slowly. In the late nineteenth century the use of large sums of money in senatorial campaigns became a public concern, as rumors circulated about bribery of state legislators during elections. In response, Congress gradually began adopting laws to regulate the way campaigns were paid for. The 1883 Civil Service Act[2] forbade coercion of contributions from federal employees, and Federal Corrupt Practices acts passed in 1910 and 1911[3] required first political committees and then House and Senate candidates to file reports of contributions and expenditures to let the public know who was paying for campaigns. The laws also placed a $10,000 limit on the amounts of their own money Senate candidates could spend on campaigns.

---

[2] 22 Stat. 403 (1883).

[3] 36 Stat. 822, Ch. 392 (1910); 37 Stat. 25, Ch. 33 (1911).

Direct Election (1913)

While the 1866 law helped to avoid some of the types of disputes that had arisen previously, it turned out not to be a panacea. Deadlocks in state legislatures continued to cause long vacancies in some Senate seats, sometimes lasting a year or more, because of a failure to complete an election. In such cases, the state was deprived of its full representation in the Senate. The number of these deadlocks increased toward the turn of the twentieth century, with a total of forty-five occurring between 1891 and 1905. According to George H. Haynes, who studied the senatorial election process, the law's fatal flaw consisted in its insistence on election by a majority rather than a plurality of the votes. Small factions were thus able to withhold their support in close races to prevent an election until a candidate met their demands. This problem, combined with an increase in the corrupting use of money in Senate elections, led progressive reformers to press for a system of direct popular election of senators.[4]

The initial steps were taken by individual states. In 1904 Oregon adopted a "direct primary nominating elections law," a popular referendum in which the voters could express a preference among Senate candidates. Although the results were not legally binding, in practice state legislators were inclined to follow the popular mandate when they formally elected a senator. When the system appeared to work effectively, other states followed suit. After years of struggle, Congress in May 1912 finally adopted the Seventeenth Amendment providing that senators be elected by the people of a state. Ratification by the states took less than a year, and the amendment became part of the Constitution in May 1913.

Campaign Finance Laws (1921–1979)

Once senators began to be elected by direct popular vote, Congress took further steps to regulate campaign financing, although for a number of years these rules could only apply to general elections, because in 1921 the Supreme Court ruled in *Newberry* v. *United States* (256 U.S. 232) that Congress had no power to regulate primary elections. This decision arose when Truman Newberry appealed his court conviction for campaign financing violations at the time the Senate was also reviewing his election (See Case 102).

The 1925 Federal Corrupt Practices Act[5] expanded the reporting requirements established by the earlier laws and set ceilings on expenditures by Senate and House candidates. It prohibited the solicitation of contributions from federal employees by either candidates or other federal

---

[4] George H. Haynes, *The Election of Senators* (New York, 1906); U.S., Congress, Senate, *The Senate, 1789-1989: Addresses on the History of the United States Senate,* by Robert C. Byrd, vol. 1, S. Doc. 100-20, 100th Cong., 1st sess., 1988, Chapter 21.

[5] 43 Stat. 1053, Ch. 368 (1925).

employees. It also forbade national banks and corporations to contribute to political campaigns. Although the law contained penalties, there were no provisions for enforcement, and the Senate only blocked the seating of members when excessive expenditures were coupled with evidence of fraud and corruption (Cases 109, 110).

The Hatch Act passed in 1939[6] prohibited federal employees from participating actively in national politics and forbade collecting political contributions from individuals receiving federal relief funds. Amendments to this act adopted in 1940[7] added federal contractors to those forbidden to contribute to campaigns and limited the amounts that could be given to a federal candidate or political committee in a single year. Ending the ban that had existed since 1921, that law also specifically authorized Congress to regulate any primary elections that nominated candidates for federal office. The Supreme Court upheld this position the next year in *United States* v. *Classic et al.* (313 U.S. 299), and in 1947 the Taft-Hartley Act[8] prohibited corporations, national banks, and labor organizations from contributing to candidates in primary as well as general elections.

In the 1970s the whole manner of regulating federal election campaigns changed with adoption of the comprehensive Federal Election Campaign Act (FECA) in 1971[9], followed by amendments in 1974 and 1976. Among its provisions, the 1971 law required House and Senate candidates to file reports of contributions and expenditures with the clerk of the House or secretary of the Senate. The 1974 FECA amendments[10] limited contributions and expenditures and created the Federal Election Commission (FEC) to enforce campaign finance laws, but two years later the Supreme Court in *Buckley* v. *Valeo* (424 U.S. 1) ruled that both spending limits and the manner of selecting the members of the FEC were unconstitutional. The 1976 amendments[11] therefore changed the way the FEC members were chosen and set limits on contributions to political action committees. Since that time, the courts and the Federal Election Commission have handled campaign financing violations, while the Senate has remained responsible for reviewing the contested elections of its members.[12]

---

[6] The Clean Politics Act, 53 Stat. 1147 (1939).

[7] 54 Stat. 767 (1940).

[8] The Labor-Management Relations Act of 1947, 61 Stat. 136.

[9] 86 Stat. 3 (1971).

[10] 88 Stat. 1263 (1974).

[11] 90 Stat. 475 (1976).

[12] In 1969 Congress passed the Federal Contested Elections Act (83 Stat. 284, Public Law 91-138), but it applied only to House races.

Senate Election Procedures and Committees

Procedures

As it considered election cases over the years, the Senate developed a series of informal precedents to guide its actions. For example, if a senator-elect arrived with credentials that appeared valid on their face and were signed by the proper state authorities, that individual would be permitted to take his seat even if a challenge to the election had been filed with the Senate.

Generally, a senator with the proper credentials against whom a challenge had been filed would be seated "without prejudice." Under this arrangement, if a committee investigation later determined that for some reason the individual was not entitled to a seat, he could be "excluded" from the Senate by a simple majority vote, as opposed to having to be expelled, which required a two-thirds majority. On six occasions, the Senate excluded by majority vote a member who had originally been seated.[13] In at least two cases (Case 91, 123), the Senate voted to require a two-thirds vote to unseat the senator, but in those instances, not even a simple majority voted in favor of exclusion. In a few such instances, election cases hovered on the edge of becoming disciplinary cases when the body considered whether the allegations were serious enough to actually expel an individual or whether only exclusion was warranted. Examples included charges of election corruption (Cases 102, 117) and complaints about the actions of a member before he entered the Senate (Case 123).

Opponents sometimes sought to block a senator's seating by filing allegations with the Senate that the member-elect had engaged in possible criminal or immoral behavior before being elected. Such charges often originated with political adversaries back in the state, and usually the Senate did no more than refer the matter to a committee for a cursory investigation, on the theory that members should only be required to meet the three basic constitutional qualifications of age, residency, and citizenship (Cases 3, 33, 60, 93, 111, 120).

The Senate did take seriously charges of bribery and corruption in a member's election. The investigations of such allegations sought not only to determine whether the transgressions occurred but also whether the senator knew about or participated in them, and whether enough votes were affected to change the outcome. If the Senate determined that the member was unaware of the bribery or if it affected only a small number of votes, the body usually permitted the individual to keep his seat.

Challengers sometimes contended that, if the winning candidate was ineligible for some reason, the runner-up should be declared the winner. As

[13] Albert Gallatin, 1794, citizenship (Case 1); James Shields, 1849, citizenship (Case 21); James Harlan, 1857, election irregularities (Case 29); John P. Stockton, 1865, election irregularities (Case 47); William Lorimer, 1912, campaign corruption (Case 95); and Smith W. Brookhart, 1926, ballot recount (Case 105).

the Privileges and Elections Committee pointed out in an 1872 case (Case 59), this was apparently true under English law, where the votes for an ineligible candidate were not counted and the candidate with the next highest number of votes was declared elected. The practice in the United States, however, was to declare such an election void, rather than to grant the seat to a competitor, and the Senate held consistently to this precedent.

On five occasions (Cases 24, 79, 109, 110, 114) a participant in an election contest who had not been seated as a senator was permitted to address the Senate (one of these did not take advantage of the permission), but setting that precedent made most members uncomfortable. In several other instances contestants were allowed seats as observers on the Senate floor (Cases 4, 137, 138).

In the period after adoption of direct popular election under the Seventeenth Amendment, the Senate faced unfamiliar types of election challenges that required different approaches, and the body gradually developed new standards for handling such cases. For example, the Senate did not wish to step in where legal action in the federal or state courts was appropriate, and it seldom took very seriously the claims of a contestant who had failed to follow these avenues of redress. Similarly, when a losing candidate demanded a recount of ballots, the Senate preferred to become involved only if the state law made no provision for such a recount or after the contestant had exhausted all recourse at the state level. Where a state was equipped to conduct the recount, the Senate left the responsibility to the state. Still, in some cases the Senate felt impelled to act, and the sealed ballot boxes were shipped to Washington, where staff members, carefully observed by representatives of both candidates, scrutinized the ballots and election records for possible irregularities (Cases 102, 103, 105, 109, 114, 132, 137).

Committees

Until the mid-nineteenth century, the Senate referred contested election cases to committees specially appointed for the purpose. Then, from the 1850s to the 1870s, the Judiciary Committee reviewed such cases. Faced with the overwhelming volume of complicated election cases during Reconstruction, the Senate in March 1871 created a Committee on Privileges and Elections, apparently to relieve the burden on the Judiciary Committee, which had legislative duties to carry out. The Senate leadership offered no reasons on the Senate floor for establishing the new committee, probably because the matter was overshadowed at the time by an intense controversy over deposing Charles Sumner (R-MA) from the chairmanship of the Foreign Relations Committee that he had held for the past decade. Because Sumner had angered President Ulysses S. Grant and the secretary of state by opposing their proposed annexation of Santo Domingo, the Republican caucus had removed Sumner from Foreign Relations and instead made him chair of the new Committee on Privileges and Elections. Sumner angrily declined to serve in that post, even though one of those recommending the change declared during the heated Senate debate that Privileges and Elections was "the most important committee in the Senate."[14] As a result, when the new committee began its work later that month, William M. Stewart (R-NV) served as chairman.

The Committee on Privileges and Elections handled most contested elections until after World War II. Originally consisting of seven members, the panel expanded to nine in the mid-1870s, and by the early 1900s it had fifteen members. While there was considerable turnover from year to year, about half the members would remain from one Congress to the next to provide continuity. Few served on the committee for more than four or five years, but George F. Hoar (R-MA) devoted more than two decades to the panel, and Eli Saulsbury (D-DE) served for twelve years.

Beginning in the 1920s and continuing until the 1950s, the Senate often expressed its concern about the way campaigns were financed by establishing a special committee to review campaign expenditures in a particular election year. Occasionally, these special committees supplemented the work of the Committee on Privileges and Elections by reviewing the financial aspects of disputed elections (Cases 109, 110, 117, 126). Although the Senate usually only reviewed cases formally brought before it by the filing of an election contest or charges of campaign irregularities from the state, the special campaign expenditure committees had authority to look into matters they learned about through such informal means as newspaper articles.

In 1947, when the Legislative Reorganization Act[15] consolidated Senate committees and jurisdictions, Privileges and Elections ceased to be a separate committee and became a subcommittee under the Committee on Rules and Administration. While the Senate abolished that subcommittee in 1977, the full committee continues to be responsible for contested election cases.

Types of Election Cases

Qualifications

In determining whether to seat a member-elect, the Senate must look not only at the credentials signed by the governor that certify the election but also at whether the individual meets the three qualifications set forth in the Constitution: to be at least thirty years old, a citizen of the United States for nine years, and an inhabitant of the state from which elected (Article I, section 3). Because these requirements are clear and straightforward, few candidates who fail to meet them have run for and won election to the Senate, but in a few instances challenges have been raised and sustained. In 1794 and again in 1849, the Senate unseated members who had not been

[14] U.S., Congress, Senate, *Congressional Globe,* 42d Cong., 1st sess., pp. 43-53.

[15] 60 Stat. 812 (1946).

U.S. citizens for the requisite nine years (Cases 1, 21). When the first black senator presented his credentials in 1871, his citizenship was challenged, but the Senate disagreed and seated him (Case 54). A variation on the citizenship theme occurred when senators presented themselves from a state that had not yet officially been admitted to the Union, as with two senators from Tennessee in 1796 (Case 4) and a senator from Minnesota in 1858 (Case 32). A residence case arose in 1870 when opponents questioned whether the former military governor of Mississippi should in fact be considered a resident of the state (Case 53).

One of the most notorious cases dealing with qualifications was that of Reed Smoot, a prominent official in the Mormon church, who was seated but forced to undergo a highly public four-year investigation into whether his position in the church should disqualify him from serving in the Senate. Calls for religious tolerance eventually won out, and Smoot was permitted to retain his seat (Case 91).

Although in the early nineteenth century three senators were sworn in before the age of thirty, no objections were raised. The only instance in which age became an issue occurred in 1935, when a senator elected at the age of twenty-nine waited to be sworn in until his thirtieth birthday several months after Congress convened, and the losing candidate unsuccessfully challenged his qualifications (Case 119). In an instance where the mental health of a member-elect was at issue, the Senate wisely avoided ruling on that question (Case 19). Occasionally, a state claimed that a senator did not meet some further requirement added by the state to represent it in the Senate, for example, a mandate that state officers wait a year after the end of their terms before accepting any other office, but the Senate rejected such claims (Cases 28, 77).

The Civil War brought a new complication when one senator also served as a general in the Union army in violation of the constitutional provision that "no Person holding any Office under the United States, shall be a Member of either House during his Continuance in Office" (Article I, section 6). Still, in the heightened patriotism of the early years of the war, the Senate winked at the breach and allowed the member to retain his seat. (Case 35)

Conduct of Election (Legislatures)

Charges of irregularities in the conduct of elections varied widely. They included allegations that state legislators were bribed, charges that one house of the legislature did not have a quorum present when the election was held, or claims that other state statutory requirements had not been met. In one challenged election (Case 13) the winning candidate, as a member of the state legislature, had cast the deciding vote for himself. In another case, the speaker of the state senate, who had succeeded to the governorship on the death of the governor, still participated in the election as a legislator and cast the deciding vote (Case 84). On several occasions, a later legislature would send a new senator to contest a seat already held by an incumbent, claiming that it, rather than its predecessor body, actually had the right to elect (Cases 14, 30). A number of senators in the late nineteenth and early twentieth century were charged with actual corruption and bribing state legislators in their elections (Cases 65, 72, 75, 86, 89, 96, 97). If the Senate found adequate proof, it had two options: to expel the miscreant or declare the election void (Cases 61, 95).

Reconstruction

Attempts to seat senators from the former Confederate states returning to the Union after the Civil War posed a series of particularly complex dilemmas for the Senate, leading to nineteen of the cases in this book (Cases 44–46, 48–59, 62, 63, 66–68). The confusing period when the rebellious states scrambled for readmission saw many contradictions and inconsistencies in Senate action. Former Confederate states, once happy to renounce any association with the Union, now argued that they had never left and insisted on restoration of all their political rights and privileges within the national government. Unionists, on the other hand, who had consistently denied the validity of secession, began to demonstrate an increasing reluctance to admit representatives from these states until their loyalty could be assured. Complex constitutional issues, intensified by political partisanship and sectional enmity, led to lengthy and heated Senate debates.

In the late 1860s, the Republican party gained power in most southern states, with strong support from the newly enfranchised black voters. Many Republican officials were "carpetbaggers" who had emigrated from northern states before, during, or after the war. Others were southern "scalawags" who had supported the Union. The debates that raged over seating the senators from the newly restored states involved a variety of issues, including questions of the individual's loyalty and activities during the war (Cases 48, 49, 59), the procedures or makeup of the state legislature that elected the claimant, and whether the state had adequately fulfilled the prerequisites for readmission. Beneath the often heated and lengthy discussions ran an undercurrent of bitter partisan and intraparty conflict over the rights of blacks and the form that Reconstruction should take.

As a result, beginning in 1868 and continuing through the 1870s, the number of contested election cases handled by the Senate exploded from one or two cases a year to as many as five or six contests to be considered simultaneously. Because of this heavy workload, many cases took as long as three or four years to resolve, and one multiple-claimant case from Louisiana (Case 63) lasted for seven years. As is noted in the text, the resolution of one case was sometimes affected by a decision reached a few days earlier in another contest, with the Senate attempting to be consistent in its actions. In several instances, the Senate ruled that, when Congress passed an act readmitting a state to representation under the Reconstruction acts, it was also approving the legislature under which the state was accepted for readmission. By upholding the make-up of a given legislature, the Senate declared, it was also retroactively accepting all actions taken by that legislature, including any senatorial elections it might have conducted before the state was formally readmitted to the Union (Cases 55 and 58).

During each of the phases of Reconstruction, former Confederates were required to swear a loyalty oath in order to hold office or vote. Under Presidents Lincoln and Johnson, the oath simply pledged future loyalty to the Constitution, thus permitting many former Rebels to hold public office. Radical Republicans in Congress, however, preferred use of the "ironclad test oath," first adopted in 1862, which required all federal officeholders, in addition to swearing future loyalty, to swear that they had never voluntarily borne arms against the United States, had given no aid or encouragement to those fighting against the Union, and had never accepted any office "under any authority in hostility... to the United States." In an 1866 case (Case 48), the Senate insisted that a member from one of the former Confederate states must be able to swear this oath, setting the pattern for the admission of senators from the remaining southern states. As a result of this determination, the 1867 Reconstruction acts required all federal officeholders to swear the ironclad oath. In the 1871 case of a former Confederate surgeon who had been a noncombatant (Case 52), the Senate made an exception to this policy and adopted a joint resolution stipulating that the member-elect could omit the part of the oath relating to past actions and simply swear future loyalty to the United States. This joint resolution, passed by the House and signed by the president, marked a unique instance in which the House played a role in the seating of a senator. When the Senate had tried a similar approach in an earlier case (Case 48), the House refused to adopt the resolution, and the Senate then decided that the individual must swear the oath.

Beginning in the early 1870s, a new series of contested elections arose in Alabama, Louisiana, and South Carolina in a backlash by white supremacist Democrats against often corrupt Radical Republican control. Amid violence, intimidation of black voters, and charges of corruption, state elections produced competing legislatures, each claiming to have elected a U.S. senator. In such cases, the Senate undertook to determine which was the legitimate legislature, a departure from its usual practice not to interfere in any matter that was a state prerogative. The topic, however, represented a dangerous quagmire, for often so many irregularities surrounded the formation of each of the two rival legislatures, that the Senate, in the words of one committee report, was forced "to choose between the form [the group that had the credentials] and the substance [those who had actually been elected]" (Case 62). Since the decisions ultimately reached were usually partisan, the nature of the outcomes varied with the gradual change in the balance of power within the Senate. In fact, the body faced a flood of these time-consuming and complex cases at a time when the Republican majority was losing its dominance. A dozen contested elections related to Reconstruction came before the body between 1869 and 1877, as the party's lead slipped from an overwhelming margin of 50 seats to only 5. Then, in 1879, the Democratic party took control of the Senate, and allegations of voter intimidation that would have blocked a senator's seating a few years before no longer proved decisive. In the early 1880s the weary members allowed the final Reconstruction contests to drift to easy conclusions that were not necessarily consistent with the more stringent actions taken earlier.[16]

As Reconstruction ended in the 1880s, the Senate returned to its previous practice of seating a challenged senator-elect whose valid credentials indicated that a recognized state legislature had conducted the election according to the procedures set forth in the 1866 election act.

Conduct of Election (Direct Election)

Although direct election ended the confusing contests arising from elections by state legislatures, there was still no shortage of contested elections. Several in the early 1920s dealt with charges of excessive campaign expenditures or fraud and corruption. The earlier allegations of bribing state legislators were replaced with complaints of stuffed ballot boxes and irregular election procedures. Other common charges included registration rolls that carried names of nonresidents and deceased persons, irregular voting and ballot-counting procedures, and failure to file required financial reports. Close elections often led to calls for ballot recounts, either by the state or by the Senate.

While the Senate's review of contested elections in most cases did not change the outcome, in several notable instances the body actually overturned the results of the election. In 1926, after conducting a full recount of ballots, the Senate unseated one senator and declared that the challenger had been elected (Case 105). Also in the 1920s, evidence of excessive campaign expenditures and pervasive corruption led the Senate to refuse to seat either contender in two cases (Cases 109, 110). Nearly half a century later in 1975, after months of partisan bickering over the results of a close New Hampshire contest, the Senate declared the seat vacant, and the state held a new election (Case 137).

Vacancies

Some of the most difficult election disputes involved senators appointed by the governors of their states to fill vacancies while the state legislatures were out of session. The seemingly straightforward language of the Constitution, "if vacancies happen . . . during the recess of the Legislature of any State, the Executive thereof may make temporary appointments until the next meeting of the Legislature, which shall then fill such vacancies"

[16] In 1884 Congress finally repealed the requirement of the ironclad oath.

(Article I, section 3), turned out in practice to be far from simple when political conflicts arose. The ambiguity of the rules left the actual practice open to the influence of politics. Opponents of a particular individual or party—either in the home state or within the Senate—could bring a procedural challenge that was often decided by a party-line vote.

Before 1913 the appointment lasted only until the next meeting of the legislature. Under direct election, the appointment lasts until a special election can be held to fill the remainder of the term. Prior to direct election, questions often arose when a legislature met and failed to elect a candidate before the commencement of a Senate term. On such occasions, the state's governor frequently appointed an individual to serve until the legislature could succeed in completing an election, so that the state would not be left without full senatorial representation. The Senate struggled for years to establish a clear precedent regarding the validity of such appointments. Between 1794 and 1893, it reviewed at least nine such cases, seating all but two of the claimants. In 1893, the Senate reversed its previous practice and refused to seat three western senators (Case 82), in part from concern about how the new members might vote on legislation pending at the time. The Senate then followed the precedent of this case in denying admission to two other appointed senators in the 1890s (Cases 85, 88).

The advent of direct election ended this particular dilemma, but questions regarding appointments continued to arise for several years, because the Seventeenth Amendment states that "the legislature of any state may empower the executive thereof to make temporary appointments." Challenges to several appointed senators hinged on whether the state's legislature had in fact adopted a measure bestowing the power on the governor (Cases 98, 99, 108). After 1926, the only challenges to appointments related to conditions in the specific case, such as the appointee's qualifications (Case 134), when an appointment should terminate (Case 120), or whether an incoming or outgoing governor had the right to make the appointment (Case 124).

II. Discipline

Procedures, Laws, and Committees

As with the contested election cases, the Senate's policies and procedures for disciplining its members evolved over the years. In the earliest disciplinary incident, in 1796, the Senate decided that investigations of charges should follow correct judicial procedures, and, since the individual, who had been charged with committing perjury before his election to the Senate (Case 3), had been neither indicted nor convicted for the offense, there was no reason to carry out an inquiry. The next year, however, the Senate established the precedent that it need not wait for any action by the courts before expelling a member (Case 5), and ten years later, the Senate further emphasized its independence of the judicial process by continuing its own investigation even after an acquittal by the courts (Case 7). During the debates on these 1797 and 1807 cases, the Senate permitted the member in question to be actively represented by defense counsel, but in subsequent cases, the Senate refused to allow nonsenators to participate in floor discussions.

In general, the Senate has taken disciplinary action against a member only for misdeeds committed while serving in the body, rather than for matters that occurred previously and has moved particularly decisively on matters that fall entirely within its jurisdiction, such as infractions of Senate rules. Sometimes, even though a senator charged in newspaper reports with wrongdoing requested a formal inquiry to clear his name, the Senate declined to refer the matter to a committee. Such incidents not referred to committee do not appear in this book but have been chronicled in the earlier editions described in the Preface.

No federal statutes specifically governed the behavior of members of Congress until 1853, when a law forbade senators and representatives to accept bribes or to receive compensation for presenting claims before federal agencies. The law also barred from public office "forever" any government official convicted of receiving a bribe.[17] An 1864 law set penalties of fine and imprisonment for members who were illegally paid for providing services before a federal agency.[18] No further laws governing senators' conduct were added until 1958 when Congress adopted a code of ethics applicable to all federal employees.[19] Although this code had no force of law, it urged officials to uphold high standards of performance and not to accept favors or benefits designed to influence the performance of their governmental duties.

During the nineteenth century, the Senate generally referred disciplinary cases to committees specially appointed for the purpose. Although most

[17] 10 Stat. 170, Ch. 81 (1853).

[18] 13 Stat. 123 (1864).

[19] H. Con. Res. 175, 85th Cong., 2d sess.

of the Civil War expulsion cases were not referred to committees at all, several went to the Committee on the Judiciary. In the twentieth century until the 1960s, the Privileges and Elections Committee (or after 1947 that subcommittee of the Rules and Administration Committee) handled most censure or expulsion cases. A major change in the modern era occurred with creation in 1964 of a permanent Select Committee on Standards and Conduct that was empowered to investigate allegations of wrongdoing without waiting for specific referral by the Senate.[20] Composed of an equal number of Republican and Democratic senators to ensure bipartisanship, the committee, in addition to handling disciplinary cases, was charged with preparing a code of conduct for U.S. senators, in order to provide a formal set of standards for senatorial behavior. The code that it drafted and that the Senate adopted in 1968 regulated outside employment and some aspects of campaign fundraising, including the purposes for which campaign contributions could be used, a topic that had caused difficulties in one case the committee handled (Case 135). The code also required senators and top staff members to file annual financial disclosure reports, although they were not to be made public.[21]

After the Watergate scandal aroused further public concern about political ethics, the Senate in 1977 adopted a new code of conduct that required public financial disclosure and restricted outside employment.[22] It also limited to 15 percent of a senator's salary the amount that could be earned in outside income (although the Senate later rescinded that provision). The outside income limit was aimed particularly at perceived conflicts of interest that could arise when senators accepted large payments of honoraria in return for speaking to organizations that had an interest in legislation before Congress. Not until 1991 did the Senate entirely ban the acceptance of honoraria.[23]

The 1977 code of conduct also replaced the Committee on Standards and Conduct with a permanent Select Committee on Ethics, whose membership would also be equally divided between the parties. The newly constituted committee established a several-stage process to be followed in each inquiry, including careful safeguards designed to protect the rights of the member in question. Credible information about a possible ethical violation could trigger a "preliminary inquiry," followed if appropriate by an "initial review" to determine whether evidence warranted moving to the next stage. If four of the six committee members voted that there was sufficient evidence, the committee could then undertake a full "investigation," which must permit the individual to appear at a hearing and call and cross-examine

[20] S. Res. 338, 88th Cong., 2d sess.

[21] S. Res. 266, 90th Cong., 2d sess.

[22] S. Res. 110, 95th Cong., 1st sess.

[23] Legislative Branch Appropriations Act, 105 Stat. 447 (1991).

witnesses. A recommendation for disciplinary action by the committee again required a vote of four committee members to ensure that the decision had bipartisan support. The committee had authority to hire an outside counsel if it determined that one was needed.

In 1978 Congress passed the Ethics in Government Act that applied the public financial disclosure requirements to all three branches of the federal government.[24] A decade later, the 1989 Ethics Reform Act restricted lobbying by former members of Congress and executive branch officials for a year after leaving office and placed limits on the value of gifts that senators and staff could accept.[25]

As it reviewed cases in the 1980s and 1990s, the Ethics Committee continued to develop and refine its procedures and may adopt further changes in the future. Some senators, for example, have expressed concern about the committee's multiple role as prosecutor, judge, and jury, but as of this writing the body has yet to agree on a better arrangement. Because the committee may conduct investigations without specific referral from the Senate, it has reviewed a substantial number of possible transgressions that have been called to its attention but have not warranted taking formal action. Even when the committee has held public hearings, *such cases are not included in this volume if the panel has issued no formal report calling for action by the full Senate.*

Types of Disciplinary Cases

In disciplining its members, the Senate has two basic forms of punishment available to it: to expel a senator by a two-thirds vote, as provided in the Constitution (Article I, section 5) or, by a majority vote, to censure a member for less serious misconduct.

Expulsion

In all its history, the United States Senate has managed to muster the necessary two-thirds vote to expel one of its members on only fifteen occasions, all of them involving disloyalty to the United States. In 1797 William Blount of Tennessee became the first senator to be expelled, because of his involvement in a conspiracy that the Senate determined to be "inconsistent with his public trust" (Case 5). The remaining fourteen expulsions occurred during the Civil War for disloyalty to the Union. Initially, when southern states began seceding in the early months of 1861, the Senate was perplexed and uncertain how to handle the unfamiliar circumstance. After the first six senators, led by Jefferson Davis of Mississippi, withdrew from the Senate in January, the body could not agree on any action, finally voting in March simply to declare the seats vacant, in order to avoid officially recognizing that it

[24] 92 Stat. 1824 (1978).

[25] 103 Stat. 1716 (1989).

was possible for a state to secede from the Union (Case 34).[26] By July, however, war was in progress, and the Senate moved quickly to expel ten other senators whose states had left the Union (Case 36). In December 1861 and January 1862, the body expelled an additional four members who were known to have taken positions in the Confederate army or appeared to have offered aid and comfort to the enemy (Cases 38, 39, 40).

The Senate has considered expulsion in an additional sixteen instances, on charges that include corruption, disloyalty, or abuse of official position but has cleared many of these members after an investigation. Ten senators have been indicted while in office, but only three were convicted (the conviction of one other was later overturned by the Supreme Court). In such instances, the Senate continued to act independently of the courts, sometimes exonerating senators before their cases came to trial (Case 104). Because of the severity of the punishment in expulsion cases, however, the Senate usually waited for the courts to act and only considered expelling those who were actually convicted, even though the body recognized that its members could be held to a higher standard than obedience to the law. In at least one instance (Case 92), the Senate even waited for the appeals process to be completed before preparing to move against the individual. In fact, the Supreme Court's 1906 decision upholding the conviction in that case specifically stated that conviction "did not operate, ipso facto, to vacate the seat of the convicted Senator nor compel the Senate to expel him or to regard him as expelled by force alone of the judgment" (*Burton* v. *United States*, 202 U.S. 344). In other words, it remained the Senate's duty to carry out its own discipline of the erring member, quite apart from any sentence imposed by the courts. Two of the senators whose convictions were not overturned chose to resign before the body could act on expulsion (Cases 92, 140).[27]

Censure

A less severe sanction employed by the Senate against its members is censure. Although this measure has no tangible effect on a senator's ability to hold his office, such a formal statement of disapproval from his peers can have a powerful psychological impact on an individual. The Senate censured nine of its members between 1811 and 1990 for transgressions ranging from breach of confidentiality to fighting in the Senate chamber and more generally for "conduct that tends to bring the Senate into dishonor and disrepute." In censure cases, the Senate has not felt as strong a need as with expulsion to wait for the completion of the judicial process before acting to express its

[26] The Senate could ignore an additional five members from seceding states because their terms had expired at the conclusion of the Thirty-sixth Congress in March 1861.

[27] The other convicted member, John H. Mitchell of Oregon, does not appear in this book because his indictment and conviction occurred during a recess of the Senate, and he died only days after the Senate convened, before the matter had been referred to a committee.

condemnation of particular behavior. In voting to censure a member, the Senate sometimes has varied the specific words employed, using "condemn" or "denounce," but the meaning and impact is essentially the same; the common factor being that the full Senate votes to censure the member. Most of those chastised in this manner have either failed to be reelected or declined to run for reelection.

Other Sanctions

During the floor debate on some censure cases, defenders of the member in question have urged the Senate to use a softer term, such as "reprimand." To date, however, the full Senate has never adopted this term, although it has been used by the House of Representatives. In fact, under its rules, the Ethics Committee may only issue a reprimand for misconduct if the individual in question agrees. In one case in the 1990s, the committee did vote to reprimand a member and presented its report on the Senate floor, but because this milder sanction did not involve action by the Senate as a whole, the case is not included in this book. The same is true of another instance in which the committee "rebuked" a senator, in that case simply announcing its decision at a press conference rather than in the Senate itself. The Ethics Committee has also employed such lesser indications of disapproval as either a public or private letter of admonition to a member regarding a particular action. In addition, the committee issues advisory opinions to members and staff who seek guidance on the appropriateness of proposed conduct.

I. Early Years: 1793–1838

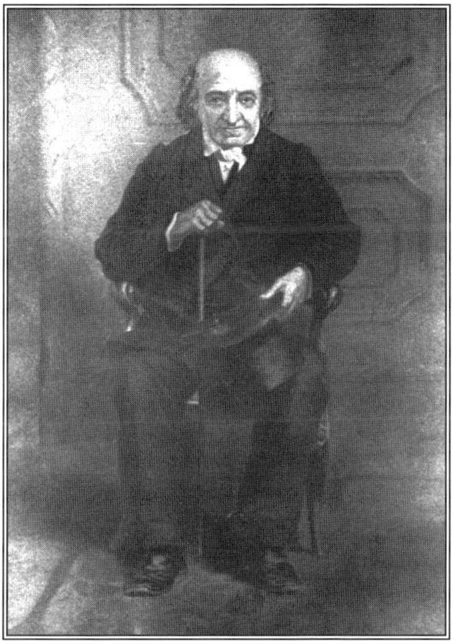

Albert Gallatin *(Case 1)*
Library of Congress

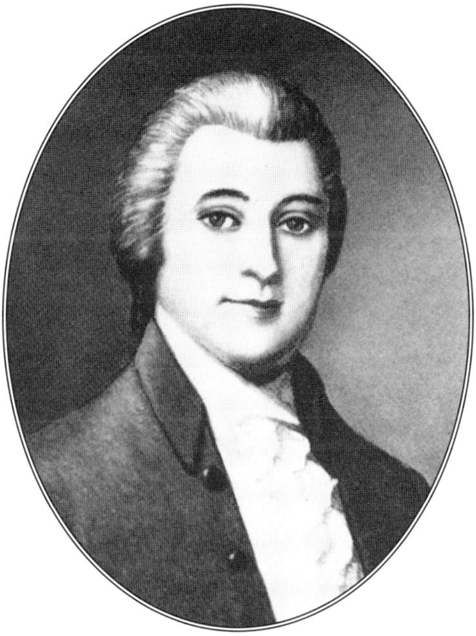

William Blount *(Case 5)*
U.S. Senate Historical Office

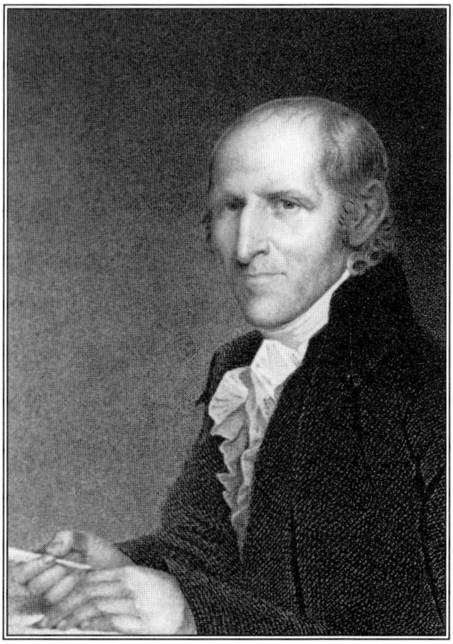

Timothy Pickering *(Case 10)*
U.S. Senate Historical Office

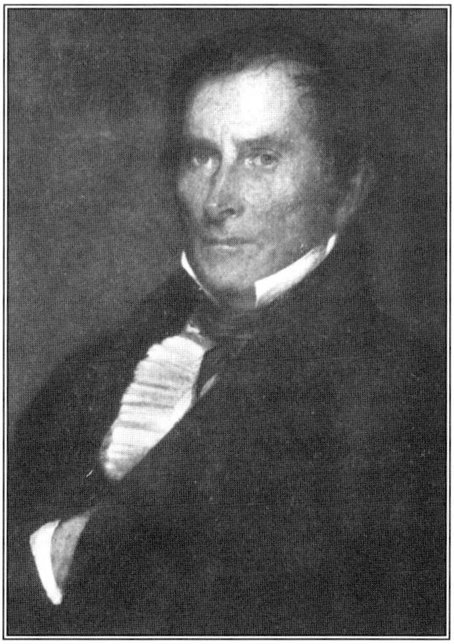

George Poindexter *(Case 15)*
U.S. Senate Historical Office

Case 1

Albert Gallatin

(1761–1849)

Pennsylvania

Election Case
December 2, 1793 to February 28, 1794

Issues
Qualifications: citizenship

Result: Unseated

Chronology:
Protest filed: Dec. 2, 1793
Referred to committee:
Dec. 11, 1793; Jan. 13, 1794
Committee report:
Dec. 31, 1793 (Federalist);
Feb. 10, 1794 (Elections)
Senate vote: Feb. 28, 1794

Background

During the nation's formative years, an increasing number of adherents to the Republican party, led by Thomas Jefferson, threatened the initial superiority of the Federalists. In 1793, Pennsylvania's Albert Gallatin, who had emigrated from his native Switzerland during the American Revolution, made a dynamic addition to Republican forces in the Senate.

Upon his election by the Federalist legislature of Pennsylvania, Gallatin unwittingly provided those same Federalists with the ammunition to reverse their earlier action. The new senator publicly questioned whether his credentials would pass the constitutional requirement of a nine-year United States residency for senators. His untimely query opened to debate the question of national citizenship, not previously an issue for members of the earliest congresses. On December 2, 1793, at the opening of the Third Congress, Gallatin took the oath of office, but that same day nineteen Pennsylvania Federalists filed a protest that Gallatin had not been a citizen for nine years at the time he was elected.

Federalist senators felt uncertain about the correctness of the election protest, since all national citizenship was still in its infancy. On the other hand, they recognized that the presence of the aggressive and outspoken Gallatin boded ill for Federalist policies. On December 11, 1793, the Senate referred the petition of protest to a committee of five Federalists.

Statement of the Case

On December 31, 1793, the Federalist committee predictably reported that Albert Gallatin failed to meet the constitutional residency requirement when he was elected to the United States Senate, citing his European birth and his continued personal ties there. In support of his position, Gallatin cited his uninterrupted United States residency of thirteen years, his substantial property holdings, his 1785 oath of allegiance to the state of Virginia, and his service in the Pennsylvania legislature.

Response of the Senate

The Federalists in the full Senate hesitated to proceed upon this report, but Gallatin's conduct soon spurred them into action. An incisive, relentless Republican and a financial wizard, Gallatin launched a complex attack upon the monetary practices of Federalist Treasury Secretary Alexander Hamilton. Fearing this powerful adversary in a Senate where they held only a slim advantage, Federalist senators activated plans to unseat Gallatin. On January 13, 1794, the Senate established a seven-member Committee of Elections to review the case. Although the committee represented both parties, Federalists controlled it by a four-to-three majority. In response to the committee's inquiries, Gallatin presented a detailed report of the events of his life, but stated that it would be prohibitively troublesome and costly for him to collect substantial evidence in his own behalf from distant sources. He also insisted that he had a right to have his case decided before the full Senate.

Propelled by Gallatin's comments and the report of the Committee of Elections on February 10, 1794, that again supported the Pennsylvania petitioners, the issue came before the full Senate for debate. The Federalists, anxious to eliminate Hamilton's troublesome opponent, appealed to a budding spirit of American nativism by suggesting that Gallatin was a sinister alien. More directly, they charged that Gallatin's Virginia oath did not satisfy naturalization laws for that state and that the new senator had not presented conclusive proof of his citizenship.

Faced with some confusion over a technical point of citizenship, Federalists saw no reason to rescue a dangerous foe. When the issue finally came to a vote on February 28, 1794, the Senate voted on party lines, 14 to 12, to unseat Gallatin. Even his Pennsylvania colleague, Robert Morris, failed him. Earlier, the mercurial Morris had declared himself neutral and had refused to present the original petition of complaint against Gallatin. Now, however, Morris shifted his position and voted with his Federalist friends.

Conclusion

The Gallatin case, in part, stemmed from a weakness in the system of choosing senators, since each state could develop its own methods for senatorial elections. The roots of Gallatin's problem lay in bitter controversy within the Pennsylvania legislature. Not until 1866, after similar contests continued to plague the Senate, did Congress enact a law to regularize state procedures for the selection of senators.

Additionally, some senators used the debate in the Gallatin dispute as an opportunity to repeat their demands that the Senate chamber be open to the public during legislative business. At that time, the Senate met behind closed doors, while the House opened its debates to those who wished to observe. Since the First Congress, efforts had been made to open the Senate's sessions. Increasingly, the state legislatures that elected senators, the press, the public, and even the president were demanding a change in the closed-door policy. Because of concerns that holding secret discussions regarding an individual senator would feed suspicions that the Senate intended to create a legislative aristocracy hidden from popular view, the Senate opened its doors for the Gallatin debate. Soon afterward, the Senate adopted a final resolution permitting open sessions and authorizing construction of public galleries, which were finally completed in 1795.

Although Gallatin's service in the United States Senate was markedly short, the episode served him well. It enhanced his already substantial reputation and gave him considerable publicity. Pennsylvania Republicans viewed him as a champion, and two years later the state's voters elected him to the House of Representatives. Later in his long and distinguished career, Gallatin served as secretary of the treasury under Thomas Jefferson, was United States delegate to the negotiations for the Treaty of Ghent, and saw diplomatic duty in France and Great Britain. Upon his retirement from public life, Gallatin moved to New York, where he headed a bank. He died on August 12, 1849.

Sources

U.S. Congress. Senate. *Annals of Congress.* 3d Cong., 1st sess. (See pp. 9–10, 19, 24, 29, 42–62.)

———. *The United States Senate, 1787–1801: A Dissertation on the First Fourteen Years of the Upper Legislative Body,* by Roy Swanstrom. S. Doc. 100–31. 100th Cong., 1st sess., 1988; reprint of 1962 edition. (See pp. 47–49.)

Johnson, Allen, and Dumas Malone, eds. *Dictionary of American Biography.* Vol. 7. New York, 1946; reprint of 1935 edition. (See pp. 103–10.)

Walters, Raymond, Jr. *Albert Gallatin: Jeffersonian Financier and Diplomat.* New York, 1957. (See pp. 50–51, 59–63.)

Case 2

Kensey Johns

(1759–1848)

Delaware

Election Case (appointment)
March 24, 1794 to March 28, 1794

Issues
Right of governor to make appointment to a term not previously filled by a legislature

Result: Not seated

Chronology:
Credentials presented: Mar. 24, 1794
Referred to committee: Mar. 24, 1794
Committee report: Mar. 26, 1794
Senate vote: Mar. 28, 1794

Background

When George Read, a signer of the Declaration of Independence from Delaware, resigned his Senate seat in September 1793, the state legislature was unable to agree upon a replacement. Not wishing to have Delaware only partially represented in the Senate, Governor Joshua Clayton appointed Read's former law student, Kensey Johns, to the seat on March 19, 1794. Johns, a Federalist of distinguished record, had participated as a "minuteman" in the American Revolution, studied law with both Read and Judge Samuel Chase, and served as a member of the Delaware Constitutional Convention. Johns' appointment provided the catalyst for a continuation of the power struggle between Federalists and Republicans in the Senate. Republicans, still smarting from the expulsion a month earlier of their colleague, Albert Gallatin, seized upon the Johns appointment as a vehicle for retaliation.

Statement of the Case

Republicans argued that Governor Clayton had violated the provision in Article I, section 3 of the Constitution that restricted gubernatorial appointments to periods when state legislatures were in recess. The Delaware legislature had met in full regular session between the resignation of Read and the appointment of Johns, giving the state ample opportunity to fill the vacancy under prescribed constitutional arrangements. Thus, the governor's actions appeared to be without legal foundation, and when Johns presented his credentials on March 24, 1794, the Senate referred the matter to the Committee of Elections. Two days later, the committee reported that Johns was "not entitled to a seat" in the Senate.

Response of the Senate

At the outset, the Federalists, although disappointed to lose an ally in the closely divided Senate, acknowledged the validity of the challenge. The clarity of the constitutional wording made it apparent that Johns had no real case. Following a short investigation, the obvious illegality of the Johns appointment brought a quick resolution on the Senate floor. With eight Federalist senators joining their Republican opponents, the Senate on March 28, 1794, by a vote of 20 to 7, agreed to the committee report and refused to seat Kensey Johns.

Conclusion

Here, the Senate first experienced the difficulties created by snarled state procedures that would continue to embroil it in election disputes throughout the nineteenth century. Impatient with the impasse in the state legislature, the Delaware governor in 1794 tried to sidestep the internal conflicts and guarantee full senatorial representation for the state.

After the Senate's action, the legislature took several more months to resolve its disagreement before finally sending Federalist Henry Latimer to the Senate in February 1795. The long delay and the bitter partisan strife hardly improved the reputation of the increasingly beleaguered Federalist party.

Kensey Johns accepted the Senate's decision and returned to Delaware, where he continued in public service. He served as the chief justice of Delaware from 1799 to 1830, when he became chancellor of the state. He died in 1848.

Sources

U.S. Congress. Senate. *Annals of Congress.* 3d Cong., 1st sess. (See pp. 73–78.)

———. *The United States Senate, 1787–1801: A Dissertation on the First Fourteen Years of the Upper Legislative Body,* by Roy Swanstrom. S. Doc. 100–31. 100th Cong., 1st sess., 1988; reprint of 1962 edition. (See pp. 49–50.)

Malone, Dumas, ed. *Dictionary of American Biography.* Vol. 10. New York, 1946; reprint of 1935 edition. (See p. 76.)

Read, William Thompson, ed. *Life and Correspondence of George Read.* Philadelphia, 1870. (See pp. 552–62.)

Case 3

Humphrey Marshall

(1760–1841)

Kentucky

Non-Category Case
February 26, 1796 to March 22, 1796

Issues
Investigation of conduct prior to a member's Senate term

Result: Senate refused to investigate

Chronology:
Letter from governor: Feb. 26, 1796
Referred to committee: Mar. 2, 1796
Committee report: Mar. 11, 1796
Senate vote: Mar. 22, 1796

Background

The intrigues of France's Citizen Genêt generated a nativist backlash that helped propel Federalist Humphrey Marshall to a Senate seat in 1795 from the Republican stronghold of Kentucky. Marshall, an aristocratic lawyer who possessed a sarcastic tongue, a great disdain for the rabble, and kinship to future Chief Justice John Marshall, had worked actively to counter both French and Spanish interests in the Kentucky area. Although Marshall won a Senate seat as a result of these anti-European activities, he also incurred the wrath of Kentucky Republican Benjamin Sebastian. An investigation, sparked by Marshall, revealed that Sebastian, a judge on the state court of appeals, had been the paid agent of the Spanish. Sebastian's lingering resentments from these frontier political clashes followed Marshall to Washington.

Statement of the Case

There was in fact no case presented against Humphrey Marshall. Kentucky's governor and delegation in the House of Representatives asked the Senate to investigate charges by Sebastian and another state judge that Marshall had committed perjury in a Kentucky lawsuit eighteen months before his election as a senator. The charges, informal in nature, reflected the bitter continuation of the feud between Federalist Marshall and the Republican majority of Kentucky. In response to the challenge, Marshall on February 29, 1796, asked the Senate to pursue the investigation, since he found himself in the awkward position of facing serious charges that had no formal basis and against which he had no systematic means of defense. The Senate on March 2, 1796, agreed to refer the matter to a committee.

Response of the Senate

The committee reported a week later that no official charges had ever been lodged against Marshall, nor did the Kentucky legislature (as reported by Kentucky members of the U.S. House of Representatives) indicate that there was any plan to do so in the future. No request to prosecute Marshall had come from either the Kentucky legislature or the governor. The report directed attention to the judicial concept that no person can be held responsible for infamous crime unless there is indictment from the grand jury. The committee concluded that Marshall must be regarded as innocent, as he had been neither charged nor convicted. This position, firmly based on both the United States Constitution and common law, superseded even Marshall's own request for an investigation.

Although the Kentucky governor's intent is unclear, apparently he hoped to cast doubt on Marshall's worthiness to retain his seat. The state's Republicans did not seem to expect the Senate to try Marshall for the alleged perjury. The Senate committee pointed out that Marshall's foes had regular legal avenues they could pursue and that the entire matter did not fall within senatorial concern. On March 22, 1796, after several days of debate, the Senate accepted the committee's recommendations and, by a vote of 16 to 8, refused to investigate the vague complaint against Marshall.

Conclusion

The case of Humphrey Marshall remains obscure in Senate history. Yet, through its decision, the Senate reinforced the basic constitutional precept that a person is innocent until proven guilty. With its refusal to consider charges that did not follow the correct judicial procedures, the Senate protected the chamber from being used by every political foe who wanted to embarrass a senatorial rival.

After Humphrey Marshall completed his Senate term in 1801, he returned to Kentucky, where he served in the state legislature and pursued agricultural interests. He also wrote the first history of Kentucky, in which he took full revenge upon his Republican enemies. In 1809, he vigorously opposed young Henry Clay's resolution to require all legislators to show their patriotism by wearing homespun suits instead of British broadcloth. Their clash resulted in a duel in which both received slight wounds. Humphrey Marshall died in 1841.

Sources

U.S. Congress. Senate. *Annals of Congress.* 4th Cong., 1st sess. (See pp. 47–60.)

———. *The United States Senate, 1787–1801: A Dissertation on the First Fourteen Years of the Upper Legislative Body,* by Roy Swanstrom. S. Doc. 100–31. 100th Cong., 1st sess., 1988; reprint of 1962 edition. (See pp. 50–51.)

Malone, Dumas, ed. *Dictionary of American Biography.* Vol. 12. New York, 1946; reprint of 1935 edition. (See pp. 309–10.)

Quisenberry, Anderson C. *The Life and Times of Hon. Humphrey Marshall.* Winchester, KY, 1892. (See pp. 57–70.)

William Blount and William Cocke

(1749–1800) (1748–1828)

Tennessee

Election Case
May 9, 1796 to June 1, 1796

Issues
Legislature's authority to elect before statehood

Result: Not seated

Chronology:
Credentials submitted: May 9, 1796
Senate vote: June 1, 1796

Background

In 1796 the Tennessee Territory, a large area of western lands ceded in 1789 by North Carolina, petitioned for admission to the Union. The ensuing congressional debate concentrated on statehood requirements as defined in the Northwest Ordinance of 1787. It also underscored the burgeoning political conflicts that the acquisition of western lands had spawned. At the heart of the discussion lay Federalist fears that the admission of a frontier region would increase the strength of the Jeffersonian Republicans. The Senate, therefore, prepared to resist the admission of Tennessee, drawing upon antistatehood arguments previously presented in House debates. The main objection centered on the procedures for conducting the census to determine whether Tennessee had the 60,000 inhabitants required for admission.

Statement of the Case

On May 9, 1796, Tennesseans William Blount and William Cocke, despite the fact that Tennessee was not yet a state, presented their credentials to the Senate. Dominated by Federalists, the Senate responded by referring the matter to a committee consisting entirely of members of that party, with the dry observation that "a paper purporting to be" the credentials had been presented.

On May 23, Blount and Cocke submitted a letter charging that Tennessee's citizens had a right to immediate senatorial representation. As Tennessee still did not rank as a state, the Senate remained unconvinced, but it did provide the two men with chairs so that they might be comfortable as spectators.

Blount consistently warned senators that denial of statehood carried high risks: threats of separation sounded in frontier Tennessee, the Spanish beckoned with political and economic inducements, and complex diplomatic negotiations with the Indians demanded attention. Relentlessly, Blount pursued senators with this message. His strategy succeeded, and Tennessee entered the Union on June 1, 1796.

Response of the Senate

In a final effort to curtail the rising power of the West and the Republicans, the Federalist Senate, by a narrow margin of 10 yeas to 11 nays, rejected the credentials of Blount and Cocke. Declaring their election by the Tennessee legislature to have been without congressional authority, the body required that the two stand for a second election held after the state's formal admission. On August 2, 1796, with Tennessee safely in the Union, the legislature again elected Blount and Cocke to be the first two senators from that state. They were seated without incident on December 6, 1796.

Conclusion

The discussion of procedures for seating senators from new states highlighted a sensitive topic, which Congress would again face in 1803 with the acquisition of the Louisiana Territory. The lack of strong governmental institutions on the frontier intensified the potential for fraud in statehood petitions. Authorities could choose to take the census at a travelers' crossroads, for example, where the chance traffic of thousands of migrants might be used to inflate the territorial population to the requisite number for admission. In the case of Tennessee, however, the Senate was anxious to secure the area for the United States against Spanish blandishments and thus readily dropped its procedural objections to statehood. Within the Senate, the case chiefly represented one more clash between political parties, as Federalists tried to undercut the growing power of the Republicans.

For Blount and Cocke the case proved to be only an episode in lives filled with adventure and accomplishment. William Cocke, a Revolutionary War veteran, continued to represent Tennessee in the Senate until 1805. After a brief retirement, he was elected to the Mississippi state legislature in 1813, and in 1814 President Madison appointed him agent to the Chickasaw nation. Cocke died in Mississippi in 1828.

William Blount, whose earlier career involved him in the North Carolina convention to ratify the United States Constitution, was the first territorial governor and superintendent of Indian affairs for the Tennessee Territory. Although Blount had worked diligently to promote the interests of frontiersmen in Tennessee, he found that his ethics and tactics in the territory were the subjects of sharp debate in the Senate. Stunned and embittered by the events surrounding the admission controversy, Blount enmeshed himself in further senatorial difficulties in 1797 (See Case 5). On that occasion, the loyal following he commanded in Tennessee rose to his support and warmly welcomed him home. He died in Knoxville in 1800.

Sources

U.S. Congress. Senate. *Annals of Congress.* 4th Cong., 1st sess. (See pp. 83, 85, 101, 103, 120–21); 2d sess. (See p. 1518.)

Johnson, Allen, ed. *Dictionary of American Biography.* New York, 1946; reprint of 1935 edition. Vol. 2 (See pp. 390–91 [Blount]); Vol. 4 (See pp. 255–56 [Cocke]).

Masterson, William. *William Blount.* Westport, CT, 1969; reprint of 1954 edition. (See pp. 294–97.)

Case 5

William Blount
(1749–1800)
Tennessee

Expulsion Case
July 3, 1797 to July 8, 1797

Issues
Disloyalty to United States

Result: Expelled

Chronology:
President's letter received: July 3, 1797
Referred to committee: July 4, 1797
Committee report: July 6, 1797
Senate vote: July 8, 1797

Background

In 1790, President George Washington appointed William Blount, a Republican, as governor of the newly formed Tennessee Territory. When Tennessee entered the Union in 1796, the legislature chose Blount as one of the state's first two United States senators (See Case 4).

Blount, who had served in the Revolutionary army, the North Carolina legislature, the Continental Congress, and the Constitutional Convention, was an active land speculator. His speculations had led him into serious financial difficulties. In an apparent effort to extricate himself, Blount concocted a scheme for Indians and frontiersmen to attack Spanish Florida and Louisiana, in order to transfer those territories to Great Britain. Unfortunately for the senator, a letter, in which Blount thinly disguised his desire to arouse the Creek and Cherokee Indians to aid his plan, fell into the hands of Federalist President John Adams.

Statement of the Case

On July 3, 1797, President Adams sent the incriminating letter to both the Senate and House, accompanied by a special message charging that Blount had sought the aid of a United States government interpreter to seize Spanish Florida and Louisiana with British and Indian help. Adams acted on an opinion from the attorney general that the letter was evidence of a crime and that Blount, a senator, was liable to impeachment under the Constitution. For the first time in the Senate's then brief history, its powers to expel and to convict in an impeachment case were to be tested.

Response of the Senate

The House and Senate promptly appointed special committees to review the matter. On July 7, the House concluded, after spirited debate, that a senator was an impeachable official and ordered the chairman of its committee to inform the Senate that the House planned to present articles of impeachment. The House also demanded that the Senate suspend Blount from his seat and guarantee his appearance to answer the charges.

In the meantime, on July 6, the Senate's committee reported in favor of expelling Blount. After having been mysteriously absent from his seat, Blount suddenly reappeared. He refused to answer questions about the notorious letter but successfully demanded the right to counsel. On July 7, the Senate received the impeachment message from the House and granted the defense counsels' request for more time to prepare the Senate case.

On July 8, after hearing two of Blount's colleagues testify that the letter was in his handwriting and listening to a response by defense counsel, the Senate took up its committee's report. The committee had cited Blount's conduct as "entirely inconsistent with his public trust" and recommended that he be expelled from the Senate. By a vote of 25 to 1, the members upheld the report in the first expulsion of a United States senator. Further, the Senate ordered Blount to appear on July 10 to answer the representatives' articles of impeachment. Although Blount gave assurances that he would appear on that date, he instead spurred his horse home to Tennessee.

Conclusion

The Senate's actions on July 8 were actually contradictory: while attempting to ensure that Blount would be present at his impeachment trial, it simultaneously declared him already guilty when it voted to expel him. In the succeeding months, the Senate unsuccessfully sought to take custody of Blount and return him to the capital. Although Blount graciously received the acting Senate sergeant at arms at his home, the unrepentant Tennessean's supporters and state authorities warned the official to make no attempt to remove their friend.

Despite Blount's absence, his impeachment trial began in the Senate on December 17, 1798, and quickly focused on the Senate's right to try an expelled senator. In a narrow vote, the Senate defeated a resolution that asserted William Blount was an impeachable officer. In this vote, the Senate failed to make clear whether its decision stemmed from a belief that no senator could be impeached or from the belief that someone who ceased to hold a "civil office" also ceased to be impeachable.

Both Republicans and Federalists found it awkward to take political advantage of the Blount case. Federalist proponents of impeachment were in the uncomfortable position of supporting a House move to impeach a senator, thus compromising the Senate's independence of the lower chamber. Republican supporters of Blount, on the other hand, faced the double dilemma of defending both the Federalist Senate and the treasonous Tennessean who had sought to benefit Great Britain, the nation the Federalists were often accused of favoring.

As for Blount, his Washington difficulties had no adverse effect on his popularity in Tennessee. Shortly after his return home, Blount won a seat in the state senate, became speaker of that body, and continued to serve there until his death in 1800.

Sources

U.S. Congress. Senate. *Annals of Congress.* 5th Cong., 1st and 2d sess. (See pp. 33–45.) An account of Blount's impeachment, as distinguished from his expulsion, is found in the *Annals*, 5th Cong., 1st and 2d sess., pp. 39–45, and 2d and 3d sess., pp. 2245–2416.

———. *The United States Senate, 1787–1801: A Dissertation on the First Fourteen Years of the Upper Legislative Body,* by Roy Swanstrom. S. Doc. 100–31. 100th Cong., 1st sess., 1988; reprint of 1962 edition. (See pp. 51–56.)

Johnson, Allen, ed. *Dictionary of American Biography.* Vol. 2. New York, 1946; reprint of 1935 edition. (See pp. 390–91.)

Masterson, William. *William Blount.* Westport, CT, 1969; reprint of 1954 edition. (See pp. 312–23.)

Turner, Frederick Jackson, ed. "Documents of the Blount Conspiracy." *American Historical Review* 10: 274, 574–606.

Case 6

Uriah Tracy

(1755–1807)

Connecticut

Election Case (appointment)
March 4, 1801

Issues
Right of governor to make appointment to a term not previously filled by a legislature

Result: Seated

Chronology:
Credentials submitted: Mar. 4, 1801
Senate vote: Mar. 4, 1801

Background

Among the most forceful of Federalist politicians, Connecticut's Uriah Tracy accumulated an impressive personal record in that state. Graced with the skills of a witty and compelling speaker, Tracy won a seat in the U.S. House of Representatives in 1793. The Connecticut legislature elected him to the Senate in 1796 to fill the remainder of a term that expired on March 3, 1801.

Statement of the Case

On March 4, 1801, a special session of the Senate convened for the inauguration of president Thomas Jefferson. Since the Connecticut state legislature had not met to select a senator for the six-year term beginning on March 4, the governor, on February 20, issued credentials appointing Tracy to continue in the seat "from the 3rd of March next until the next meeting of the legislature of said state." Jeffersonian Republicans immediately challenged the validity of the credentials. Superficially, this challenge appeared to be yet another dispute over state elections and the appointive power of governors. In reality, Republicans and Federalists challenged each other almost automatically when the slightest procedural technicalities arose.

Response of the Senate

In a controversy remarkable for its brevity, the Senate voted 13 to 10 to accept the credentials of Uriah Tracy for the special session of March 4 and 5. Immediately after this vote, Thomas Jefferson arrived in the Senate chamber and delivered his famous, "We are all Republicans, we are all Federalists," inaugural speech.

Conclusion

Despite this brief flurry of opposition, Uriah Tracy continued to serve in the Senate. The Connecticut legislature in May 1801 elected him to the full term, and he returned with his credentials at the beginning of the regular session in December 1801. Widely regarded as a hard-working senator, Tracy remained the intimate political confidant of all the leading Federalists, who routinely sought his shrewd advice. Tracy remained in the Senate until his death in 1807.

Sources

U.S. Congress. Senate. *Annals of Congress.* 6th Cong., spec. sess. (See p. 763.)

Malone, Dumas, ed. *Dictionary of American Biography.* Vol. 18. New York, 1946; reprint of 1935 edition. (See pp. 624–25.)

Case 7

John Smith

(1735–1816)

Ohio

Expulsion Case
November 27, 1807 to April 9, 1808

Issues
Senate's power to expel in the absence of an indictment

Result: Not expelled

Chronology:
Resolution introduced: Nov. 27, 1807
Referred to committee: Nov. 27, 1807
Committee report: Dec. 31, 1807
Senate vote: April 9, 1808

Background

John Smith, Ohio Republican and strong supporter of President Thomas Jefferson, ended his Senate career implicated in the messy frontier political scandal that erupted when Aaron Burr concocted a plot to lead the western territories in rebellion. Although the degree of his involvement remained murky, Smith, a champion of frontier interests who lobbied intensely for internal improvements for the West, was accused of participating in the scheme. A United States senator since 1803, Smith would have been a valuable collaborator for Burr, because of his extensive political contacts and his business as a contractor supplying provisions for the army. During an 1805 visit to Ohio, when he stayed with John Smith, Burr expressed interest in promoting a canal around the Falls of the Ohio River and leading a military expedition against the Spanish in Florida if the United States declared war on Spain. Again, in September 1806, Burr visited Smith for several days, claiming on that occasion that he was escorting a group of settlers to his lands in the Louisiana Territory. Smith later contended that he had believed Burr's explanations of the reasons for his visits to Ohio.

In December 1806, however, President Jefferson issued an alert, charging that Burr's actual purpose was an invasion of Mexico and calling on the western states to help suppress the scheme. Smith responded patriotically by financing weapons to be used by the militia who were preparing to defend against the Burr expedition and even delivered the arms himself to New Orleans. As a result, he did not arrive in Washington until January 1807, missing much of the Senate session. This apparent dereliction of duty led the Ohio legislature to request his resignation. Indignant, Smith refused.

While in the Louisiana Territory on business in the summer of 1807, Smith learned that he had been indicted by a court in Richmond, Virginia, on charges of participating in Burr's conspiracy. In September 1807, after first traveling to West Florida, Smith surrendered to the governor of the Mississippi Territory, who sent him to Richmond for trial. Before Smith could reach Virginia, however, he learned that the court there had acquitted Aaron Burr in August 1807, on the grounds that some evidence was inadmissible. The prosecutor, therefore, had also dropped the charges against the Ohio senator. Smith then journeyed to Washington to attend the Senate session.

Statement of the Case

On November 27, 1807, a resolution in the Senate requested that a committee be appointed to investigate whether Smith's association with Burr rendered him ineligible to retain his seat. Smith claimed to welcome the investigation as a means to establish his innocence. On December 31, the committee, chaired by John Quincy Adams (F-MA), returned a report unfavorable to Smith, stating, "The conspiracy of Aaron Burr and his associates against the peace, union, and liberties of these States is of such a character, and . . . its existence is established by such a mass of concurring and mutually corroborative testimony, that it is incompatible, not only with the honor and privileges of this House, but with the deepest interests of this nation, that any person engaged in it should be permitted to hold a seat in the Senate of the United States." Still, the committee continued, "whether the facts, [as shown by the evidence collected by the committee] are sufficient to substantiate the participation of Mr. Smith in that conspiracy or not will remain for the Senate to decide." Those who believed in Smith's complicity contended that he must have known far more than he admitted about Burr's plans.

Since the bills of indictment against Smith had been identical to those against Burr, whose acquittal rested more on a legal technicality than on proof of his innocence, the committee recommended that John Smith, as an accomplice to the conspiracy, should be expelled from the Senate.

Response of the Senate

The full Senate discussed the matter from January 13 to 20, 1808, and again in mid-March before agreeing to Smith's request to allow him more time to gather evidence and postponing debate until April 1. On that date, John Smith, represented on the floor by prominent Baltimore attorneys Francis Scott Key and Robert Goodloe Harper, faced a full Senate debate on a resolution to expel him for participation in the Burr conspiracy. During its consideration of the case, the Senate called and examined witnesses as well as considering a large number of depositions.

Although Smith's attorneys sought to explain away his moves as those of a naive but hospitable patriot, the accuracy of the charges against Smith was not the only issue. Rather, much of the debate centered on previous expulsion cases before the Senate—those of William Blount of Tennessee (See Case 5) and Humphrey Marshall of Kentucky (See Case 3). In the case of Marshall, the Senate dismissed charges because they were not supported by formal indictments. Now, in the case of John Smith, the Senate reversed its earlier position and asserted that the body could expel a member, even in the absence of legal prosecution, on the theory that the expulsion authority represented a political power to be exercised when necessary to preserve "the purity of the Senate." Smith's lawyers, Key and Harper, contended that the Senate had no jurisdiction "to discharge the duties of a court" simply because the appropriate court had neglected such duties. John Pope (D-KY) dismissed this argument, asserting that a person who accepts membership in a legislative body becomes to some extent responsible to that institution for his conduct.

Despite the weight of circumstantial evidence that John Smith had possessed detailed information about the true purpose of Burr's expedition, more than a third of the senators agreed with the view of William B. Giles (D-VA). Giles maintained that Smith had no reason to question Burr's political integrity until the arrival of President Jefferson's proclamation denouncing the planned rebellion, after which he had moved promptly to help prevent it. These senators apparently accepted the possibility that Smith's only crime was a weak perception of human character. By a vote of 19 yeas to 10 nays, only one short of the two-thirds required, the Senate on April 9, 1808, failed to adopt the resolution of expulsion.

Conclusion

Through the debate in the Smith case, the Senate broadened and clarified its definitions of senatorial jurisdiction in expulsion cases. Smith's attorneys argued that "the power of expulsion is confined to acts done in the presence of the Senate" or that, in indictable cases, the Senate "must wait for an indictment before it can expel." The Senate rejected both of these arguments on the premise that the Constitution, either in letter or in spirit, imposed no limitation upon the authority of the Senate in the conduct of its own affairs. In addition, John Smith, by insisting on an investigation, had reinforced the legitimacy of the Senate role, for, as John Quincy Adams pointed out, "Acquittal implies the jurisdiction of the tribunal as much as conviction."

Smith escaped the disgrace of expulsion, but in Ohio and Washington sentiment against him ran high. Aware that he could not expect any future political support, Smith on April 25, 1808, resigned his seat in a letter to the governor of Ohio, rather than communicating directly with the president of the Senate. In a lengthy justification of his behavior, Smith explained that he chose the unusual resignation method because he could express his political sentiments and motivations more freely in a letter than in the formal atmosphere of the Senate chamber. Complaining that he had suffered political betrayal by President Jefferson and his party, he urged "every man [to] cast off the vassalage of party." Smith returned to Ohio, but his misadventures destroyed him both politically and financially. Forced into bankruptcy, he moved to Louisiana Territory, where he lived in poverty, carrying out a few duties as a Baptist clergyman until his death in 1824.

Sources

U.S. Congress. Senate. *Annals of Congress.* 10th Cong., 1st sess. (See pp. 82–98, 163–70, 178–80, 184–331.)

Malone, Dumas, ed. *Dictionary of American Biography.* Vol. 17. New York 1946; reprint of 1935 edition. (See p. 296.)

Wilhelmy, Robert W. "Senator John Smith and the Aaron Burr Conspiracy." *The Cincinnati Historical Society Bulletin* 28 (Spring 1970).

Case 8

Samuel Smith

(1752–1839)

Maryland

Election Case (appointment)
May 29, 1809 to June 6, 1809

Issues
Right of governor to make appointment to a term not previously filled by a legislature

Result: Retained seat throughout session

Chronology:
Request for ruling: May 29, 1809
Senate vote: June 6, 1809

Background

Samuel Smith (R-MD), a Baltimore merchant first elected to the United States Senate in 1803, increasingly found himself at odds with his political party during Jefferson's presidency. In spite of somewhat strained relations, Smith campaigned actively for Jefferson's heir apparent, James Madison. On the eve of the Madison administration, the association soured when Smith and his faction learned that the president-elect planned to appoint an arch-foe, Albert Gallatin, as secretary of state. Threatened with an intraparty rupture, Madison sought to pacify the rivals by retaining Gallatin as treasury secretary, the position he held under Jefferson, and naming Samuel Smith's brother, Robert, as secretary of state. Gallatin, his feelings bruised, saw a chance for revenge in March 1809 when Samuel Smith's term expired.

Statement of the Case

In commerce-minded Maryland, sentiment against Jefferson's Embargo Act had created an unexpected groundswell of support for the Federalist party, so that by 1809 the Maryland house of delegates passed to Federalist control, while the Republicans dominated the senate. Early in the year, the legislature deadlocked over a second term for Smith. The house refused to agree to his nomination, and the senate refused to consider any other candidate. A Gallatin colleague, Maryland Republican Joseph Hopper, added to the stalemate by accusing the Smith brothers of criminal wrongdoing. With the house controlled by the opposition and members of his own party charging him with corruption, Smith failed to gain reelection. The assembly then adjourned without choosing a Maryland senator. This prompted the state's Republican governor, on March 4, 1809, to give Smith interim credentials for the Senate term that began that day. Aware of the controversy surrounding him, Smith sought to avoid criticism from both Federalist and Republican foes by asking the Senate to clarify his status. He specifically inquired whether his special credentials extended through the entire regular session of the Senate scheduled to begin on May 22, 1809, or if they terminated on the opening of the next session of the Maryland legislature on June 5, 1809.

Response of the Senate

Smith's question was presented to the Senate on May 29, 1809. On June 6, William B. Giles (R-VA), a close friend of Smith's, offered a resolution specifying that Smith be allowed to retain his seat during the session of the Maryland legislature, unless the assembly named a successor during that session. Joseph Anderson (R-TN) countered with a resolution citing the constitutional provision that a senator who holds his seat by executive appointment cannot continue in that seat when his state legislature is again in session. This motion was immediately defeated, and the original resolution was adopted by a vote of 19 to 6.

Conclusion

The technical issue raised in Smith's query to the Senate underscored the problems inherent in the original process for choosing senators. By accepting Smith's credentials until he was properly elected or replaced, the Senate in this instance managed to prevent the threatened break in Maryland's representation caused by the state's own assembly. Political rivalries at the state level interfered with representation in the U. S. Senate so often that, as the nineteenth century progressed, it became increasingly evident that the system for selecting senators needed revision.

Throughout the summer of 1809, Smith's foes in Maryland, encouraged by Gallatin, continued their assault on the senator, even though an investigation had cleared the Smith brothers of any misuse of government money. Smith responded to these tactics by launching an aggressive campaign across the state. The senator entertained Maryland voters at huge outdoor barbecues and then treated them to rousing political speeches. Thanks to his efforts, the Republicans regained control of the Maryland house of delegates that fall, ensuring Smith's reelection on November 16, 1809. Samuel Smith served in the Senate until 1815, and again from 1822 to 1833. He was elected mayor of Baltimore in 1837 and died two years later.

Sources

U.S. Congress. Senate. *Annals of Congress.* 11th Cong., 1st and 2d sess. (See pp. 15–25.)

Cassell, Frank A. *Merchant Congressman in the Young Republic: Samuel Smith of Maryland, 1752–1839.* Madison, WI, 1971.

Malone, Dumas, ed. *Dictionary of American Biography.* Vol. 17. New York, 1946; reprint of 1935 edition. (See pp. 341–42.)

Case 9

Stanley Griswold

(1763–1815)

Ohio

Election Case (credentials)
June 2, 1809 to June 15, 1809

Issues
Qualifications: residency

Result: Seated

Chronology:
Credentials presented: June 2, 1809
Referred to committee: June 9, 1809
Committee report: June 15, 1809
Senate action: June 15, 1809

Background

Stanley Griswold's early careers as a Connecticut clergyman and a New Hampshire editor both suffered because of his outspoken manner. An articulate Republican, Griswold did not hesitate to plunge into controversy and appalled his Federalist neighbors with his intense support of the French Revolution. In 1805 President Thomas Jefferson rewarded his staunch follower with an appointment as secretary of the Michigan Territory. In 1808, Griswold clashed with the governor of that territory, and the peripatetic Republican resigned and moved to Ohio. Less than a year after his arrival in Ohio, Griswold received a gubernatorial appointment to fill the Senate seat of Edward Tiffin, who had resigned while the Ohio legislature was in recess.

Statement of the Case

On June 2, 1809, Stanley Griswold presented his credentials and was seated. On June 9, James Hillhouse, a Connecticut Federalist, entered a resolution to challenge the credentials of Griswold, charging that the new senator had not fulfilled the residency requirements for Ohio. The Senate appointed a five-member Committee of Elections, with Hillhouse as chair, to review the matter.

Response of the Senate

On June 15, 1809, the committee returned a report favorable to Griswold. The committee based its recommendations on the fact that neither the United States Constitution nor the state laws of Ohio specified residency requirements. Therefore, the Senate accepted the certification of the governor of Ohio that Griswold was an inhabitant of Ohio.

Conclusion

Griswold served in the Senate only until December 11, 1809, when he resigned because the legislature had elected a successor to serve out the remainder of Tiffin's term. On March 16, 1810, he was appointed circuit judge for the newly formed Illinois Territory. Although he possessed little legal training, Griswold spent the next five years traveling through that frontier land, where he administered the law and encouraged opportunities for religious worship. He died in 1815.

Sources

U.S. Congress. Senate. *Annals of Congress.* 11th Cong., 1st sess. (See pp. 23, 27, 34, 37.)

Johnson, Allen, and Dumas Malone, eds. *Dictionary of American Biography.* Vol. 8. New York, 1946; reprint of 1935 edition. (See p. 12.)

Case 10

Timothy Pickering

(1745–1829)

Massachusetts

Censure Case
December 31, 1810 to January 2, 1811

Issues
Violation of injunction of secrecy

Result: Censured

Chronology:
Resolution introduced: Dec. 31, 1810
Senate vote: Jan. 2, 1811

Background

Massachusetts Federalist Timothy Pickering built an impressive record of public service before he entered the United States Senate in 1803. He served as postmaster general of the United States from 1791 to 1795, as secretary of war in 1795, and as secretary of state from 1795 to 1800. In the latter position, he developed an intense animosity toward France growing out of the events of the French Revolution. He feared that France was seeking to undermine American independence and the result would be mob rule. One biographer concluded that "for more than twenty years his views of French influence and policy constituted an obsession which warped his judgment, weakened his political scruples, and involved him in sundry transactions which clouded his reputation and obscured his great services." While serving as secretary of state under John Adams, he conspired against the president's efforts to settle difficulties with France, leading Adams to dismiss him in May of 1800. Although Pickering was considered, with Alexander Hamilton, a major leader of the Federalist party, his actions greatly weakened that party's public standing. Federalist friends worried over his excesses; Republican enemies repudiated him in effigy and caricature.

In 1810, Pickering found himself one of a tiny minority in the Senate, as Republicans swept that year's elections in the northeastern states. When he returned to Washington in December 1810, he searched desperately for an issue by which he could demonstrate that the Republican leaders were charlatans. He found that issue in the seizure, six weeks earlier, of West Florida by a group of American settlers who declared that region independent of Spain and sought annexation by the United States. President James Madison immediately took possession of the region, claiming that it was a part of the Louisiana Purchase. In the words of a biographer, "Pickering, who thought the seizure an unconstitutional act of aggression against a friendly power, sensed an opportunity to embarrass the government."

Statement of the Case

During the Senate debate about the adminstration's action on December 31, Pickering introduced a letter written by French Foreign Minister Talleyrand that President Thomas Jefferson had submitted to the Senate five years earlier. Talleyrand had pointed out that the United States had no legitimate claim to the West Florida region under the Louisiana Purchase. Although Pickering had prepared a long speech, he got no further than reading the minister's letter before Samuel Smith (R-MD) interrupted to inquire whether the letter had ever been made public. To his dismay, Pickering realized that he had broken a Senate rule by reading an executive document before the injunction of secrecy had been officially removed. Senate Republicans were delighted to have caught their foe in such an indiscretion. That same day, Henry Clay introduced a resolution of censure.

Response of the Senate

On January 2, 1811, the Senate debated the resolution to censure Pickering. A few Federalists argued weakly that Pickering meant no deliberate harm and that the rule of secrecy had not always been followed perfectly. But when Henry Clay (R-KY) spoke, the temper of the Senate became instantly clear. Clay noted that, if the Senate failed to indicate a sharp disapproval of Pickering, there could be little hope of restraining such violations in the future. The fact that transgressions had occurred in the past did not excuse Pickering's action but rather intensified the necessity for a strong reprimand. Timothy Pickering, unrepentant throughout, insisted that he saw no indiscretion in his conduct. The Senate disagreed and passed Henry Clay's resolution of implied censure on a 20 to 7 vote in which Federalists joined Republicans. Passage of the resolution, which stated that Pickering's reading of the letter represented "a palpable violation of the rules of this body," made Pickering the first person to be censured in the history of the Senate.

Conclusion

Senators accepted the argument of Maryland's Samuel Smith that the president relied on the honor of the Senate to hold certain communications in confidence. The failure of one member to do so jeopardized the system of presidential communication and the Senate's constitutional power to advise and consent. Pickering's action in reading a secret message, even such an outdated one, threatened the future relationship between the Senate and the chief executive. For the good of the whole Senate, it was necessary to reprimand Pickering. In addition, supporters of the administration were glad to divert attention from the constitutional issues raised by President Madison's decision to seize West Florida without prior congressional authorization.

Pickering created his own difficulties in the Senate, vigorously insulting Federalist colleagues as well as Republican opponents. Had he modified his manner, his party could have justified giving him fuller support during the debate. Defeated for reelection in 1811, Pickering later returned to Washington to serve in the House of Representatives from 1813 to 1817. He then retired to his home in Massachusetts, where he devoted himself to agriculture. He died in 1829, a fervent Federalist to the end and one of the last members of that political party.

Sources

U.S. Congress. Senate. *Annals of Congress.* 11th Cong., 3d sess. (See pp. 66–83.)

Clarfield, Gerald. *Timothy Pickering and the American Republic.* Pittsburgh, 1980. (See pp. 245–49.)

Malone, Dumas, ed. *Dictionary of American Biography.* Vol. 14. New York, 1946; reprint of 1935 edition. (See pp. 565–68.)

Case 11

Jesse Bledsoe

(1776–1836)

Kentucky

Election Case
January 20, 1815

Issues
Termination of service after resignation

Result: Seat declared vacant

Chronology:
Request for ruling: Jan. 20, 1815
Senate vote: Jan. 20, 1815

Background

Jesse Bledsoe acquired a reputation as an active frontiersman in the founding days of Kentucky. As a sickly youngster, he had moved from Virginia to the Kentucky region with an older brother. Once his health improved, Bledsoe vigorously pursued a career in law and public office. He was elected to the Kentucky state legislature, and in 1808 he served as that commonwealth's secretary of state. From 1813 to 1815, Jesse Bledsoe represented Kentucky in the United States Senate.

Statement of the Case

On December 24, 1814, Jesse Bledsoe (R) offered his resignation to the governor of Kentucky. He requested that the Kentucky legislature, which was then in session, be informed of his decision and a successor elected. The governor replied that he planned to hold the resignation in hopes of convincing the senator to change his mind. If, by the end of December, Bledsoe still could not be persuaded to retain his seat, then the governor agreed to notify the state legislature. On January 20, 1815, Bledsoe submitted to the Senate a letter inquiring about his status. Since the legislature had subsequently proceeded to name a successor, Bledsoe wished to know whether the Senate still recognized his right to the seat or declared it vacant.

Response of the Senate

The Senate devoted little time to this question. After Bledsoe's letter had been read, Jonathan Roberts (PA), a fellow Republican, submitted a resolution stipulating that Bledsoe's seat not be declared vacant. New York Federalist Rufus King countered with an amendment to declare the seat vacant, which was adopted, and the amended resolution then carried by a vote of 27 to 6. Bledsoe's seat, therefore, went to his elected successor, Republican Isham Talbot, who took his seat on February 2, 1815.

Conclusion

The Senate's decision in the Bledsoe case reinforced the existing procedures for naming senators. The Constitution clearly limited appointments by governors to times when state legislatures were in recess. The Senate recognized that a written resignation from Bledsoe gave the Kentucky legislature, then meeting in regular session, full authority to name a new senator. At the same time, the episode represented one more in an increasing number of election disputes generated by a complex and inefficient system for selecting senators.

Bledsoe returned to Kentucky, serving in the state legislature from 1817 to 1820 and later as a circuit judge and professor of law at Transylvania University. In 1833, he moved to Mississippi and then to Texas, where he died in 1836.

Sources

U.S. Congress. Senate. *Annals of Congress.* 13th Cong., 3d sess. (See pp. 175–76, 207.)

Case 12

James Lanman

(1769–1841)

Connecticut

Election Case (appointment)
March 4, 1825 to March 7, 1825

Issues
Right of governor to make appointment to a term not previously filled by a legislature

Result: Not seated

Chronology:
Credentials presented: Mar. 4, 1825
Referred to committee: Mar. 5, 1825
Committee report: Mar. 7, 1825
Senate vote: Mar. 7, 1825

Background

After a distinguished career in public service in Connecticut, James Lanman was elected as a Democrat to the United States Senate in 1819. In the Senate, Lanman served on the Committee for Commerce and Manufactures, where he supported the interests of the New England trade bloc.

Statement of the Case

When his term expired on March 3, 1825, Lanman presented credentials from the governor appointing him to a second term. They were "to take effect immediately after the 3d day of March 1825, and to continue until the next meeting of the legislature," which was scheduled for May of that year. The Senate immediately challenged these credentials because the governor of Connecticut had pre-issued them on February 28, 1825. Once again, the question centered on whether the failure of the state legislature to choose a senator gave the governor the right to do so. The arguments assumed a regional tone as Horatio Seymour (D-VT) supported Lanman, while Littleton Tazewell (D-VA) opposed acceptance. Lanman, apparently surprised by the turn of events, requested time to prepare a reply. He had little reason to expect any difficulty since in four similar cases no significant challenges had been raised. After a lengthy floor discussion about procedures, the Senate on March 5 agreed to refer the matter to committee. In addition, it accepted the proposal by Martin Van Buren (D-NY) that Lanman be granted time to speak for himself when the committee report was returned.

Response of the Senate

On March 7 the committee, composed of Tazewell, John Eaton (D-TN), and Henry Edwards (D-CT), reported that they had reviewed all the previous cases that bore upon the Lanman situation and had found that a governor could fill a vacancy if the legislature was not in session. An existing Connecticut statute reinforced this view by specifically authorizing the governor to fill a vacancy caused by "expiration of the term of service of a senator" if the legislature was not in session. Based on that information, and citing the precedent in the case of Uriah Tracy (See Case 6), Edwards introduced a resolution permitting Lanman to take his seat. John Holmes (D-ME) argued in opposition that under the Constitution a governor lacked authority to issue credentials in advance of a vacancy. The Senate agreed, rejecting the committee's recommendation by a vote of 18 yeas to 23 nays, thus denying Lanman his second term.

Conclusion

The rejection of James Lanman's credentials represented a pivotal case in the evolution of senatorial election challenges. It highlighted the increasingly complex task the Senate faced when forced to rule on contested elections, the local circumstances of which often remained obscure to the national legislature. Although the Senate apparently denied Lanman his seat because a state executive had no authority to anticipate a vacancy, this doctrine had not been observed in earlier cases, nor was it maintained several years later in the 1837 challenge to Ambrose Sevier's credentials (See Case 16). In that instance, the committee made the distinction that the vacancy in the Lanman case was not "unforeseen" but merely represented the expiration of a regular term.

The meaning of the Lanman case was extensively discussed by the Senate half a century later in the 1879 case of Charles H. Bell (See Case 71), in which it was cited as a precedent both for and against seating Bell. The source of the difficulty lay in the vague outline of the discussion contained in *Niles' Weekly Register*, the only source—both now and in 1879—for the actual debate on the case.

Perhaps behind the facade of constitutional arguments lay southern feelings bruised by Lanman's pro-New England votes on the Committee of Commerce and Manufactures and northern memories of Lanman's vote with the South on the Missouri Compromise of 1820.

Lanman retired to his home in Connecticut. There he continued his public career, first as a judge in the state courts and then as the mayor of Norwich. He died in 1841.

Sources

U.S. Congress. Senate. *Journal.* 18th Cong., 2d sess. (See pp. 272, 281.)

Niles' Weekly Register 28. (See pp. 31–32.)

Case 13

Ephraim Bateman

(1780–1829)

New Jersey

Election Case
February 26, 1827 to May 22, 1828

Issues
Conduct of election (legislator voting for himself)

Result: Retained seat

Chronology:
Credentials presented: Feb. 26, 1827
Referred to committee: May 6, 1828
Committee report: May 22, 1828
Senate action: May 22, 1828

Background

After spending several years as a tailor, a teacher, and a physician, Ephraim Bateman entered the New Jersey legislature in 1808. From 1815 to 1823, he served in the U.S. House of Representatives, after which he returned to the state legislature. In November 1826, following the death of Joseph McIlvaine (Adams-NJ), Bateman was the chairman of the joint meeting of the state legislature responsible for selecting a new United States senator. Originally, four candidates were nominated, but two withdrew, narrowing the race to Ephraim Bateman of the Adams party and Theodore Frelinghuysen of the Anti-Jackson party. With Bateman voting for himself, the joint meeting, by a vote of 29 to 28, elected Bateman to the senatorial seat for the remainder of McIlvaine's term and for a new term beginning March 4, 1827. On February 26, 1827, Bateman presented his credentials for the new term.

Statement of the Case

In February 1827, in the final days of the Nineteenth Congress, several members of the New Jersey legislature and other citizens challenged the legality of Ephraim Bateman's election. Their petition accused Bateman of illegal and improper conduct when he presided over the joint meeting and cast the deciding vote for himself in the contest for the Senate seat. The Senate tabled the petition, and when the Twentieth Congress convened on December 3, 1827, Ephraim Bateman was sworn in and took his seat.

In April 1828, after Bateman had already been serving in the Senate for several months, a group of the original petitioners asked John Eaton (J-TN) to bring their protest before the Senate. In response, Eaton, on May 6, 1828, introduced a resolution proposing that the February 1827 petition against Bateman be referred to a select committee, and the Senate agreed.

Response of the Senate

On May 22, 1828, the committee filed a report recommending that Bateman's election be declared legal and that the Senate take no further action. Witnesses had testified that, during the joint meeting of the New Jersey legislature, Ephraim Bateman stepped down from the chair and asked his colleagues to vote on the acceptability of his continued presence. When the joint meeting deadlocked on the question, Bateman resumed the chair.

In a review of the procedures followed in Bateman's election, the Senate committee determined that New Jersey had observed all constitutional directives relating to senatorial elections by state legislatures. It happened that Bateman was a duly elected and competent member of the legislature that designated him the senator-elect. Preferring not to comment upon the propriety of a man voting for himself, the senators dismissed the petition of the New Jersey citizens without further consideration. In effect, the Senate committee announced that it did not wish to address gray areas of right and wrong that had no direct relationship to constitutionally prescribed procedures.

Conclusion

In this instance, the Senate reaffirmed the responsibility of state legislatures to establish qualifications for their members, limitations on their actions, and definitions of the "interests" that would disqualify a member. No such restrictive precepts existed under New Jersey law. As a duly elected member of the legislature, Bateman had a right to vote for U.S. senator; the Senate, therefore, saw no reason to deny Bateman his seat and declined to judge the "moral" question of whether it was appropriate for the candidate to vote for himself.

Ephraim Bateman served only a brief time in the United States Senate. He resigned his seat on January 12, 1829, due to ill health, and died on January 28.

Theodore Frelinghuysen (AJ), the defeated candidate in this contest, won the other New Jersey Senate seat in 1829 and served one six-year term.

Sources

U.S. Congress. Senate. *Journal*. 19th Cong., 2d sess., 1826–1827. (See p. 238.) 20th Cong., 1st sess., 1827–1828. (See pp. 364, 451.)

———. *Senate Documents*. No. 202. 20th Cong., 1st sess., 1827–1828.(See pp. 1–21.)

Case 14

Elisha R. Potter v. Asher Robbins

(1764–1835) (1757–1845)

Rhode Island

Election Case
December 2, 1833 to May 27, 1834

Issues
Determination of which of two legislatures had the authority to elect

Result: Robbins retained seat

Chronology:
Credentials presented: Dec. 2, 1833
Referred to committee: Dec. 9, 1833
Committee report: Mar. 4, 1834
Senate vote: May 27, 1834

Background

The political atmosphere of Rhode Island, a state founded in the 1630s on the principle of tolerance, had evolved two hundred years later to a climate of conflict and distrust. After the American Revolution, Rhode Island had failed to adopt a state constitution and, instead, continued to use King Charles' Charter of 1663 with only occasional amendments. The awkward arrangement of applying a document from a seventeenth-century monarchy to an eighteenth- and nineteenth-century democracy guaranteed political troubles for Rhode Island.

The problems surfaced nationally with the election of Asher Robbins (AJ) to a second term in the Senate. On January 28, 1833, Governor Lemuel H. Arnold issued Robbins' credentials for the Congress scheduled to convene December 2, 1833. Before the latter date, however, political shifts in Rhode Island brought a new legislature to power. In October 1833, that body declared Robbins' election void and elected Elisha R. Potter, a former U.S. representative and current member of the state legislature, as a replacement. A new governor, John Brown Francis, then issued Potter's credentials.

Statement of the Case

When Congress convened on December 2, 1833, the Senate administered the oath of office to Asher Robbins, although Elisha Potter was also present with credentials. Faced with two claimants, both holding papers of executive certification, the Senate on December 9, referred the contest to a select committee.

The committee needed to resolve three major questions: did Asher Robbins have the requisite constitutional qualifications to be a senator; did his commission comply with the laws of Rhode Island; and was his selection made by the legitimate state legislature or by a rump group of Rhode Island dissidents? The supporters of Potter claimed the issue hung upon the last question. They asserted that the powers of the state legislature and Governor Lemuel H. Arnold had expired in 1832, the assembly and the executive had continued to hold office illegally, and their selection of Robbins in 1833 represented an invalid election.

Response of the Senate

On March 4, 1834, George Poindexter (AJ-MS) reported the committee's finding that Asher Robbins had been duly and constitutionally elected a senator from Rhode Island and was entitled to his seat. Both Robbins' qualifications and his executive credentials passed scrutiny. In the matter of whether Robbins' election had been conducted by the legitimate state legislature, the committee members referred to the Rhode Island charter of 1663, as amended by subsequent legislation. They argued that an amendment adopted in 1832 was specifically designed to carry out the intention of the charter that officials should continue in office beyond the ends of their terms until their successors were chosen. The committee concluded that the U.S. Senate did not have the right to cast doubt on the recognized domestic policy of the state.

Silas Wright (J-NY) filed a lengthy minority report in which he complained that the committee overlooked the history of Rhode Island elections. Wright charged that the charter, although antiquated and awkward, was nonetheless the fundamental law of Rhode Island. It clearly limited terms of office in the state to one year, and any attempt by the agencies of the Rhode Island government to extend their authority was a direct violation. Based on that interpretation, Wright concluded that the 1832 amendment permitting the Rhode Island legislators and chief executive to continue in office until their successors were elected was contrary to the terms of office set in the charter. Thus, the legislators who had elected Asher Robbins in January 1833 retained their offices illegally, and the election was invalid. On the other hand, no one questioned the validity of the state legislature that elected Elisha Potter.

Consideration of the reports dragged through several postponements until May 27, 1834, when the Senate voted 27 to 16 to recognize Asher Robbins' claim to the seat.

Conclusion

This dispute marked the first time two senators with conflicting credentials, each set correct in form, appeared on the same day. By its action in seating Robbins, the Senate recognized the individual who presented the valid credentials bearing the earlier date. The credentials of a second claimant went to a select committee.

On June 23, 1834, by a narrow vote of 20 to 19, the Senate agreed to pay Potter his travel expenses and a per diem allowance for the time he had spent in Washington. Potter returned to Rhode Island, where he continued to serve in the state legislature until his death in September 1835. Asher Robbins remained in the Senate until 1839. He became postmaster of Newport, Rhode Island, in 1841 and died in 1845.

Continued conflicts over the severe limitations upon suffrage and the unjust nature of apportionment finally prompted Rhode Island to draft and ratify a much-needed state constitution in the 1840s.

Sources

U.S. Congress. Senate. *Register of Debates in Congress.* 23d Cong., 1st sess. Vol. 10, Part. 1, 1833–1834. (See pp. 2–11, 13–14, 19, 804–7, 1229–30, 1252–57). Part 2. (See pp. 1813, 2021, 2037–38.)

———. *Congressional Globe.* 23d Cong., 1st sess. (See pp. 1, 13, 127, 214–15, 282–83, 287, 289, 301, 405, 436, 464, 468.)

Case 15

George Poindexter

(1779–1853)

Mississippi

Censure Case
February 23, 1835 to March 2, 1835

Issues
Allegations of conspiracy

Result: Not censured

Chronology:
Request for investigation: Feb. 23, 1835
Referred to committee: Feb. 23, 1835
Committee report: Mar. 2, 1835
Senate vote: Mar. 2, 1835

Background

Senate opposition to President Andrew Jackson intensified during the 1830s. Criticism of Jackson's fiscal policies and his use of presidential power escalated until Henry Clay (AJ-KY) submitted two resolutions of censure against the president on December 26, 1833. While these resolutions were debated, the political feud between the chief executive and the Senate took on an increasingly personal tone. On March 28, 1834, the Senate adopted Clay's censure resolutions.

One of the most rancorous battles flared after "Old Hickory" clashed with his former friend and ally, George Poindexter (AJ-MS). The enraged Poindexter, a feisty character given to vitriolic excesses, abandoned the president and threw his political support to Jackson's bitterest opponents, Clay and John C. Calhoun (N-SC).

In this unpleasant political climate, Jackson attended a funeral in the House of Representatives chamber on January 30, 1835. As Jackson started to leave, Richard Lawrence, an unemployed English house painter, stepped forward and fired two weapons at the startled president. Both pistols misfired, Lawrence was apprehended, and Jackson continued with his appointments for the day.

Statement of the Case

Lawrence turned out to be mentally deranged, for under questioning, the would-be assassin insisted that Jackson had blocked his family's legal right to the English throne. The case appeared to have no connection to U.S. domestic political arguments, yet rumors soon spread that George Poindexter had helped to engineer the attack. When Jackson, who suspected Poindexter of complicity in the affair, refused to silence the accusatory reports in the pro-Jackson *Washington Globe,* the truculent Mississippian turned to the Senate for vindication. On February 23, 1835, Poindexter asked to have a committee investigate and, if the charges were found to be true, that he be expelled from the Senate. The Senate referred the matter to a select committee.

Response of the Senate

After hearing testimony from forty witnesses, the committee reported on March 2, 1835, that the only evidence against Poindexter came from two disreputable men, David Stewart and Mordecai Foy. No witness spoke in defense of the despicable Stewart, who had convinced Foy, a severe alcoholic, to swear that Poindexter and Lawrence had been observed in conversation several days before the assault. The "affidavits" of Stewart and Foy, which formed the basis for the charges against Poindexter, proved to be so flimsy that ultimately even the *Washington Globe* admitted their fraudulence.

A political undercurrent that the committee addressed only in the most circumspect language concerned the role that Jackson played. Jackson clearly had contacts with Charles Coltman, a member of the city council, who controlled Stewart and attempted to recruit other "witnesses." Coltman, a candidate for construction superintendent on the planned new treasury building, denied that he had hoped his endeavors for Jackson would secure his appointment. The Senate committee expressed courteous sympathy for the president's safety concerns but obliquely condemned the questionable tactics used against a political opponent. The committee reported that there was no evidence against Poindexter, and the forty-one senators present to hear the report voted unanimously to accept the recommendation to dismiss the charges.

Conclusion

Although exonerated in this instance, George Poindexter did not conclude his Senate career on a positive note. A man of intemperate habits who was vilified in his home state, Poindexter lost his bid for reelection in 1834, as his reputation steadily declined. He moved to Kentucky and then returned to Mississippi, where he died in 1853.

This relatively minor episode reveals the political and personal vindictiveness of which Andrew Jackson was capable when crossed. The occasion also marked the first attempt upon the life of a chief executive and the first Senate committee investigation of an attack upon a president. It would not be the last.

Sources

U.S. Congress. Senate. *Journal.* 23d Cong., 2d sess. Vol. 25. (See pp. 183, 196, 215, 226.)

———. *Congressional Globe.* 23d Cong., 2d sess. (See p. 315).

———. Senate Report No. 148. 23d Cong., 2d sess., 1834–1835.

Miles, Edwin A. "Andrew Jackson and Senator George Poindexter." *The Journal of Southern History* 24 (February 1958): 62–63.

Remini, Robert V. *Andrew Jackson and the Course of American Democracy, 1833–1845.* New York, 1984. (See pp. 151–59, 228–30.)

Rohrs, Richard C. "Partisan Politics and the Attempted Assassination of President Andrew Jackson." *Journal of the Early Republic* 1 (1981).

Case 16

Ambrose H. Sevier

(1801–1848)

Arkansas

Election Case (appointment)
February 27, 1837 to March 8, 1837

Issues
Right of governor to make appointment to a term not previously filled by a legislature

Result: Seated

Chronology:
Credentials presented: Feb. 27, 1837
Referred to committee: Mar. 6, 1837
Committee report: Mar. 7, 1837
Senate vote: Mar. 8, 1837

Background

Political events of the 1830s developed an increasingly acrimonious tone as sectional division over slavery intensified. The admission of Arkansas, a proslavery territory, provided an opportunity for new sectional clashes in Congress. Surprisingly, no one challenged the credentials of the new state's two incoming senators, and the two Jacksonians, Ambrose H. Sevier and William S. Fulton, took their seats without incident on December 5, 1836.

Statement of the Case

Ambrose Sevier, who had supported the statehood effort during his eight years as delegate to Congress from the Arkansas Territory, was assigned by lottery to the class of senators whose terms expired on March 3, 1837. In order to prevent any interruption in Arkansas' senatorial representation, the state's governor on January 17, 1837, appointed Sevier for the Senate term that would begin on March 4, and William Fulton, on February 27, presented the new credentials for Sevier.

In a Senate highly charged with regional and partisan divisions, Daniel Webster (AJ-MA) moved quickly to protest the legality of presenting credentials for a Senate seat when no vacancy yet existed. There followed a tersely polite exchange between Webster and Sevier in which each disclaimed any personal bias about the outcome of the challenge.

Response of the Senate

In response to Webster's protest, the chair ruled that, because one Congress could not judge the qualifications for a future Congress, the matter could not be reviewed until March 4, 1837. On that day, Ambrose Sevier appeared and presented his credentials dated February 25, 1837. Two days later, the Senate ordered the Judiciary Committee, chaired by Felix Grundy (J-TN), to consider Sevier's predated credentials.

The Judiciary Committee, dominated by sympathetic Jacksonians, returned its report to the Senate the following day. Not surprisingly, the committee members argued that their party colleague should be seated. The report focused on the power of state executives to appoint senators during periods of legislative recess. Because the Arkansas legislature had recessed before Sevier drew the lot for his senatorial class assignment, the state assembly was unaware of the expiration date and the need to select a new senator. The committee also noted that a review of earlier challenges to predated credentials turned up no case similar to this one. In the cases it did find, all such senators had been seated, with the exception of James Lanman, whose credentials had been rejected by the Senate in 1825 (See Case 12). That case had involved merely the expiration of a regular Senate term, rather than an unforeseen vacancy like that in the Sevier case. The committee, therefore, recommended that Sevier be seated. The Senate agreed, 26 to 19, voting largely on sectional and party lines, and Ambrose Sevier took his seat on March 8, 1837.

Conclusion

This case represented a continuation of the confusing problems caused by the senatorial selection process. Such challenges repeatedly forced the Senate to grapple with United States constitutional requirements, individual state procedural laws, and senatorial precedents. In ambiguous cases, the Senate vote was usually partisan.

Ambrose Sevier served as chairman of the Committee on Foreign Relations and the Committee on Indian Affairs, and as president pro tempore of the Senate. He resigned from the Senate in March 1848 to become the U. S. minister to Mexico and helped to negotiate the treaty after the Mexican War. He died in 1848.

Sources

U.S. Congress. Senate. *Journal*. 24th Cong., 2d sess. (See pp. 358, 366–67.)

———. *Congressional Globe*. 24th Cong., 2d sess. (See pp. 1, 262.)

Malone, Dumas, ed. *Dictionary of American Biography*. Vol. 16. New York, 1946; reprint of 1935 edition.(See pp. 601–2.)

Case 17

John Ruggles

(1789–1874)

Maine

Censure Case
February 21, 1838 to April 25, 1838

Issues
Allegations of corruption

Result: Not censured

Chronology:
Request for investigation: Feb. 21, 1838
Referred to committee: Feb. 21, 1838
Committee report: April 12, 1838
Senate action: April 25, 1838

Background

John Ruggles (D-ME), a distinguished lawyer and jurist, came to the Senate in 1835. In addition to his legal expertise, Ruggles maintained a keen interest in mechanical science and the advancement of technology. An occasional inventor, Ruggles prepared the 1836 bill to reorganize the United States Patent Office. His acquaintance with patent specifications caused him some difficulty in 1838.

Statement of the Case

Henry C. Jones, a New Jersey inventor, charged that Ruggles offered to use his senatorial influence to secure an advantageous decision on Jones' patent for a mailbag lock. Additionally, Jones asserted that Ruggles promised to pressure the postmaster general, Amos Kendall, to grant a contract for use of the Jones lock on all United States mailbags. Jones insisted that Ruggles wanted a one-quarter interest in the patent in return for his assistance. When Ruggles learned of these charges through a New York newspaper, the annoyed senator brought the matter to the attention of his Senate colleagues. On February 21, 1838, they referred the subject to a select committee chaired by Hugh L. White (W-TN).

Response of the Senate

During the committee's hearings, John Ruggles was not only present but dominated the interrogation of Henry C. Jones. The senator acknowledged having a legitimate business agreement to prepare patent specifications for Jones, in lieu of payment for which he would receive an interest in the patent. Ruggles' legal skills quickly destroyed Jones' credibility. Repeatedly, Ruggles focused on the details of his transactions with Jones to show that their contact had been entirely legal and in keeping with acceptable lobbying practices of the day. Testimony from other witnesses revealed Jones to be a person of questionable integrity and unpredictable humor. Jones reinforced these impressions by blatantly asking one witness to limit the scope of his testimony. As his muddled and contradictory case collapsed around him, Jones informed the committee that business matters called him home, and he left Washington. On April 12, 1838, the committee reported to the Senate that it found no evidence to sustain the charge by Jones and therefore considered it "inexpedient" to pursue the matter further. On April 25, the Senate agreed.

Conclusion

Ruggles failed in his bid for reelection in 1840 and returned to his home in Maine, where he practiced law and pursued his interest in inventions. He died in 1874. Amos Kendall, the object of Jones' most abusive and vulgar vilification, stepped down as postmaster general in 1840.

Sources

U.S. Congress. Senate. *Congressional Globe,* 25th Cong., 2d sess. (See pp. 302–3, 333.)

———. Senate Report No. 377, 25th Cong., 2d sess., 1838.

II. Mid-Century: 1844–1858

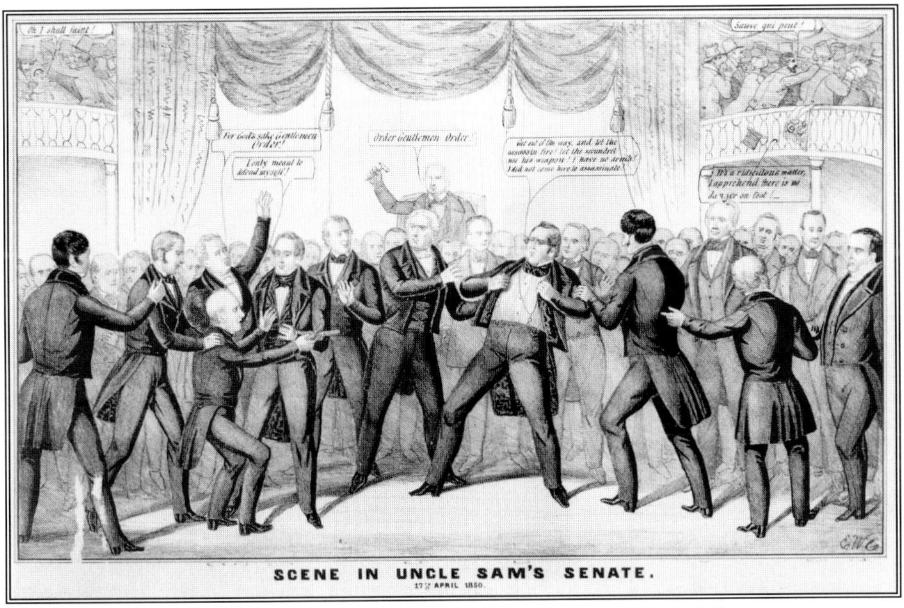

Henry S. Foote and Thomas Hart Benton *(Case 22)*
Library of Congress

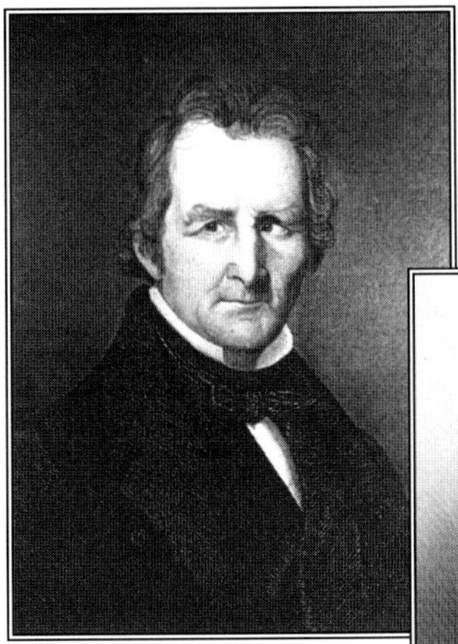

Benjamin Tappan
(Case 18)
Library of Congress

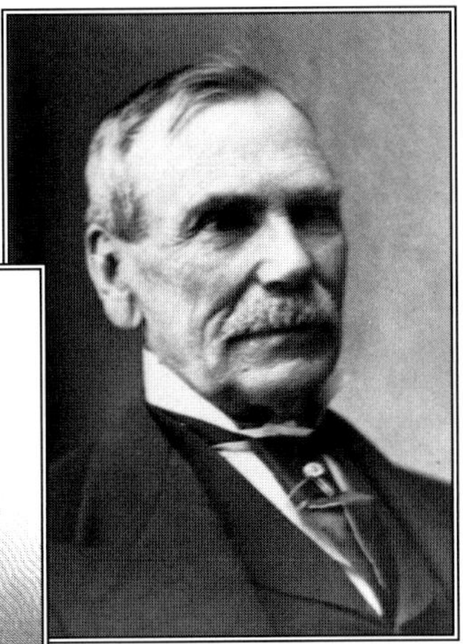

James Shields
(Cases 21, 32)
U.S. Senate Historical Office

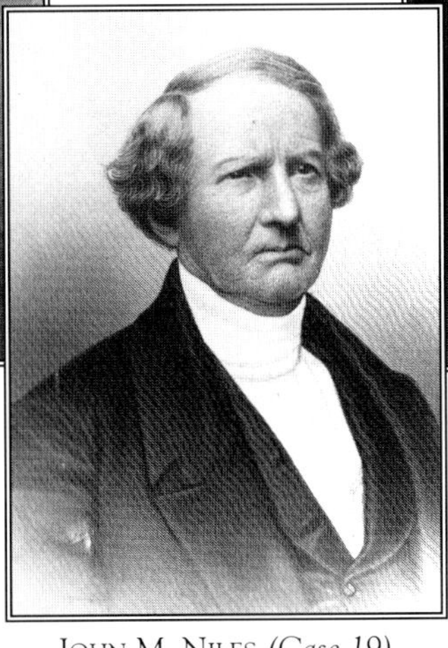

John M. Niles *(Case 19)*
Connecticut Historical Society, Hartford, CT

Case 18

Benjamin Tappan

(1773–1857)

Ohio

Censure Case
April 29, 1844 to May 16, 1844

Issues
Violation of injunction of secrecy

Result: Censured

Chronology:
Request for investigation: April 29, 1844
Referred to committee: April 29, 1844
Committee report: May 8, 1844
(Proceedings made public: May 16, 1844)

Background

Newly independent Texas first petitioned the United States for annexation in 1837. In the following years, the issue remained mired in political disagreements tied to the slavery controversy. By 1844, as the question of annexation moved toward a congressional confrontation, both northern and southern leaders freely used partisan newspapers to reveal the strategy of the opposition and to inflame sectional sentiment.

On April 22, 1844, President John Tyler sent to the Senate a message in which he outlined the terms of an annexation agreement with Texas. This communication was protected by the confidentiality of a Senate executive session. Still, some senators objected to the secret nature of the president's negotiations about the agreement, as well as to his attempts to pass the annexation accord without Senate discussion.

Statement of the Case

Five days after President Tyler's confidential message arrived in the Senate, the *New York Evening Post* printed the document. On April 29, 1844, a perturbed William S. Archer (W-VA), who was responsible for managing the treaty materials as chairman of the Senate Foreign Relations Committee, asked that a select committee investigate the circumstances under which the *Post* had secured the document. The Senate unanimously approved Archer's resolution and appointed him chairman of the select committee.

The committee subpoenaed William G. Boggs, editor of the *New York Evening Post,* but before that testimony could be heard, Benjamin Tappan (D-OH), a seventy-year-old first-term senator, notified the committee of his involvement in the matter. Tappan, the audacious, sharp-witted, and sarcastic elder brother of ardent abolitionists Arthur and Lewis Tappan, readily admitted that he gave his copy of the treaty materials to a messenger with instructions to deliver the items to the editors of the New York paper. The testimony of the messenger, Jonathan D. Stevenson, and the editor, William Boggs, corroborated Tappan's admission. When the committee reported back to the Senate on May 8, Archer submitted a resolution calling for the expulsion of Benjamin Tappan for violating the Senate's order that the treaty materials remain confidential.

Response of the Senate

From May 8 to 10, the Senate in closed session debated two resolutions in the Tappan matter. The first would have expelled Tappan for flagrant violation of Senate Rule 38, which provided that "all confidential communications, made by the President of the United States to the Senate, shall be by the members thereof kept secret." A substitute introduced by Thomas F. Bayard, Sr. (D-DE) called for censure rather than expulsion. On May 10 the Senate adopted Bayard's substitute resolution of censure by a vote of 38 to 7. Archer then offered another resolution that declared, since Tappan had apologized and acknowledged his wrongdoing, no further action of censure should be taken against him. The Senate passed this measure by a vote of 39 to 3 and then approved a proposal by the committee adding to the Senate's rules a provision that "disclosing for publication" materials "directed by the Senate to be held in confidence" would be grounds for expelling a member.

Subsequently, on May 16, at Archer's instigation, the Senate made public its proceedings in the Tappan matter, which had been conducted in secret. This action was apparently designed to embarrass Tappan and further emphasize the Senate's disapproval of his conduct.

Conclusion

Tappan, a ferociously independent man, had not joined in the antislavery activities of his brothers and had refused to enter abolitionist petitions from citizens of Ohio. Yet he was among those senators offended by President Tyler's conduct in the Texas negotiations. Tappan's revelations to the *New York Evening Post,* although a violation of Senate rules, reflected the accommodating relationship many of his senatorial colleagues maintained with journalists. Recognition of this fact, coupled with Tappan's prompt confession, weakened the expulsion efforts of William Archer. Tappan served out the remaining months of his Senate term, which ended on March 3, 1845. He died in 1857.

Sources

U.S. Congress. Senate. *Senate Journal.* 28th Cong., 1st sess. Appendix. (See pp. 426, 438–43.)

Filler, Louis. *The Crusade Against Slavery: 1803–1860.* New York, 1960. (See pp. 179–80.)

Malone, Dumas, ed. *Dictionary of American Biography.* Vol. 18. New York, 1946; reprint of 1935 edition. (See pp. 200–201.)

Ratcliffe, Donald J., ed. "The Autobiography of Benjamin Tappan," *Ohio History* 85 (Spring 1976): 109–57.

Case 19

John M. Niles

(1787–1856)

Connecticut

Election Case (qualifications)
April 30, 1844 to May 16, 1844

Issues
Whether the Senate should examine other than the constitutionally mandated qualifications

Result: Seated

Chronology:
Credentials presented: April 30, 1844
Referred to committee: April 30, 1844
Committee report: May 16, 1844
Senate action: May 16, 1844

Background

John M. Niles (D), Connecticut lawyer and editor, served in the Senate from 1835 to 1839. In 1843, the Connecticut legislature elected Niles to another term in the Senate, but before he could take his seat, a severe mental and physical illness overtook him. He entered a private resort at Utica, New York, for treatment that lasted over a year. Unable to galvanize himself into action on his return, Niles continued to procrastinate about his Senate responsibilities. Finally, in April 1844, Niles' physician advised him that the best road to complete recovery would be to assume his duties in the Senate. Niles then moved into a Washington boardinghouse and eventually appeared in the Senate on April 30, 1844. John Fairfield (D-ME) presented the senator-elect's credentials and announced that Niles was in the chamber and ready to take his oath of office.

Statement of the Case

Before the Connecticut Democrat could take his oath in the Whig-controlled Senate, Spencer Jarnagin (W-TN) rose to protest. Jarnagin argued that the Senate could not be ignorant of the circumstances surrounding the long delay in Niles' presentation of his credentials. Rumors circulated in Washington that Niles suffered from complete insanity, politely described in Jarnagin's speech as an "alienation of the mind." Based on these reports, Jarnagin asked that a committee be appointed to determine whether the senator-elect's afflictions rendered him ineligible to hold his seat. Jarnagin questioned only Niles' mental competency and did not challenge the validity of his credentials.

Response of the Senate

The resolution as introduced asked for a committee to investigate the election returns and qualifications of John Niles and "his capacity at this time to take the oath." There followed some uneasy discussion about whether to add the term "mental competency." Some senators thought that such an inquiry would not only exceed the powers of the Senate but could set a precedent that might expose future members to a dangerous kind of scrutiny. Others expressed uncertainty about the wisdom of pursuing such a personal medical issue at a time when many members were away from Washington attending the Democratic nominating convention in Baltimore. When the Senate decided to adopt the resolution in its original form with no direct reference to Niles' mental state, the issue moved from the uncomfortable realm of medicine to the safer arena of senatorial qualifications. The committee could define "qualifications" either as mental ones or as those clearly expressed in the Constitution under age and residence. The senators appointed to the committee that day included Jarnagin.

On May 16, 1844, the committee members reported that they found the credentials to be in perfect order. Discussions with Niles had convinced them that, although he had suffered from an extreme illness, the senator-elect was "not of 'unsound mind' in the technical sense." Agreeing with Niles' physician, the Senate committee recommended a daily dose of Senate business as the best remedy for any lingering malaise. The Senate concurred, by voice vote, and John Niles took his oath of office that same day.

Conclusion

The Senate demonstrated a wise caution in hesitating to undertake a formal medical evaluation of a fellow member. A precedent for investigations into mental competency could have haunted future Senates, when any rival would have been free to hurl the charge of insanity at an opponent and members would have been compelled to consider the allegations. Although the committee members did in fact consider the state of Niles' mental and physical health in meeting with him and incorporating a letter from his physician into their report, the official mandate of the committee referred only to his "capacity." Thus the Senate avoided setting what might prove to be a dangerous precedent while establishing its authority to define and interpret the scope of its own procedural power.

John Niles served in the Senate until 1849. At the end of his Senate term, he retired to Connecticut, where he devoted himself to horticulture. When he died in 1856 without heirs, he bequeathed his personal library to the Connecticut Historical Society and a large part of his monetary worth to the needy of the city of Hartford.

Sources

U.S. Congress. Senate. *Congressional Globe.* 28th Cong., 1st sess. (See pp. 564–65, 592, 602–3, 636.)

Malone, Dumas, ed. *Dictionary of American Biography.* Vol. 13. New York, 1946; reprint of 1935 edition. (See pp. 522–23.)

Case 20

John M. Clayton

(1796–1856)
Delaware

Spencer Jarnagin

(1792–1853)
Tennessee

Walter T. Colquitt

(1799–1855)
Georgia

Censure Case
March 12, 1846 to March 16, 1846

Issues
Allegations of disloyalty

Result: Not censured

Chronology:
Referred to committee: Mar. 12, 1846
Committee report: Mar. 16, 1846
Senate vote: Mar. 16, 1846

Background

At the beginning of 1846, the United States and Great Britain were locked in a bitter dispute over the location of a permanent boundary for the Oregon Territory. The rapid migration of American farmers into the region after 1842 increased the importance of settling this longstanding dispute. Prominent Whigs, including Daniel Webster (MA), who in 1842 had negotiated a settlement for the Maine boundary, urged that the Oregon boundary should run along the forty-ninth parallel. Expansionists in the Democratic party countered with demands that the entire territory north to 54° 40' be taken by force if necessary. This latter goal became part of the 1844 Democratic party platform, and President James K. Polk, a Democrat, displayed an unyielding attitude in pursuit of the whole territory in his first message to Congress in December 1845. The resolution to terminate joint United States-British occupation of the territory sparked a two-month Senate filibuster at the beginning of 1846.

In this climate, the first issue of the *Washington Daily Times*, under the editorship of Hiram H. Robinson, appeared on February 2, 1846. In a bid to win administration printing patronage, Robinson took as his primary issue the acquisition of Oregon and devoted editorials and long articles to the Oregon debate in Congress. Early in March, the *Times* published allegations that a cabal of Whigs and anti-administration Democrats was plotting with the British minister to force the president into a compromise over Oregon. "LOOK TO THE SENATE," Robinson's editorials warned repeatedly, without identifying individual senators suspected of traitorous activity.

Statement of the Case

Amid charges that some of its members were guilty of treason, the Senate on March 12 responded to Robinson's demand for an investigation by appointing a committee under the chairmanship of Spencer Jarnagin (W-TN). Three specific areas emerged as concerns of the committee. The *Times* charged that, during a dinner at the residence of the British minister, several senators had engaged in improper conversations about the Oregon negotiations. Additionally, John Clayton (W-DE), seated at the host's table, was said to have detailed the strength of the pro-British group by a "count of their noses." The third charge specified that, shortly before the English steamer *Cambria* departed for home, the British minister met with a group of Whigs in the Capitol and discussed how soon the Senate could vote on the Oregon question.

The *Times*' evidence rested on the testimony of several witnesses. The committee summoned Robinson and publisher Jesse Dow to prove their accusations. Surprisingly, the two journalists decided to divulge their sources. According to Historian Donald A. Ritchie, "it was a foolish decision, since each of the witnesses they called—a naval officer, a Senate doorkeeper, lobbyists, and other journalists—had everything to lose and nothing to gain by corroborating the *Times*' allegations against the Senate." Under oath, each witness denied knowledge of a plot. Dow and Robinson's case and credibility immediately collapsed.

Response of the Senate

After Chairman Jarnagin stepped aside because he was implicated along with Clayton and Walter Colquitt (D-GA), Thomas Hart Benton (D-MO) drafted the committee's report, which was presented on March 16. Although Robinson had suggested several names, the committee identified only three senators. It refused to call the others but sent each a letter explaining that the Times had mentioned them in the allegations.

Based on denials by various Whig senators, Benton's report dismissed the charge that a group met with the British minister in the Capitol. Further, when the Whigs withdrew a motion to hasten the Oregon debate, it appeared unlikely that party members were seeking to force a Senate decision by a date promised to the British.

The committee noted that, while Robinson admitted writing all the articles, he had no personal knowledge of the truth of any of the events. Convinced that all the charges were journalistic inventions, the committee recommended that editor Robinson, publisher Dow, and all their reporters be suspended from the Senate gallery. Daniel S. Dickinson (D-NY) protested, not for the newspaper, but in defense of freedom of the press, wryly noting that "no senator had ever been slain by a paper bullet." Regardless, the Senate on March 16 accepted the recommendation of the committee.

Conclusion

The episode appeared to have no significant impact upon the careers of the individual senators involved. Walter Colquitt resigned in 1848. He died in Macon, Georgia, in 1855. Spencer Jarnagin lost a bid for reelection and returned to Tennessee to practice law. He lived in Memphis until his death in 1853.

John Clayton resigned from the Senate in 1849 to assume the office of secretary of state. In 1853, when Clayton returned to the Senate, his enemies once again raised cries of "sell out to the British" for the former secretary's controversial management of the Clayton-Bulwer Treaty. Clayton died in 1856 before completing his Senate term.

Permanent expulsion of the *Times* from the Senate gallery ended any hope that it might obtain vital government printing patronage. Within a few days of the Senate's decision, Jesse Dow announced the demise of his month-old newspaper.

Sources

U.S. Congress. Senate. *Journal.* 29th Cong., 1st sess. (See pp. 194–97.)

———. *Congressional Globe.* 29th Cong., 1st sess. (See pp. 488, 500–502.)

Johnson, Allen, ed. *Dictionary of American Biography.* Vol. 4. New York, 1946; reprint of 1935 edition. (See p. 316 [Colquitt]; pp. 185–86 [Clayton].)

Ritchie, Donald A. *Press Gallery: Congress and the Washington Correspondents.* Cambridge, MA, 1991. (See p. 27.)

Case 21

James Shields

(1806–1879)

Illinois

Election Case
March 2, 1849 to March 15, 1849

Issues
Qualifications: citizenship

Result: Unseated (election voided)

Chronology:
Credentials presented: Mar. 2, 1849
Referred to committee: Mar. 6, 1849
Committee report: Mar. 13, 1849
Senate vote: Mar. 15, 1849

Background

James Shields, an Irish immigrant of vigor and style, arrived in the United States about 1826. He settled in Illinois, where he studied law and began a career in politics, winning a variety of posts ranging from state auditor to judge of the supreme court. Named federal land commissioner in Washington, D.C., in 1845, he resigned from that position to lead an Illinois regiment in the Mexican War. His military successes, plus a near-fatal wound that he turned to political advantage, won him considerable fame. In 1849, shortly after his return to Illinois, he was elected as a Democrat to the United States Senate, defeating incumbent Democrat Sidney Breese. This incident led one prominent Whig to attribute Shields' victory to "that Mexican bullet" and to observe: "What a wonderful shot that was! The ball went clean through Shields without hurting him, or even leaving a scar, and killed Breese a thousand miles away."

Statement of the Case

Dissatisfaction with the victory gained by the vain and dramatic Shields over the colorless Breese divided the Illinois state Democratic leadership and led Shields' opponents within the party to question the status of his citizenship. Despite his many years of active civic involvement, Shields had not applied for naturalization until October 21, 1840. His foes could thus challenge his credentials, presented on March 2, 1849, on the basis that the nine-year constitutional residency requirement for senators could not be fulfilled until October 20, 1849. On a motion by Shields' colleague and friend Stephen A. Douglas (D-IL), Shields was seated on March 6, during the brief special session, while his credentials were referred to a select committee.

Response of the Senate

On March 13, the committee recommended that Shields' election be declared void. Although Shields accepted the committee's decision and emphasized that he did not seek a postponement or further consideration, the Senate launched into a complicated procedural debate.

The discussion centered on whether the constitutional residency requirement must be met at the time of election or at the beginning of Senate duties. Henry S. Foote (D-MS) offered a compromise suggestion that the question be postponed until the regular session began in December, when the matter would become moot, but this approach attracted little support.

The core of the debate apparently concerned the balance of power between Whigs and Democrats in the Senate. Foote charged that the rejection of Shields represented an attempt to increase the influence of Senate Whigs, then in the minority. Douglas added that the manner of the rejection significantly assisted this strategy. If Shields could resign and his seat be declared vacant, then the governor could appoint a replacement promptly. If, however, the Illinois election was declared void, then no replacement could be named until the next regular session of the state legislature in eighteen months. This ploy, the Democrats argued, could effectively limit their number in the Senate.

Despite the lengthy and often heated debate, the fact remained that Shields' residency fell short of the nine-year requirement. On March 15, the Senate declared the Illinois election void.

Conclusion

Convinced that Sidney Breese had instigated the residency inquiry, Shields offended the Senate by sending his predecessor a highly emotional and threatening letter. When his indiscretion was revealed, Shields made a passionate speech of apology to the Senate and declared that he would return to Illinois to seek the endorsement of his constituents.

An intense political debate ensued in Illinois over the constitutionally proper means of filling the vacancy. Some held that the governor had the power to appoint a replacement, while others insisted that that power lay only with the legislature in special session. Stephen Douglas argued that the Constitution defined the appointive power of the governor in language "sufficiently broad and comprehensive to include every description of vacancy which might occur during the recess of the Legislature." He believed that the framers of the Constitution had intended to ensure that each state was fully represented and thus the governor could fill such vacancies. Despite Douglas' advice, the governor, choosing to avoid what he considered a touchy political dilemma, called the legislature into special session several months later, in October 1849. The legislature, on the twenty-first ballot, again elected James Shields, who had by then been a citizen for the requisite nine years.

This incident proved to be but one phase of Shields' varied and dynamic career. Defeated for reelection in 1855, he moved to Minnesota. Shields became one of that state's first two senators in 1858 (See Case 35), serving until March 1859. Twenty years later, in 1879, he served briefly as a senator from Missouri, thus becoming the only person successively to represent three states in the United States Senate. He died in 1879.

Sources

U.S. Congress. Senate. *Congressional Globe.* 30th Cong., 2d sess. Appendix. (See pp. 326–51.)

Johannsen, Robert W. *Stephen A. Douglas.* New York, 1973. (See pp. 257–61.)

Malone, Dumas, ed. *Dictionary of American Biography.* Vol. 17. New York, 1946; reprint of 1935 edition. (See pp. 196–97.)

Case 22

Thomas Hart Benton

(1782–1858)

Missouri

Henry S. Foote

(1804–1880)

Mississippi

Censure Case
April 17, 1850 to July 30, 1850

Issues
Breach of comity

Result: Not censured

Chronology:
Incident in chamber: April 17, 1850
Referred to committee: April 23, 1850
Committee report: July 30, 1850
Senate action: July 30, 1850

Background

In 1850, sectional attitudes toward slavery were clearly defined, and regional opponents in Congress frequently abandoned accepted standards of legislative decorum in heated exchanges that became decidedly personal.

Henry S. Foote (D-MS) and Thomas Hart Benton (D-MO) became increasingly hostile toward one another, their animosity often erupting on the floor of the Senate. Foote repeatedly attacked Benton for his failure to support the South on the slavery issue. For days during consideration of the Compromise of 1850, Benton endured Foote's far-fetched accusations of treason, scornful comparisons to "that degenerate Roman senator, Catiline," and sarcastic references to the "nasality" of his intonation. Finally, on April 17, 1850, Benton lost patience with the feisty, diminutive Mississippian. The tall, husky Missouri senator rose and advanced toward Foote, whose shrill voice and contorted face promised yet another insulting harangue. Confronted by Benton's unmistakable fury, the startled Foote hastily retreated toward the vice president's chair, brandishing a loaded pistol. Benton, who had been about to turn away, became further incensed at the sight of the weapon. He strode in the direction of Foote, shouting: "I have no pistols! Let him fire! Stand out of the way! Let the assassin fire!" The chamber erupted in loud disorder as onlookers ducked for shelter or tried to separate the two foes. Both participants were restrained, Foote gave up his pistol, and Benton returned to his seat.

Statement of the Case

Although the Senate was accustomed to political tensions created by sectional conflict, its members could not tolerate the appearance of weapons and the threat of violence in the chamber. Nor would an angry Benton permit the matter to be ignored. On April 23, 1850, after a short debate, the senators agreed to appoint a committee to investigate the matter. Chaired by James A. Pearce (W-MD), the committee included such prominent Whig senators as Daniel Webster of Massachusetts and John Bell of Tennessee.

Response of the Senate

After hearing the witnesses that the combatants paraded before it, the committee issued its report on July 30, 1850. Sensitive to the tinder-box atmosphere in the chamber as sectional tensions multiplied, the panel sought to defuse rather than exacerbate the crisis and therefore issued a general rebuke to the whole Senate. The committee determined that the roots of the turbulent scenario lay in the Senate's neglect of its own rules of order. The Foote-Benton clash represented only the most excessive of several such incidents of disregard for correct procedure. Sharply critical of any resort to insults and violence on the floor, the panel hoped that its condemnation would deter any further outrageous behavior. Regarding the particular altercation, the committee absolved Foote of any intent to assassinate Benton but acknowledged that he had "without any sufficient provocation, indulged in personalities toward Mr. Benton of the most offensive character, such as were calculated to rouse the fiercest resentment in the human bosom. These were suffered by Mr. Benton for the longest time with great forbearance." While the committee recommended no action by the Senate, it did conclude its report with a warning: "Should . . . similar scenes of violence again occur, they cannot doubt that the Senate will enforce prompt, stern, and effectual punishment." The Senate tabled the committee's report and took no further action on the matter.

Conclusion

The incident underscored the growing intensity of feeling between ideological supporters and opponents of slavery. Their verbal exchanges in the Senate continued to be hostile and inflammatory until the southern states seceded in 1860–1861.

Thomas Hart Benton, after nearly thirty years of consecutive service in the Senate, was defeated in 1851. As the storm clouds of the Civil War approached, Benton still remained a unifying symbol for the foes of slavery, serving in the House of Representatives from 1853 to 1855. For the remainder of his life, until his death on April 10, 1858, he continued to follow the latest political developments and occupied himself with his writing.

Henry S. Foote concluded his Senate career in 1852, when he resigned to become governor of Mississippi. He lived briefly in California but returned to Mississippi before the Civil War. After the war, he practiced law and wrote several books. At the time of his death on May 19, 1880, Foote was superintendent of the federal mint at New Orleans.

Sources

U.S. Congress. Senate. *Congressional Globe.* 31st Cong., 1st sess. (See pp. 366, 762–64, 769, 1153, 1479–81.)

Coleman, James P. "Two Irascible Antebellum Senators: George Poindexter and Henry S. Foote." *The Journal of Mississippi History* 46 (February 1984): 17–27.

Johnson, Allen, ed. *Dictionary of American Biography.* New York, 1946; reprint of 1935 edition. Vol. 2. (See pp. 210–13 [Benton].) Vol. 6. (See pp. 500–501 [Foote].)

Smith, E. B. *Magnificent Missourian: The Life of Thomas Hart Benton.* Philadelphia, 1958. (See pp. 269–72.)

Case 23

Robert C. Winthrop

(1809–1894)

Massachusetts

Election Case (appointment)
February 4, 1851 to February 8, 1851

Issues
Time limits on appointment by governor (appointed senator held office only until the legislature elected a successor)

Result: No action required

Chronology:
Request for ruling: Feb. 4, 1851
Referred to committee: Feb. 4, 1851
Committee report: Feb. 5, 1851
Senate action: Feb. 8, 1851

Background

In 1828, shortly after his graduation from Harvard, Robert C. Winthrop entered the law offices of Daniel Webster. Twenty-two years later, the Massachusetts governor selected Winthrop to succeed his former associate, "Black Dan" Webster, when the latter resigned from the Senate to become secretary of state. Winthrop, a Whig who had served as Speaker of the U.S. House of Representatives during the previous Congress, began his Senate duties on July 30, 1850.

Statement of the Case

On February 1, 1851, the Massachusetts state legislature elected Robert Rantoul, Jr. (D) to fill the remainder of Webster's unexpired term that was due to end on March 3 of that year. On February 4, Winthrop petitioned the Senate for a clarification of his status. He wished to know precisely when his term expired and Robert Rantoul's began, thus raising the prickly problem of the time limits on an interim Senate appointment made by a state executive. Winthrop emphasized that he did not wish either to abandon his responsibility to the Commonwealth of Massachusetts prematurely or to remain in the Senate one moment longer than he was entitled to. Earlier related precedents, Winthrop commented, did not provide any firm rulings on the proper conduct for an interim appointee.

Response of the Senate

The Senate agreed to consider Winthrop's request, and the Judiciary Committee took up the issue of the duration of interim appointments. On February 5, the committee returned its report. Citing the 1809 case of Maryland's Samuel Smith (See Case 9), the committee declared that a senator appointed by a governor was entitled to hold his seat until the state legislature filled the vacancy, the Senate was officially informed of that election, and the new senator's credentials were presented.

On February 7, Robert Winthrop announced he had received through the mail the credentials of Robert Rantoul. Meanwhile, Rantoul, who had been absent from Massachusetts and not consulted by the legislature prior to his election, had accepted his new post and was en route to Washington. Winthrop, adamant that he would not continue beyond his constitutional right, submitted Rantoul's credentials and retired from the Senate.

Although there had as yet been no floor debate on the report of the Judiciary Committee, Winthrop's withdrawal prompted Henry Clay (W-KY) to object both to the committee report and to Winthrop's retirement. His remarks generated a lengthy, complicated discussion about the meanings of "vacancy," "temporary appointment," "original power," "limits of power," "acceptance," and a variety of other constitutional terms. The exchanges dragged on, and tempers frayed.

Finally, on February 8, John P. Hale (FS-NH) chided members for straying far afield. There was, he said, "nothing on earth before the Senate but a mere abstract question. There is nobody that claims a seat. Mr. Rantoul is not here, and Mr. Winthrop has gone." He warned the Senate that outsiders would decide that the United States Senate had an abundance of leisure and misused its time discussing an irrelevant question. Jarred by Hale's scolding, the Senate set aside the topic of appointed senators.

Conclusion

Robert Rantoul served for the remaining month of Daniel Webster's term. Later that year, he was elected to the U.S. House of Representatives and died in office in 1852. Robert Winthrop sought to win a full term in the Senate in 1851 but was defeated by Charles Sumner. During the remainder of his long life, he earned a modicum of fame as a public speaker. He died in 1894.

Sources

U.S. Congress. Senate. *Congressional Globe.* 31st Cong., 2d sess. (See pp. 425–26, 437, 459–67, 477–78.)

———. Senate Report No. 269. 31st Cong., 2d sess., 1851.

Baxter, Maurice G. *One and Inseparable: Daniel Webster and the Union.* Cambridge, MA, 1984. (See pp. 484–85.)

Donald, David Herbert. *Charles Sumner and the Coming of the Civil War.* Chicago, 1960. (See pp. 185, 191–92, 195, 201–2.)

Malone, Dumas, ed. *Dictionary of American Biography.* Vol. 20. New York, 1946; reprint of 1935 edition. (See pp. 416–17.)

Winthrop, Robert C., Jr. *Memoir of Robert Charles Winthrop.* Boston, 1897.

Case 24

David L. Yulee v. Stephen R. Mallory

(1810–1886) (1813–1873)

Florida

Election Case
March 8, 1851 to August 27, 1852

Issues
Right of losing candidate in contested election to address the Senate

Result: Mallory retained seat

Chronology:
Notice of contest: Mar. 8, 1851
Referred to committee: Dec. 1, 1851
Committee report: Aug. 21, 1852
Senate vote: Aug. 27, 1852

Background

David Levy and Stephen R. Mallory, each born in the West Indies, migrated to Florida and entered local politics. In 1845, with the admission of Florida to the Union, Levy (D) became one of the state's first senators, having served previously as the territorial delegate. Early in 1846, at Levy's request, the Florida state legislature officially changed his name to David Levy Yulee. In 1851 the state general assembly failed to reelect Yulee when, on three ballots, the 58 members repeatedly divided their votes 29 to 29. One-half of the legislature voted for David Yulee, but the other half registered blank votes. Two days later, 31 members voted for Stephen R. Mallory (D) and 27 voted for Yulee. The Florida assembly declared Mallory the victor.

Statement of the Case

Early in March 1851, during the brief special session, the Senate received a letter of contest from Yulee, but on December 1, 1851, at the beginning of the regular session of the Senate, the body seated Stephen Mallory. It then referred his credentials and Yulee's letter to a specially appointed committee for review.

Yulee maintained that Mallory's election violated Florida election rules but that the complexity of the local political regulations restricted the ability of non-Floridians to grasp the meaning of the state laws. Yulee asked that the election be turned back to the Florida legislature as the only body capable of interpreting the intent of the law.

Response of the Senate

The committee reported more than a year later on August 21, 1852, recommending that the Senate adopt a resolution stating that Stephen Mallory had been duly elected. During the Senate debate on August 27, James A.

Bayard, Jr. (D-DE) objected to the requests of Yulee's supporters that he be heard on the floor of the Senate. Bayard argued that further debate only obstructed the completion of public business in a session that was rapidly drawing to a close. His remarks precipitated a lengthy debate over Yulee's right to floor time. Yulee's opponents protested that, if the contestant gained the floor, precious time would be wasted.

The tardiness with which the committee had completed the Yulee report added weight to the senator's cause. Stung by these criticisms, Jesse D. Bright (D-IN) explained that Chairman John M. Berrien (W-GA) had been called home for a "domestic affliction" and that upon his return Bright himself left Washington. Once the committee finally assembled, Bright explained, it was his understanding that both Florida contestants preferred to defer the decision until after the national political conventions. This may have been true of David Yulee, who orchestrated Stephen Douglas' attempt to capture the 1852 Democratic presidential nomination, but Mallory denied vehemently that he had requested any postponement. To emphasize his desire for a speedy resolution, Mallory urged the Senate to give Yulee two hours to speak and promised to say nothing in reply.

Finally given his opportunity to address the Senate, and with Edwin M. Stanton as his counsel, Yulee reiterated his argument that only the Florida legislature could understand the complexities of an election resolution passed in 1845. In addition, he asserted that the 29 blank votes actually had been cast in his favor. Yulee's opponents countered that the current Florida legislature was not the same as that involved in the election dispute and questioned how a blank vote assumed the character of assent. On the subject of the blank votes, one senator noted that, after each of the three failed ballots, the president of the Florida joint meeting announced "no election." Had any of the Florida legislators intended that the blank vote be an aye, ample opportunity had existed for individuals to note the mistake. Clearly, the purpose of the blank votes had been to show that the Florida legislature had a quorum for an election, thus avoiding any future challenges by Yulee on that procedural point.

The Senate unanimously voted to reject Yulee's claim to the seat and recognize Mallory as the duly elected Florida senator.

Conclusion

On March 17, 1853, the Senate voted to grant Yulee per diem and mileage for the period when he was contesting the seat.

Florida returned David Yulee to its other Senate seat in 1855. He and Mallory represented the state together until they both withdrew with other southern senators on January 21, 1861. During the Civil War, Mallory served as secretary of the navy for the Confederacy. He practiced law in Florida after the war and died in 1873. Yulee served in the Confederate Congress and was a prisoner of state briefly when the South was defeated. In 1880 Yulee moved to Washington, DC. He died in 1886.

Sources

U.S. Congress. Senate. *Congressional Globe.* 32d Cong., 1st sess. (See p. 2488, Appendix, pp. 1170–77). 2d sess. (See pp. 280–83.)

Malone, Dumas, ed. *Dictionary of American Biography.* Vol. 12. New York, 1946; reprint of 1935 edition. Vol. 12. (See pp. 224–24 [Mallory]) Vol. 20. (See pp. 638–39 [Yulee].)

Case 25

Archibald Dixon

(1802–1876)

Kentucky

Election Case (appointment)
December 6, 1852 to
December 20, 1852

Chronology:
Credentials presented: Dec. 6, 1852
Senate vote: Dec. 20, 1852

Issues
Right of governor to make appointment to fill a vacancy only for a limited time; right of legislature to elect to fill a vacancy that would occur in the future

Result: Seated

Background

In December 1851, the ailing Henry Clay resigned his Senate seat, effective the first Monday of September 1852. On December 30, 1851, the Kentucky legislature elected Archibald Dixon, a Whig and political friend of Clay, to serve the remainder of the term from September 1852 to March 1855. Shortly after this vote, the Kentucky legislature adjourned.

Clay's health deteriorated rapidly and he died on June 29, 1852. Within a few days, Democratic Governor Lazarus Powell appointed Democrat David Meriwether to be senator until the date of Clay's intended resignation in September. Meriwether took his seat on July 15, 1852, and served for seven weeks until Congress adjourned on August 31, 1852.

Statement of the Case

When the Senate reconvened in December, the status of David Meriwether and Archibald Dixon appeared clear. Meriwether, the senator appointed to fill the vacancy caused by the death of Henry Clay, had left the Senate by the date of Clay's intended resignation in September 1852. Archibald Dixon, elected for the term beginning on Clay's planned date of resignation, arrived to take his seat on December 6, 1852. Although no Kentuckians challenged these procedures, William M. Gwin (D-CA) protested Dixon's seating. He insisted that, when the Senate recessed in August, Kentucky had two senators and that no new vacancy had been created.

Response of the Senate

James C. Jones (W-TN), who had presented Dixon's credentials, pointed out that Meriwether was not contesting the seat. Gwin countered that there was no need for a contestant since no vacancy existed. He noted that he had questioned the validity of Meriwether's credentials the previous July, because of the time limit the Kentucky governor had placed on Meriwether's tenure. Supporters of Dixon observed that Kentucky's actions represented harmonious cooperation between an executive and a legislature. After the legislature selected a successor for Clay's post-resignation term, the governor, with the state assembly adjourned, exercised his proper authority to appoint an interim senator for the seat unexpectedly vacated by Clay's death. Other senators agreed, adding that the conditions of Meriwether's appointment were fully known and recognized by the Senate when his credentials were accepted in July.

As the debate continued over several days, subsequent responses from a variety of senators made it evident that the Kentucky credentials matter had become yet another pretext for debate on states' rights. Theoreticians began analyzing the source of final authority in the structure of American government. The supporters of states' rights charged that Kentucky was entitled to two senators because the states were sovereign, while the opponents argued that Kentucky was entitled to two senators by virtue of the limited sovereignty granted states by the United States Constitution.

The wide-ranging debate rambled on until December 20, when George E. Badger (W-NC) interjected a bit of humor by suggesting that he could make a very good fifteen-minute speech on the topic but that, in the tradition of the Senate, he would continue for forty-five minutes. "Our speeches here," Badger contended, "will convince nobody in the Chamber, if they convince any one outside." His colleagues agreed the time had come to terminate the argument and voted 27 to 16 to seat Dixon.

Conclusion

By seating Archibald Dixon the Senate responded affirmatively to three questions: could a state legislature fill a vacancy before it actually occurred; could the governor limit the duration of a term; and could there be one vacancy caused by death and three months later a second vacancy caused by resignation, both for the same man?

The Senate voted mileage and per diem until December 20, 1852, for David Meriwether, who had waited in Washington for the outcome.

Archibald Dixon did not seek reelection to his Senate seat in 1854. He resumed the practice of law in Kentucky, where he died in 1876.

Sources

U.S. Congress. Senate. *Congressional Globe*. 32d Cong., 1st sess. (See pp. 1783–84; 2d sess., pp. 1–5, 12–19, 24, 43–47, 58–62, 69–76, 90–96.)

Case 26

Samuel S. Phelps

(1793–1855)

Vermont

Election Case (appointment)
January 4, 1854 to March 16, 1854

Issues
Whether appointment expires when the legislature next meets or only when the legislature elects a successor

Result: Senate ruled term expired

Chronology:
Request for ruling: Jan. 4, 1854
Referred to committee: Jan. 4, 1854
Committee report: Jan. 16, 1854
Senate vote: Mar. 16, 1854

Background

After graduating from Yale in 1811 and serving in the War of 1812, Samuel Phelps entered a career in public service in Vermont. He was first elected to the United States Senate as a Whig in 1838 and was reelected in 1844. Phelps, an outspoken and forceful orator, delivered a powerful anti-slavery speech in 1848. At the completion of his term, Phelps returned to Vermont, but on January 17, 1853, the governor of the state appointed him to fill the Senate vacancy created by the January 14 death of William Upham. On January 19, 1853, Phelps took the oath of office and was seated.

Statement of the Case

As the Vermont legislature reached no agreement on a permanent replacement for Upham when it met in October and December 1853, Phelps returned to the Senate when the new Congress convened in December. On January 4, 1854, William H. Seward (W-NY) inquired whether Phelps, as an executive appointee, could continue to hold his seat even though the Vermont assembly had already met in two regular sessions. Seward wondered whether the existence of an intervening legislature, even if it failed to fill a senatorial vacancy, terminated the appointment of a senator named by the governor. The Senate referred the question of Phelps' status to the Judiciary Committee.

Response of the Senate

On January 16, 1854, the committee returned majority and minority reports. The former contended that, although clear limitations restricted the gubernatorial power to appoint during a legislative recess, the executive nomination continued in force until superseded by the action of the legislature or until the Senate term expired. The majority report therefore supported Phelps' claim to the seat, citing the precedent established in the 1809 case of Samuel Smith of Maryland (See Case 8).

In a minority report, Andrew P. Butler (D-SC) and James A. Bayard, Jr. (D-DE) countered that, once a legislature met and had the opportunity to make a selection, a gubernatorial appointment would automatically terminate, even if the body did not use its power to elect a successor. Therefore, they asserted, Phelps had no right to continue in office.

Phelps, who was known for his violent temper, argued valiantly, if bitterly, that nothing in the phraseology "make appointments" implied duration. He grumbled that frequent postponements and delays had successfully fragmented his arguments, then complained of the "empty desks . . . the chills of winter, the approach of old age, and the infirmities which beset me." Although he believed his position to be well supported by earlier contests, he explained that he felt too feeble to read the corroborating selections from *Congressional Globes* stashed under his desk. At this, Henry Foote (D-MS) "cheerfully" hauled forth the volumes and read the passages for him.

The arguments for and against the beleaguered senator dragged on until March 16, 1854. Then, perhaps encouraged by Phelps' remark that the best favor the Senate could do was to retire him from all responsibility, the members, by a vote of 12 yeas to 26 nays, rejected the committee majority's recommendation in favor of Phelps and determined that he was not entitled to a seat in the Senate. They then unanimously voted to pay him mileage and per diem to the date of the vote.

Conclusion

The confusion surrounding gubernatorial appointments heightened as the number of challenges increased. Opposing sides, often influenced by the escalating sectional conflict of the 1850s, took advantage of the contests for their own political convenience. Each new challenge further underscored the awkwardness of the senatorial election process.

The Phelps case was no exception, and the exchanges during the almost two months of debate were notable for their caustic unpleasantness. As a result of this stalemate, Vermont lacked full Senate representation from March 16 to October 14, 1854, when the legislature finally elected a new senator to fill the remaining months of the vacancy. Phelps died the year after he left Washington.

Sources

U.S. Congress. Senate. Senate Report No. 34. 33d Cong., 1st sess., 1854.

———. *Congressional Globe.* 33d Cong., 1st sess. (See pp. 103, 115–17, 250–52, 303–4, 610, 630–32, 639–46, 676, Appendix, pp. 356–69.)

Case 27

Jared W. Williams

(1796–1864)

New Hampshire

Election Case (appointment)
July 25, 1854 to August 4, 1854

Issues
Whether appointment expired when the legislature met or only when it elected a successor

Result: Senate ruled term expired

Chronology:
Request for ruling: July 25, 1854
Referred to committee: July 25, 1854
Committee report: Aug. 2, 1854
Senate vote: Aug. 4, 1854

Background

Following his graduation from Brown University in 1816, Jared W. Williams devoted himself to public service. He held positions in both houses of the New Hampshire legislature, as judge of the probate court, and as governor of New Hampshire. He also served in the U.S. House of Representatives from 1837 to 1841. On November 29, 1853, after Senator-elect Charles Atherton died of a stroke before he could take office, the New Hampshire governor named Jared Williams (D) to the seat. On December 12, 1853, Williams presented his credentials and was seated without incident.

Statement of the Case

On July 25, 1854, Stephen R. Mallory (D-FL) submitted a resolution questioning the eligibility of Williams to retain his seat, since the New Hampshire legislature had met that June in regular session. Having failed to elect a successor to the deceased Charles Atherton, the legislature had adjourned until the following May. Because Mallory's challenge raised an often-disputed constitutional point, the Senate referred the status of Jared Williams to the Judiciary Committee.

Response of the Senate

On August 2, 1854, the committee, chaired by Andrew P. Butler (D-SC), returned a report largely based upon a communication from the New Hampshire governor and on the state's constitution. From this information, the committee concluded that, once the governor dissolved the legislature, it had no power to reassemble until called at its regular constitutional time. Although the committee acknowledged that the governor had the authority to convene a special session of the state legislature, it doubted that this would fulfill the requirement that the selection of a senator be made in the regular meeting of the assembly. The committee therefore labeled the Williams case identical to that of Samuel Phelps of Vermont the previous year (See Case 26) and declared the appointment expired.

In the early morning hours of August 4, during an all-night session shortly before adjournment, the Senate voted to accept the committee's recommendation. Then, later that morning, as the Senate raced to finish its business, Augustus C. Dodge (D-IA) pointed out that Williams, in feeble health, had left the Senate the previous evening assured that the subject of his eligibility would not soon come to a vote. Dodge, despite the complaints of several colleagues, prevailed in his request that the Senate reconsider its action and give Williams floor time to defend his case.

When Williams took the floor later that same morning, he told an impatient and unfriendly Senate that it had misunderstood the circumstances in New Hampshire, where he denied the legislature had ever disbanded. He asked for a postponement to enable representatives of the state of New Hampshire to present their view of the case. Responding to opponents who charged he was seeking to delay a decision only in order to collect extensive mileage and per diem fees, Williams declared, "I am anxious to disabuse the minds of those who entertain the opinion... that I am a hanger-on here for place and pay." He insisted that his concern was for his duty to New Hampshire. The Senate, unmoved by his arguments, refused either to postpone the case or to ask the Judiciary Committee for additional review. It first voted against postponement, 11 yeas to 37 nays, then, after brief debate, accepted the Judiciary Committee report that declared Williams' term expired.

Conclusion

The case of Jared Williams, essentially identical to that of Samuel Phelps, occurred so soon after that of the Vermont senator that the resolution was certain to be the same. During the brief debate following the Judiciary Committee's report, James C. Jones (W-TN), perhaps more prophetically than he intended, remarked, "If we have not settled this question by the whole action of the Senate for the last twenty years, we never shall, never can settle it." Another sixty years would pass before the nation would abandon the Constitution's awkward and challenge-prone system for electing senators.

Jared Williams returned to New Hampshire, where he died in 1864.

Sources

U.S. Congress. Senate. *Congressional Globe*. 33d Cong., 1st sess. (See pp. 2208–11.)

———. Senate Report No. 385. 33d Cong., 1st sess., 1854.

Case 28

Lyman Trumbull

(1813–1896)

Illinois

Election Case (qualifications)
December 3, 1855 to March 5, 1856

Issues
Right of state to impose additional eligibility requirements for senators

Result: Retained seat

Chronology:
Credentials presented: Dec. 3, 1855
Referred to committee: Dec. 20, 1855
Committee report: Feb. 27, 1856
Senate vote: Mar. 5, 1856

Background

After holding a series of public offices in Illinois, Lyman Trumbull (D) won election in 1848 to the state supreme court. Although reelected to that post in 1852 for a term running until 1861, he resigned in May 1853, shortly after beginning his new term, citing poor health and his inadequate salary. In the spring of 1854, Congress passed the Kansas-Nebraska Act. This measure, sponsored by Stephen A. Douglas (D-IL) effectively repealed the 1820 Missouri Compromise that had banned slavery in the northern territories. In the outcry that followed, the Illinois Democratic party split into pro- and anti-Nebraska Act factions. Trumbull, enraged at Douglas for sponsoring the measure so hateful to the free-soil forces, ran for the United States House of Representatives, winning election in November 1854 to a term beginning in December 1855.

Trumbull did not enter the House, however, because early in 1855 he was drawn into a heated race for the United States Senate seat held by James Shields (D). On February 8, after ten ballots in the state legislature, Trumbull won election to the Senate. In the process, he defeated Whig candidate Abraham Lincoln and the pro-Douglas Democratic forces that had first supported James Shields and then popular Governor Joel A. Matteson, who remained untainted by the Kansas-Nebraska Act.

Statement of the Case

The regular Democrats, furious at Trumbull's election, quickly decided to harass him. On February 21 they published a "legal opinion" that found Trumbull ineligible for the Senate seat under a provision of the state constitution that required state officers to wait a year after the end of their terms before accepting any other office. By their calculation, Trumbull would not be eligible until 1862. Trumbull responded that he had resigned from the state supreme court—and a successor had been chosen—eighteen months before his election to the Senate. He therefore contended that the provision of the state constitution did not apply in this case.

When the Senate convened for its new session on December 3, 1855, Trumbull presented only partial credentials. Since Democratic Governor Matteson had refused to sign his election certificate, Trumbull could only offer the statement of the legislative vote as certified by the Illinois secretary of state. Immediately, Lewis Cass (D-MI) submitted a protest to Trumbull's seating signed by forty-two members of the one-hundred-member Illinois legislature. In accordance with normal procedure, Trumbull was seated pending further investigation but received no committee assignments and was prohibited, by custom, from participating in any Senate business except that which related to his seating. On December 20, the Senate referred the matter to the Judiciary Committee.

Response of the Senate

On February 27, 1856, the Judiciary Committee, reporting that it was hopelessly deadlocked, urged the full Senate to resolve the matter. Pro-Douglas forces then introduced a resolution declaring the seat vacant. Trumbull supporters countered with a proposal that he be declared seated. John J. Crittenden (OP-KY) argued that Lyman Trumbull met every constitutional requirement for admission to the United States Senate and that no state had the power to add new qualifications or disqualifications. He noted that, although restrictive provisions had crept into a number of state constitutions, it was his understanding that the Senate had never regarded these as binding upon itself. Convinced that Trumbull's credentials fulfilled all the constitutional requirements, Crittenden requested that the election be declared valid.

George E. Pugh (D-OH), a Douglas lieutenant, responded that the language of the Constitution was that of exclusion, and not of qualification. He agreed that the states could not alter the language of the United States Constitution but contended that, since a senator acted as both a federal agent and an officer of the state, individual legislatures could add state qualifications. Drawing upon a series of precedents set in earlier challenges, Pugh constructed an argument for states' rights, concluding that a favorable resolution for Trumbull "would be yet another stride, longer than any stride yet taken, towards that consolidation of powers in the federal government, which has already grown to an inordinate degree, and... now threatens us."

On March 4, 1856, committee chairman Butler, at the request of his colleagues, addressed the question, expressing support for Trumbull. Although he had long supported states' rights, he said, he believed that doctrine did not apply in this case. "I am not so far a states-rights man," he declared, "as absolutely to forget the honor, and the justice... of compacts." Although legislators had a dual responsibility both to their federal and state constitutions, he maintained that the states had relinquished the power of determining the qualifications of senators and could not therefore change those qualifications. A colleague agreed, asserting, "It belongs to us to judge the qualifications prescribed by the Constitution of the United States . . . the state tribunals are the exclusive judges of the qualifications required by their own constitution."

On March 5, satisfied that Trumbull's judicial resignation more than a year before his Senate election had passed the scrutiny of the Illinois legislature and convinced that no state could add stipulations to the United States Constitution, the Senate, by an overwhelming vote of 35 to 8, upheld Trumbull's claim to his seat.

Conclusion

The challenge to Lyman Trumbull's credentials became one more excuse for the Senate to argue heatedly the nature of states' rights. Additionally, it demonstrated once again that the method of electing senators continued to create time-consuming dilemmas for the national legislature.

Lyman Trumbull served in the Senate until 1873. In 1856 he joined the newly formed Republican party, remaining there throughout the Civil War. Then, after he voted for acquittal in Andrew Johnson's 1868 impeachment trial, his Republican colleagues scorned him and he drifted away from the mainstream of the party. After leaving the Senate, Trumbull returned to the Democratic party, failing in 1880 to capture the governorship of Illinois. Trumbull died in Chicago in 1896.

Sources

U.S. Congress. Senate. *Congressional Globe.* 34th Cong., 1st sess. (See 58, 343, 466–68, 514–15, 547–52, 562–67, 579–84.)

———. Senate Report No. 15. 34th Cong., 1st sess., 1856.

Johannsen, Robert. *Stephen A. Douglas.* New York, 1973. (See pp. 462–64, 469.)

Krug, Mark M. *Lyman Trumbull: Conservative Radical.* New York, 1965. (See pp. 94–114.)

Malone, Dumas, ed. *Dictionary of American Biography.* Vol. 19. New York, 1946; reprint of 1935 edition. (See pp. 19–20.)

Roske, Ralph J. *His Own Counsel: The Life and Times of Lyman Trumbull.* Reno, NV, 1979. (See pp. 13–33.)

Case 29

James Harlan

(1820–1899)

Iowa

Election Case
December 3, 1855 to January 12, 1857

Issues
Conduct of election

Result: Unseated

Chronology:
Credentials presented: Dec. 3, 1855
Referred to committee: Dec. 15, 1856
Committee report: Jan. 5, 1857
Senate vote: Jan. 12, 1857

Background

Passage of the Kansas-Nebraska Act early in 1854 effectively opened territories to slavery and sparked a thunderous political explosion. Antislavery Whigs and Democrats combined with free-soilers and abolitionists to establish an anti-Nebraska party, which subsequently became the Republican party. The accompanying political shock waves were felt in numerous Senate election contests (See Case 28).

In Iowa thirty-five-year-old James Harlan (OP) quickly emerged as a strong candidate in a crowded field to challenge incumbent Democratic Senator Augustus Caesar Dodge, whose term was to expire in March 1855. The politically astute Harlan avoided being pinned down on positions by the many factions that jockeyed for control within each party. Refusing to respond in writing to a questionnaire, he agreed to meet personally with anyone who wanted an elaboration of his views. He expressed his platform as follows: "If elected to the Senate of the United States, in all Constitutional questions that might arise, I would expect to be guided in my action by the decisions of the Supreme Court and the well settled principles of constitutional law—in all questions of Legislative Expediency, by the views and wishes of the legislature and people of Iowa—and in all questions of Conscience by the Bible."

The legislature of Iowa, which was required to elect senators in joint session, met on December 21, 1854, and January 5, 1855, and failed to make a choice. On Saturday, January 6, 1855, the state house convened and sent a message to the senate that it was ready to meet in joint convention to elect a senator but was informed that the senate had already adjourned to the following Monday. Since the session had been announced when the convention adjourned the preceding day, some senators, but not the senate's president, arrived in the house chamber ready to continue the election. The speaker of the house convened the joint convention, which elected new officers and sent the sergeant at arms to inform the absentees that the convention was ready to proceed with the election. A vote for U.S. senator was then taken, with a majority of the house and of the whole legislature present, but not a majority of the senate. Harlan received 52 votes—a bare majority of the votes cast—to win a seat in the United States Senate. When the Iowa senate met the following Monday, it protested that the election was not legal since a majority of senators had not been present.

Statement of the Case

Although Harlan's opponents in Iowa challenged the legality of his selection, the U.S. Senate on December 3, 1855, administered the oath to Harlan. Despite attempts by his Democratic Iowa colleague, George W. Jones, to call up the matter in August 1856, the Senate permitted the question to lie on the table for a year. On December 15, 1856, when Jones again moved to take up the petition challenging Harlan's election, Harlan offered records of the state legislature and letters from Iowa supreme court justices to support his claim to the seat. Convinced that the subject no longer generated any concern in Iowa, Harlan cheerfully accepted the reference of his case to the Judiciary Committee. He observed in passing, however, that the panel contained not one political friend, as each member opposed him on every current national issue. Although he hastened to soften the impact of that observation by adding that he never intended to question the impartiality of any committee member, for he had learned early in his Senate career that such cases were always adjudicated fairly, Harlan's remark irritated his opponents. Andrew P. Butler (D-SC), chairman of the Judiciary Committee, suggested that, if the Senate had a Committee on Privileges and Elections composed of the oldest senators, such cases could be dispatched without these charges of bias.

Response of the Senate

On January 5, 1857, the Judiciary Committee, having reviewed the proceedings of the Iowa legislature in 1854, returned a report recommending that Harlan's seat be declared vacant. The recommendation gave rise to lengthy partisan explanations of the fine points of the Iowa constitution. In supporting Harlan, William H. Seward (OP-NY) argued that the United States Senate required that a person's credentials show election by the state legislature, whose transactions, once it merged into a common body, superseded individual characteristics. The debate meandered through wordy definitions of "quorum," "majority," and "united votes," until a weary James A. Bayard, Jr. (D-DE) remarked, "I am not sure that it would not have been wiser if it had pleased the convention that framed the federal Constitution to delegate the power to the respective states to elect their two senators by a popular vote instead of choosing them by the legislatures. I do not see any evil that could have followed from it."

In the face of the passionate exchanges, the initial good humor of the senators evaporated, replaced by heated clashes and near insults. The acrimonious debates concluded on January 12, 1857, when the Senate voted 28 to 18 to declare the seat vacant.

Conclusion

Five days after the Senate's action, the Iowa legislature elected Harlan as a Republican. Reelected in 1861, Harlan served as a delegate to the peace convention held that year as a last effort to avoid the coming war. At the close of the Civil War, he resigned from the Senate to become secretary of the interior for Andrew Johnson, returning in 1867 to serve a full term. Harlan died at his Iowa home in 1899.

Cases like Harlan's demonstrated the need for the federal law that was finally passed a decade later in 1866, setting forth procedures for state legislatures to follow in electing U.S. senators. That act specifically provided that, in the joint assembly of both houses, a majority of all the votes of the joint assembly would be sufficient to elect if a majority of members of both houses were present, the condition that had existed for Harlan's 1855 election.

Sources

U.S. Congress. *Congressional Globe.* 34th Cong., 1st sess. (See pp. 2098, 2129–30.) 3d sess. (See pp. 112–17, 238–57, 260–70, 287–99.)

———. Senate Report No. 300. 34th Cong., 3d sess., 1857.

Brigham, Johnson. *James Harlan.* Iowa City, IA, 1913. (See pp. 79–107.)

Johnson, Allen, and Dumas Malone, eds. *Dictionary of American Biography.* Vol. 8. New York, 1946; reprint of 1935 edition. (See pp. 268–69.)

Case 30

Henry S. Lane v. Jesse D. Bright
(1811–1881) (1812–1875)

and

William M. McCarty v. Graham N. Fitch
[dates unknown] (1809–1892)

Indiana

Election Case
February 9, 1857 to February 14, 1859

Issues
Conduct of election; whether a Senate vote in a contested election was final or could be reversed

Chronology:

Fitch and Bright
Credentials presented:
Feb. 9, 1857; Mar. 4, 1857
Referred to committee:
Feb. 10, 1857; Dec. 17, 1857
Committee report: May 24, 1858
Senate vote: June 12, 1858
Result: Fitch and Bright seated

Lane and McCarty
Credentials presented: Jan. 24, 1859
Referred to committee Jan. 24, 1859
Committee report: Feb. 3, 1859
Senate vote: Feb. 14, 1859
Result: Upheld first decision

Background

As the Republican party gained strength in northern Indiana, its members in the state legislature engaged in increasingly acrimonious clashes with Democrats from the southern part of the state. The opening of the 1857 legislative session brought the hostilities to a rowdy climax when boisterous, reportedly armed Republicans milled about the halls and the floor of the senate, disrupting attempts by the Democratic lieutenant governor to call the roll. The disorderly behavior of the Republicans included the illegal installation of their own "chair" who "swore in" party colleagues, whose election credentials might otherwise have been challenged.

The senate Republicans then employed tactics learned from state Democrats in earlier years and refused to go into joint session with the house for the election of United States senators. Through this device, the Republicans vainly hoped to stall the selection of senators until their party controlled a majority of both houses of the legislature. For their part, the Democrats simply ignored the state law that required a joint resolution for the legislature to hold an election and met to take a senatorial vote. Since both U.S. Senate seats were open to election—one for a full term held by incumbent Democrat Jesse D. Bright, and one that had been vacant since 1855—the rivalry was exceptionally keen.

Statement of the Case

This chaotic election returned the powerful and outspoken veteran Jesse Bright, who had served as Senate president pro tempore, to Washington for a full term. Graham N. Fitch, a physician and former member of the House of Representatives, won the second seat. Republicans, however, showed no inclination to let the matter fade, even after Bright presented Fitch's credentials on February 9, 1857, and the Senate seated Fitch. On the following day, at the request of Lyman Trumbull, an Illinois Democrat who joined the Republican party in 1857, and Thomas J. Rusk (D-TX) the Senate referred Fitch's credentials and supporting papers to the Judiciary Committee. On March 4, 1857, the opening day of a brief special session of the Thirty-fifth Congress, Jesse Bright was seated for his new term. Then, when Congress convened in December of that year, the Senate referred the credentials of both Fitch and Bright to the Judiciary Committee.

Response of the Senate

On May 24, 1858, the Judiciary Committee issued a report that upheld the right of Fitch and Bright to their seats, but Republicans and Bright's Democratic opponents continued to charge that the composition of the committee, five Democrats and two Republicans, precluded a just decision. Supporters of Bright and Fitch countered that the Indiana Democrats had violated no rules, because, for a joint session to conduct a valid election, only a majority of the total membership needed to be present, rather than a quorum from each house. After a lengthy discussion, the Senate on June 12, 1858, voted down a motion, 23 to 30, to deny Fitch and Bright their seats and then by voice vote agreed that they held their seats legally.

By 1858, Indiana Republicans had gained control of both houses of the state legislature. Dissatisfied with the Senate's acceptance of Bright and Fitch, the state assembly elected two new senators. On January 24, 1859, Republicans Henry S. Lane and William M. McCarty appeared and presented duly signed credentials designating them senators from Indiana.

Jesse Bright was an expansionist who supported the admission of Kansas under the proslavery Lecompton Constitution in 1858. In doing so, he gained the enmity of his former Democratic ally in the Senate, Stephen A. Douglas of Illinois, who strongly opposed admitting Kansas as a slave state. Thus, Douglas joined one of Bright's Republican adversaries, William H. Seward of New York, in moving quickly to legitimize the status of Lane and McCarty and pressing to grant the claimants seats on the floor. A decision on that resolution was postponed while the credentials went to the Judiciary Committee for review. Less than two weeks later, on February 3, 1859, the committee reported that the Indiana legislature was attempting to reverse a decision made by the Senate under its constitutional authority to judge the qualifications of its own members. It therefore determined that the elections of Lane and McCarty were invalid since no vacancies existed. A short minority statement by Jacob Collamer (R-VT) contended that the Senate's decision was not necessarily final and could be reversed. Unswayed by this argument, the Senate on February 14, 1859, voted 30 to 15 to uphold the opinion that the June 12, 1858, judgment was irreversible. The votes of southerners pleased by Fitch and Bright's stance on Lecompton, made the difference.

Conclusion

The Indiana election represented the worst example of how local party battles could consume inordinate amounts of time in the national legislature. Despite the intense partisan unrest created by the formation of the new Republican party, the Senate jealously guarded its own constitutional prerogative to judge the qualifications of its members.

Graham Fitch completed his term in 1861. Following service as an officer in the Civil War, he returned to the practice of medicine. He died in 1892.

Jesse Bright had a political past replete with charges of misconduct and "bossism," and his career after the election challenge would include more of the same. In 1862, the Senate expelled Bright for a wartime indiscretion (See Case 40).

Sources

U.S. Congress. Senate. *Congressional Globe.* 34th Cong., 3d sess. (See pp. 1034–40, Appendix, pp. 193–215, 385–86, 392–97.)

———. *Congressional Globe.* 35th Cong., 1st sess. (See pp. 567–70, 698–710, 720–24, 1658–59, 2923–49.) 2d sess. (See pp. 534–35, 599–602, 957–59, 1014–19, Appendix, pp. 128–48.)

———. Senate Report No. 2. 35th Cong., special sess., 1857.

———. Senate Report No. 19. 35th Cong., 1st sess., 1858.

———. Senate Report No. 275. 35th Cong., 1st sess., 1858.

———. Senate Report No. 368. 35th Cong., 2d sess., 1859.

Johnson, Allen, ed. *Dictionary of American Biography.* New York, 1946; reprint of 1935 edition. Vol. 3. (See pp. 45–46 [Bright]) Vol. 10. (See pp. 574–75 [Lane].)

Murphy, Charles B. "The Political Career of Jesse D. Bright." *Indiana Historical Society Publications* 10 (1931): 101–45.

Summers, Mark W. *The Plundering Generation: Corruption and the Crisis of the Union, 1849–1861.* New York, 1987. (See p. 264.)

Simon Cameron

(1799–1889)

Pennsylvania

Election Case
March 6, 1857 to March 13, 1857

Issues
Election irregularities; electoral misconduct

Result: Seated

Chronology:
Petition received: Mar. 6, 1857
Referred to committee: Mar. 9, 1857
Committee report: Mar. 11, 1857
Senate vote: Mar. 13, 1857

Background

Starting as a newspaperman, Simon Cameron became wealthy by engaging in a variety of businesses, including railroad construction, banking, and insurance. He was also politically active and influential, although his tactics often provoked criticism. When serving as a commissioner for the Winnebago Indians, for example, Cameron gained notoriety by adjusting their claims through notes paid on his own bank. Despite such scandals, the Pennsylvania legislature in 1845 elected Cameron to fill the Senate vacancy created by the resignation of Democrat James Buchanan. Defeated for reelection in 1848, Cameron abandoned the Democrats in 1854, and in 1856 the state legislature returned him to the Senate as a Republican.

Statement of the Case

Cameron's controversial past and his separation from the Democrats guaranteed a challenge to his election. On March 6, 1857, two days after Cameron took his oath, sixty-nine members of the Pennsylvania legislature requested a Senate investigation. They based their protest upon charges that a majority of each branch of the state legislature did not favor Cameron's election, that the state senate failed to meet statutory requirements, and that "corrupt and unlawful means" had been used to influence votes in his favor.

Response of the Senate

On March 9, 1857, Cameron asked that the petition from the Pennsylvania legislature be sent to the Judiciary Committee. After two days of inquiry, the committee reported that it saw no need to consider the matter further.

The committee found that the full state legislature had assembled for the senatorial election and that Cameron received a majority vote. An investigation into the statutory protest showed that the appointment of the state senate's teller occurred on the day of the election, instead of one day previously as directed by state law. The committee considered this procedural violation to be so minor that it in no way invalidated the election. The committee dismissed as vague the charges of corruption in Cameron's selection.

Committee member George E. Pugh (D-OH) in a minority report attacked his colleagues for refusing to investigate allegations of corruption submitted by a responsible source, an insinuation that brought a swift denial from others on the Judiciary Committee. Chairman Andrew P. Butler (D-SC) insisted that the appropriate arena for settling the dispute lay not with the United States Senate, but with the state. He defended the committee's judgment, saying, "Let the members who have been charged with corruption be tried by their peers. It would be . . . unsafe . . . for us to send out a roving commission. . . . I am a State-rights man; and I say that the vicinage try the man, and when they . . . bring out the evidence, I will . . . expel the member."

Cameron expressed amazement at the entire episode, assuring the Senate that in Pennsylvania the protest was regarded "as a mere piece of humbug." Senators chuckled in amusement when Cameron remarked that several petitioners confided they had only signed to avoid offending Pennsylvania officials who had the power to make political appointments. Cameron declared, "I come here to add to my fame, to my character, to my reputation . . . ; and that cannot be done by money." Chairman Butler reiterated that it was up to the Pennsylvania legislature, rather than the U.S. Senate, to determine whether corruption had been involved in Cameron's election. Apparently the Senate agreed. On March 13, 1857, the members voted to discharge the Judiciary Committee from any further consideration of Cameron's right to his seat.

Conclusion

Simon Cameron served in the Senate until 1861, when he resigned to become secretary of war, but his questionable management of war contracts led the House of Representatives to censure him. In 1862, Cameron served briefly as minister to Russia, and in 1867 he was again elected to the United States Senate, remaining there until 1877. Adroit in behind-the-scenes political manipulation, Cameron built a powerful Republican machine in Pennsylvania that he passed along to his son, who succeeded him in the Senate. Cameron died in Pennsylvania in 1889.

Sources

U.S. Congress. Senate. *Congressional Globe.* 34th Cong., 3d sess. (See Appendix, pp. 385–91.)

Johnson, Allen, ed. *Dictionary of American Biography.* Vol. 3. New York, 1946; reprint of 1935 edition. (See pp. 437–39.)

Case 32

James Shields

(1806–1879)

Minnesota

Election Case
February 25, 1858 to March 4, 1858

Issues
Senator's right to be seated before statehood

Result: Not seated

Chronology:
Credentials presented: Feb. 25, 1858
Referred to committee: Feb. 25, 1858
Committee report: Mar. 4, 1858
No Senate action

Background

In 1855, the peripatetic James Shields (D), formerly a senator from Illinois (See Case 21), moved to the Minnesota Territory. Shields, an active Roman Catholic, saw the frontier as an ideal place for poor Irish immigrants to build prosperous lives through planned communities. Although his grand plans for Catholic colonization in the West never materialized, Shields had some success with a small town he helped to organize in Minnesota. In December 1858, as Minnesota was preparing for admission to the Union, the legislature selected Shields as one of the state's first two senators.

Statement of the Case

On February 25, 1858, John J. Crittenden (Am-KY) read a letter from Shields requesting that he be sworn in as senator, on the theory that Minnesota had become a state through the Enabling Act of 1857, even though Congress had not yet given its final approval. Arguing that political divisions were either territories or states and that the Constitution had no provision for an intermediary stage of a "state out of the Union," Shields contended that the ratification of the Minnesota state constitution and the selection of representatives to the national legislature gave the citizens a right to have their delegates seated. Robert W. Johnson (D-AR) immediately challenged Crittenden. He insisted that, since Minnesota had not yet been admitted to the Union, Shields was not entitled to take his seat as a senator.

Johnson's objection launched a procedural debate over whether a territory automatically entered the Union as soon as it met the conditions of an enabling act. If Minnesota had the rights of a state, then Shields had a right to his seat; if the enabling act did not confer statehood, then Johnson's challenge was valid. The Senate agreed that, for Shields to be seated, Minnesota had to be a state. The question of the political status of Minnesota was referred to the Judiciary Committee.

Response of the Senate

On March 4, 1858, the committee reported, rejecting the theory that compliance with an enabling act granted statehood. Stating that admission to the Union rested finally on formal recognition from the United States Congress, the committee ruled that Minnesota was not a state. The Senate ordered the report printed but took no other action on it. James Shields was therefore not seated.

Conclusion

On May 11, 1858, Minnesota entered the Union. The following day James Shields and Henry M. Rice (D) presented their credentials. In spite of an objection that the Minnesota election predated statehood and that the legislature should vote again (See Case 33), the Senate decided to seat Shields and Rice.

Shields drew a seat in the class of senators whose terms would expire on March 3, 1859, and he failed in his bid for reelection. In 1860 he moved to California, served as a brigadier general in the Union army during the Civil War, and finally moved to Missouri. There, shortly before his death in 1879, Shields was elected to represent a third state in the United States Senate, the only person to achieve this distinction. He died unexpectedly while on an 1879 lecture tour in Iowa.

Sources

U.S. Congress. Senate. *Congressional Globe.* 35th Cong., 1st sess. (See pp. 861–67, 2076–77.)

Condon, William H. *Life of Major-General James Shields.* Chicago, 1900.

Case 33

Henry Mower Rice

(1816–1894)

Minnesota

Election Case
May 12, 1858 to June 9, 1858

Issues
Legislature's authority to elect before statehood; allegations of corruption prior to Senate service

Result: Retained seat

Chronology:
Credentials presented: May 12, 1858
Referred to committee: May 15, 1858
Committee report: June 9, 1858
Senate vote: June 9, 1858

Background

The charming and personable Henry M. Rice, a native Vermonter who moved to Minnesota as a young man, understood the broad spectrum of frontier entrepreneurship and parlayed his knowledge into a variety of financial and political successes. A land surveyor, fur trader, and Indian negotiator who had represented the territory as a delegate in Congress, Rice was an obvious choice for the United States Senate when Minnesota Territory became a state in 1858. Rice (D) and James Shields (D) were elected by the Minnesota legislature in 1857 but could not take their seats until May 12, 1858, the day after Congress voted to admit Minnesota as a state (See Case 32).

Statement of the Case

Upon the presentation of Rice's credentials, Albert G. Brown (D-MS) objected that the Minnesota legislature had elected the senators prematurely. Brown argued that a legislature could only elect senators after the territory officially became a state. This attack generated little support. When Brown contended that the Minnesota case resembled that of Tennessee in 1796 (See Case 4), other senators reminded him that Tennessee had acted before passage of an enabling act. The two Minnesotans were then permitted to take the oath of office.

Of greater concern were charges by James Harlan (R-IA) that Minnesota citizens accused Rice of fraud in the exercise of his duties as a land agent for the Fort Crawford reservation. Although several senators sharply criticized the Iowan for presenting the charges, the Senate on May 15, 1858, instructed the Committee on Military Affairs and the Militia to conduct an inquiry.

Response of the Senate

On June 9, 1858, the Committee on Military Affairs returned its report. The investigation revealed that the basis for the citizens' complaints lay in the methods Rice used to sell the land at Fort Crawford. Settlers testified that, although they had expected to pay $1.25 an acre for the land, Rice charged $1.50 per acre. He justified the additional 25 cents as a tax to cover surveying, advertising for the sale, and miscellaneous expenses; but he only gave settlers receipts for the $1.25 per acre. The disgruntled settlers, angered by the short notice given for the sale, argued that it would have been cheaper to make the trip to the regular land office. Rice's witnesses insisted that adequate advance notice had been given and the purposes for the surcharge had been openly stated. The land office registrar suggested that settlers were annoyed because Rice's system denied them the opportunity to earn profits ranging from $2.00 to $5.00 an acre through illegal dealings with the Indians.

The committee therefore asserted that it found no evidence to disqualify Rice and asked to be discharged from further consideration of the matter. Even though committee member Preston King (R-NY) dissented from the report and sharply condemned the management of the land sale, the Senate unanimously adopted the committee's report with its recommendation that Henry Rice was entitled to his seat.

Conclusion

Land transactions in the West were notoriously shady. Whether the fault lay with Rice and his surveyor, the War Department, or the settlers, the Senate chose not to delve too deeply into the murky business. Several senators had known and liked Rice for many years and seemed personally unwilling to question his conduct.

After completing his Senate service, Rice continued to be active in public matters, especially in treaty negotiations with several Indian tribes. Rice died in San Antonio, Texas, in 1894.

Sources

U.S. Congress. Senate. *Congressional Globe.* 35th Cong., 1st sess. (See pp. 2075–79, 2123, 2163, 2823.)

———. Senate Report No. 314. 35th Cong., 1st sess., 1858.

Malone, Dumas, ed. *Dictionary of American Biography.* Vol. 15. New York, 1946; reprint of 1935 edition. (See pp. 540–41.)

Marshall, William R. "Henry Mower Rice." *Minnesota Historical Society Collections* 9 (1901): 654–58.

III. Civil War: 1861–1865

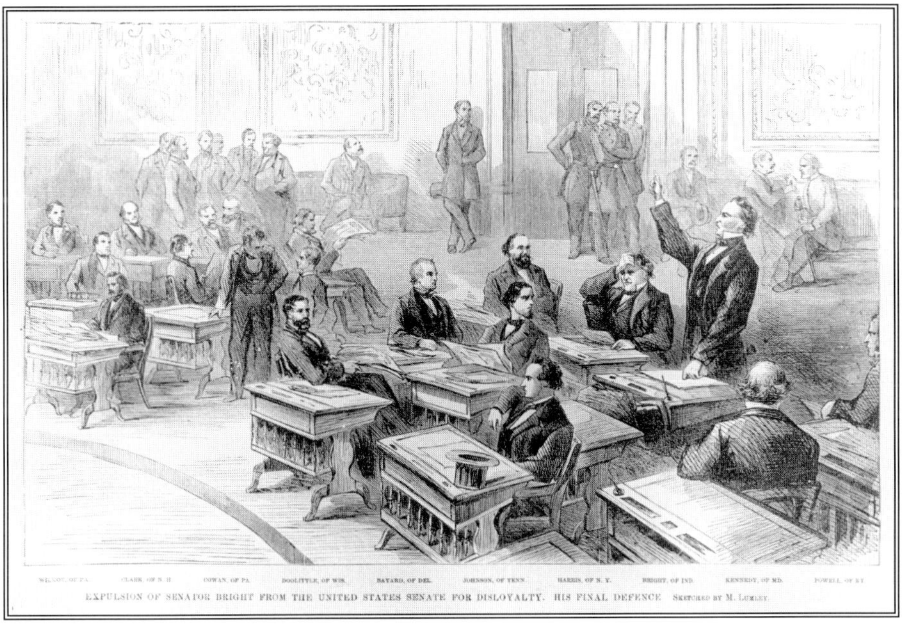

JESSE D. BRIGHT *(Case 40)*
U.S. Senate Collection

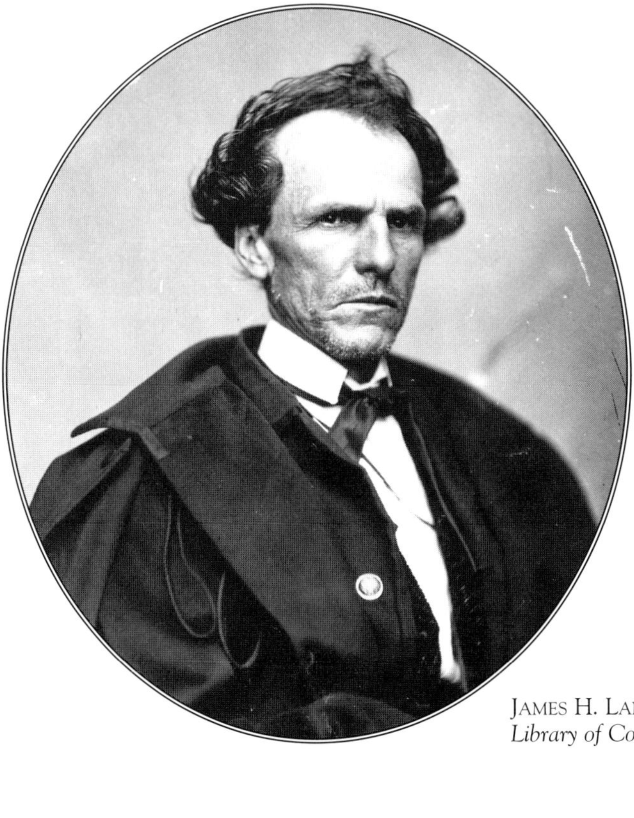

JAMES H. LANE *(Case 35)*
Library of Congress

Case 34

Clement C. Clay, Jr.
(1816–1882)
Alabama

Robert A. Toombs
(1810–1885)
Georgia

Jefferson Davis and Albert G. Brown
(1808–1889) (1813–1880)
Mississippi

Stephen R. Mallory
(1813–1873)
Florida

Judah P. Benjamin
(1811–1884)
Louisiana

Expulsion Case
January 21, 1861 to March 14, 1861

Issues
Disloyalty to Union

Result: Seats declared vacant

Chronology:
Statements of withdrawal: Jan. 21, 1861
Senate vote: March 14, 1861

Background

With the election of Abraham Lincoln in 1860, the states of the Deep South—South Carolina, Mississippi, Florida, Alabama, Georgia, and Louisiana—prepared to secede from the Union. Southern sentiment was fragmented: some citizens favored immediate secession by individual states, some preferred cooperative action by all states in the South, and others opposed secession altogether. By mid-January 1861, however, South Carolina, Mississippi, Florida, and Alabama had voted to secede, and the Democratic senators from these states agreed to withdraw from Congress and return to their homes. On January 21, at the conclusion of the Senate's routine morning business, Florida's David Yulee rose to lead the statements of withdrawal. Stephen Mallory of Florida and Clement Clay and Benjamin Fitzpatrick of Alabama followed. Mississippi's Albert Brown had already withdrawn from the Senate on January 12 and was no longer in Washington. His ailing colleague Jefferson Davis delivered the final oration that ended with the courteous observation, "I see now around me some with whom I have served long; there have been points of collision; but I . . . carry with me no hostile remembrance . . . it only remains for me to bid you a final adieu." Georgia seceded on January 19, and on the twenty-eighth Alfred Iverson added his name to those who departed. On February 4, following Louisiana's secession on January 26, John Slidell and his colleague Judah Benjamin also withdrew after bidding the Senate an emotional farewell.

Statement of the Case

On January 22, 1861, confusion abounded as those remaining in the Senate tried to define the events of the previous day. They grappled with at least four principal issues: the difference between withdrawal and resignation; the permanent or impermanent quality of the withdrawals; the subsequent status of committee memberships; and the underlying uncertainty over the legality of secession. They also debated whether the official Senate *Journal* should record the withdrawals. That not all southern senators acted in the same manner or at the same time compounded the difficulty. One Georgia senator, Robert Toombs, withdrew without sending formal notification to the Senate. The South Carolina senators, James H. Hammond and James Chesnut, announced their plans through home state newspapers but never communicated with the Senate itself.

Several of the southern senators whose states would soon secede were still present on January 22 and participated in the discussion. Judah Benjamin of Louisiana especially stressed the view that secession was possible, that the senators had withdrawn rather than resigned, and that the Senate's *Journal* should report the secessions and the withdrawal of the senators. Although perplexed members sought to use the language of the Constitution as a guide for identifying the proper responses to the peculiar situation, no common agreement emerged in the constitutional interpretations, and the senators continued to flounder for definitions of the action that had been taken. The Senate sidetracked both motions designed to address the problem: Benjamin's to correct the *Journal* to reflect the senators' announcement that, since their states had seceded, they were withdrawing from the Senate; and a substitute stating that the senators "announced that they were no longer members of the Senate, and withdrew." The latter approach, indicating that the senators had simply resigned, was preferred by those who objected to in any way officially acknowledging that secession had occurred. The Senate took no further action on the motions before the close of the Thirty-sixth Congress on March 3.

Response of the Senate

On March 4, 1861, a new Republican majority assumed control of Congress, but it, too, demonstrated no clear notion about how to handle the secession crisis. When the Senate on March 14 again considered the dilemma of the southern senators, so much anger and sadness permeated the speeches that a troubled James A. Bayard, Jr. (D-DE) advised, "All I ask... is, to leave the question undisturbed... unless it be the desire of... the Senate to complicate the affairs of the country, already sufficiently complicated; to irritate passions already sufficiently aroused; and to afford additional chances for the utter destruction of the Union, when it is already sufficiently endangered." The Senate, however, rejected both Bayard's substitute resolution stating that the senators had withdrawn because their states had seceded and another stating that they had "ceased to be members of the Senate." Instead, the Senate simply voted to pronounce the seats vacant and to direct the secretary of the Senate to omit those names from the roll. This resolution applied to Albert G. Brown, Jefferson Davis, Stephen R. Mallory, Clement Clay, Robert Toombs, and Judah Benjamin. It did not apply to David Yulee, Benjamin Fitzpatrick, Alfred Iverson, James Hammond, or John Slidell, because their Senate terms expired before the new Republican Congress convened. The Senate waited until July 1861 to deal with the case of James Chesnut (See Case 36).

Conclusion

The debate over senatorial withdrawal marked only the first of many constitutional disputes surrounding the major issue of secession. The southern senators justified their withdrawals by the argument that, when a state left the Union, the need for senatorial representation ended. The Senate, however, did not wish to acknowledge the legitimacy of secession. By merely declaring the seats vacant and implying that a new senator with legitimate credentials could represent that state, the Senate in effect denied the act of secession.

All the southern senators involved in the withdrawal dispute returned to their home states and participated in the Confederacy. At the close of the war, Jefferson Davis, who led the Confederacy as president, was imprisoned for two years, as were Clement Clay and Stephen Mallory for shorter periods. Robert Toombs sought refuge in Havana and London for two years. After the war, most turned to agricultural pursuits or the practice of law. Only Judah Benjamin, who fled to England in 1865, remained publicly prominent, carving out a prestigious postwar career there as a prominent barrister. Jefferson Davis spent a quiet retirement in Mississippi and died in New Orleans in 1889.

Sources

U.S. Congress. Senate. *Congressional Globe.* 36th Cong., 2d sess. (See pp. 352, 484–487, 500–505, 589, 720–22, 1454–56.)

Davis, William C. *Jefferson Davis: The Man and His Hour.* New York, 1991. (See pp. 294–96.)

Durkin, Joseph T. *Confederate Navy Chief: Stephen R. Mallory.* Columbia, SC, 1987. (See pp. 121–24.)

Evans, Eli N. *Judah P. Benjamin: The Jewish Confederate.* New York, 1988. (See pp. 110–12.)

McPherson, James M. *Ordeal by Fire: The Civil War and Reconstruction.* New York, 1982.

Case 35

Frederick P. Stanton v. James H. Lane

(1814–1894) (1814–1866)

Kansas

Election Case
July 4, 1861 to January 16, 1862

Issues
Qualifications: senator also serving as general

Result: Lane retained seat

Chronology:
Credentials presented: July 4, July 12, 1861
Referred to committee: July 12, 1861
Again referred to committee: Dec. 18, 1861
Committee report: Jan. 6, 1862
Senate vote: Jan. 16, 1862

Background

In 1855, James H. Lane, a supporter of slavery, arrived in the Kansas territory to be a political lobbyist for the Stephen Douglas wing of the Democratic party. In the subsequent regional disorders, Lane found himself abandoned by his Democratic patrons and left to face the complicated territorial politics alone. Bitterly disappointed at this treatment, Lane, a flamboyant and compelling orator, transferred to the Republican party, where his arrival was greeted with cool suspicion. Despite a turbulent political career and an equally stormy personal life that included the murder of a business opponent, Lane managed to capture one of the first Senate seats when Kansas entered the Union in April 1861.

Statement of the Case

Lane, who embraced Republicanism as fervently as he had once denounced it, arrived in Washington at the start of the Civil War. When he heard that the life of President Abraham Lincoln was threatened, Lane immediately organized a small band called the "Frontier Guard" and posted it briefly at the White House. Lane's enthusiastic defense of the new president launched a close friendship that ultimately made him one of the chief executive's most intimate military confidants.

Before the extraordinary session of Congress called by President Lincoln convened in July, Lane disbanded the Frontier Guard and hurried back to Kansas to organize a volunteer army. Although some citizens in Kansas regarded Lane's military behavior as self-serving, irrational, and opportunistic, his spirited conduct impressed Lincoln, who, on June 20, 1861, appointed him brigadier general of the Kansas volunteers. Lane announced his appointment in the Kansas newspapers, delegated responsibility for recruitment to a fellow officer, and returned to Washington for the congressional session.

On July 4, 1861, James Lane's credentials were presented to the Senate, and he fulfilled a longstanding ambition by taking his oath of office. Then, on July 12, Frederick P. Stanton appeared in the Senate with credentials signed by Lane's archfoe, Kansas Governor Charles Robinson. Contending that Lane's Senate seat became vacant upon his appointment as brigadier general, the governor had appointed Stanton, a Democrat and former governor of Kansas Territory, to fill the alleged vacancy. The Senate referred the conflict to the Committee on the Judiciary.

Response of the Senate

Surprised and outraged, Lane refused even to appear before the committee, which on August 2, 1861, returned a report favorable to Stanton. Committee members considered that when Lane accepted President Lincoln's military appointment on June 20, 1861, the Kansas seat became vacant. As evidence, the committee cited Lane's announcement in a Leavenworth newspaper that "the president . . . has been pleased to place in my hands the honor of leading the gallant sons of the youngest State of the Union." Lane challenged this interpretation for, he insisted, he merely wrote the statement and did not affix his name to it as a brigadier general.

The Senate adjourned without settling the issue. Lane promptly returned to Kansas, where he did not permit his cloudy senatorial status to deter him from his military activities. While Lane and his enemy, Governor Robinson, each used the war as an excuse for securing personal military control of the state, the senator continued to enhance his reputation in Washington by sending a steady stream of informative military bulletins to the War Department. From September to November 1861, Lane skirmished around the Kansas countryside with an army that became infamous for its depredations.

In November, Lane interrupted his military campaign to travel to Washington for the new Senate session. He began an impassioned attempt to convince the Union that a decisive winter assault employing a substantial army of black soldiers could cripple the Confederacy. As Lane battled for approval of an aggressive war effort, his Senate colleagues deliberated about Stanton's claim to the Kansas seat. Then, in December, at Lane's request, the question was resubmitted to the Judiciary Committee, together with Lane's defense. The Kansas senator stated that he had gone to the commanding general soon after receiving the appointment and learned that he could not formally become a brigadier general until he resigned his Senate seat. He had responded to the general that in that case he would not accept the appointment.

On January 6, 1862, a divided committee returned a new report that, despite a brief letter of explanation from President Lincoln, still supported Stanton. The committee did not share the commanding general's view and instead maintained that Lane had virtually resigned his seat by accepting the military position. In the debate that followed, Lane's supporters developed two lines of reasoning. One group argued that Congress had not yet passed the enabling legislation when Lincoln made the June 1861 appointment; therefore, since no official position of brigadier general existed before a congressional act of July 22, Lane was legally seated on July 4. The second group preferred Lane's explanation that he himself had never actually accepted the commission or received any pay for the position but had merely said he intended to accept.

After further debate, the Senate on January 16 rejected the Judiciary Committee's recommendation and voted, 24 to 16, that Lane was entitled to his seat. Stanton received the compensation of a senator for the period spent contesting the seat. The following day, Lane met with President Lincoln, General George C. McClellan, and newly appointed Secretary of War Edwin M. Stanton to discuss plans for his military campaign in Kansas.

Conclusion

Lane's attempts to maintain two official positions clearly violated the constitutional provision that "no Person holding any Office under the United States, shall be a Member of either House during his Continuance in Office" (Article I, section 6). His difficulties, however, may have stemmed as much from the extreme political rivalries in Kansas and the bitter enmity of Charles Robinson as from constitutional concerns. After all, Oregon Senator Edward D. Baker was an officer of the Union army who often appeared in the Senate chamber in his uniform, even though he had promised the Oregon legislature for months that he would resign his Senate seat. The death of the immensely popular Baker at the Battle of Ball's Bluff in October 1861 may have influenced the Senate not to penalize the emotional and zealous Lane for his dramatic commitment to the Union cause.

Following the resolution of his Senate status, Lane again traveled to Kansas, where he continued to participate in the military management of the state. After frequent clashes with other Kansas military leaders thwarted a planned expedition, Lane in February 1862 notified the state legislature that, contrary to his recent promises, he would not resign his Senate seat. Reelected in 1864 after a tumultuous campaign, Lane remained a senator until his death by suicide in July 1866.

Sources

U.S. Congress. Senate. *Congressional Globe.* 37th Cong., 1st sess. See pp. 82, 406–7, 438–41, 450–52.) 2d sess. (See pp. 127–30, 222–27, 290–97, 336–44, 359–64, 376–79.)

———. Senate Report No. 1. 37th Cong., 1st sess., 1861.

Bailes, Kendall E. *Rider on the Wind: Jim Lane and Kansas.* Shawnee Mission, KS, 1962.

Connelley, William E. *James Henry Lane.* Topeka, KS, 1899.

Spring, Leverett W. "The Career of a Kansas Politician." *American Historical Review* 4 (October 1898): 80–104.

Stephenson, Wendell. *Political Career of James H. Lane.* Publications of the Kansas Historical Society 3, 1930.

James M. Mason and Robert M. T. Hunter

(1798–1871) (1809–1887)

Virginia

Thomas L. Clingman and Thomas Bragg

(1812–1897) (1810–1872)

North Carolina

James Chesnut, Jr.

(1815–1885)

South Carolina

A.O.P. Nicholson

(1808–1876)

Tennessee

William K. Sebastian and Charles B. Mitchel

(1812–1865) (1815–1864)

Arkansas

John Hemphill and Louis T. Wigfall

(1803–1862) (1816–1874)

Texas

Expulsion Case
July 10, 1861 to July 11, 1861

Issues
Disloyalty to Union

Result: Expelled

Chronology:
Resolution introduced: July 10, 1861
Senate vote: July 11, 1861

Background

In April 1861 any hope of reconciliation between the North and the South evaporated when the Confederates fired upon Fort Sumter and President Abraham Lincoln called for 75,000 volunteers to suppress the insurrection. No longer could the United States Senate hope that the southern legislatures would appoint new senators to fill the vacant seats in the chamber. Following Lincoln's 1860 election, most senators from southern states had not returned to Washington. Many of those who were in the capital had, in varying ways, withdrawn from the Senate during January and February of 1861. At the beginning of the Thirty-seventh Congress in March, the new Republican-dominated Senate voted to declare their seats vacant and to omit reading their names on the roll (See Case 34). No action was taken regarding those whose terms had just expired at the end of the previous Congress. One Tennessee senator, Andrew Johnson, a staunch Unionist, refused to follow the secessionists and served in the Senate until he resigned in 1862 to become the military governor of the state at President Lincoln's request.

In March, Louis Wigfall of Texas declared to the Senate that he understood that Texas had seceded from the Union and that, if this was the case, he was now a foreigner and owed no allegiance to the United States. He announced his intention to remain in Washington to carry out his duties in the Senate until he received official confirmation of the secession. This announcement sparked an effort to expel him. In the ensuing debate, a number of the southern senators who remained in Washington contended that expulsion was a punitive action created to deal with actual wrongdoing and that it should not be taken against a member simply for expressing the political opinion that secession was possible. Led by Thomas Clingman of North Carolina, the southerners claimed that, if Texas had indeed seceded, the proper approach would be to adopt a resolution stating that, since Texas was no longer one of the United States, "she is not entitled to be represented in this body." They also pointed out that none of the senators who had already withdrawn had been expelled, but the Senate had simply declared their seats vacant.

The debate over expelling Wigfall highlighted the conflicting views held by senators regarding the nature of the Union, with southerners asserting that they owed their allegiance to their states, and to the Union as a whole only through their states. Once their state seceded, they had no further obligation to the United States. On March 12, 1861, the Senate referred the matter to the Judiciary Committee, which returned no report on its deliberations.

By the time Congress reconvened in July 1861, open warfare was in progress, and the Senate faced the unresolved problem of the remaining southern senators, who had now left Washington but had not formally withdrawn their membership. Still murky was the status of William Sebastian and Charles C. Mitchel of Arkansas, Thomas Clingman and Thomas Bragg of North Carolina, South Carolina's James Chesnut, Tennessee's A. O. P. Nicholson, Texas' John Hemphill, and James M. Mason and Robert M. T. Hunter of Virginia. Also included in this group was Louis Wigfall of Texas.

Statement of the Case

In order to clarify the status of the ten southern senators who had not been dealt with during the March session, Daniel Clark (R-NH) on July 10, 1861, submitted a resolution asking for their expulsion from the Senate. Clark cited the failure of these senators to appear in the chamber and their active involvement in the Confederate government as evidence that they had participated in a conspiracy against the peace and union of the United States government. The resolution he introduced stated:

> Whereas a conspiracy has been formed against the peace, union, and liberties of the people and Government of the United States; and in furtherance of such conspiracy a portion of the people of the States of Virginia, North Carolina, South Carolina, Tennessee, Arkansas, and Texas, have attempted to withdraw those States from the Union, and are now in arms against the Government; and whereas [the senators from those states] have failed to appear in their seats in the Senate and to aid the Government in this important crisis; and it is apparent to the Senate that said Senators are engaged in said conspiracy for the destruction of the Union and Government, or, with full knowledge of such conspiracy, have failed to advise the Government of its progress or aid in its suppression: Therefore,
>
> *Resolved,* That the said Mason, Hunter, Clingman, Bragg, Chesnut, Nicholson, Sebastian, Mitchel, Hemphill, and Wigfall be, and they hereby are, each and all of them, expelled from the Senate of the United States.

Response of the Senate

As he had in the March debates, James A. Bayard, Jr. (D-DE) rose to the defense of the southern senators and urged moderation. Bayard opposed the expulsion measure, arguing that the southern senators followed the directions of their states and that no senator individually had conspired against the government. Bayard suggested that the expulsion rule should be reserved for individual acts of misconduct, since formal expulsion of the southern senators would only exacerbate an already inflamed situation. Milton S. Latham (D-CA) supported Bayard because he believed expulsion implied moral turpitude, a stain upon the personal character of the individuals that most would agree was unjust.

But the passions of war produced more fervent arguments from their opponents. Daniel Clark retorted that he failed to admire the "openness" of the absent senators, and he hoped the Senate would not repeat its action of the March session. Clark declared, "They have taken up arms against the Government; . . . their guns are now within sound of your capital; and shall we sit here in the Senate and deliberate and doubt whether we shall turn out of this Senate the very men who are ready to explode those guns against your capital? . . . let them be ejected from the councils of the nation." Near the conclusion of the arguments, James A. McDougall (D-CA) derided the cautions of his California colleague Latham when he dryly noted that there might be no moral turpitude in their actions because, "Treason was always a gentlemanly crime. . . . However, it is none the less a crime. . . . No man has a right to a place on this floor who espouses a cause adverse to the Government."

The angry mood prevailed, and on July 11, 1861, the Senate voted 32 to 10 to expel the ten senators.

Conclusion

The wholesale expulsion of ten senators represented but one in a series of events unique to the Civil War. For such an extraordinary decision, the Senate debate lasted a remarkably short time. The brevity of the discussion reflected the intense acrimony generated in a war where friends and neighbors became bitter foes. The firing upon Fort Sumter had dashed any lingering leniency among senators toward their opponents in the Confederacy. On some occasions the Senate might be in a tolerant and forgiving humor, but not in the heat of civil conflict.

Nine of the expelled senators participated actively in the Confederacy as senators, military officers, or diplomats. Most returned to private life after the war, although James Chesnut and Thomas Clingman attended the National Democratic Convention in New York in 1868. Robert M.T. Hunter, a delegate to the Hampton Roads peace conference with Abraham Lincoln in 1865, was imprisoned briefly at the close of the war. After the end of Reconstruction in 1877, he secured positions in the Virginia state government. A.O.P. Nicholson served as chief justice of the Tennessee supreme court from 1870–1876.

Only William K. Sebastian did not engage in confederate politics or military service. He returned to his home in Arkansas, resumed the practice of law, and did not support the Confederacy. Shortly before his death in 1865, Sebastian moved to Memphis, Tennessee. In 1877, the Senate, convinced by Sebastian's passive demeanor before and during the Civil War that he was not an active conspirator against the Union, revoked the expulsion order and gave full compensation to his children.

Sources

U.S. Congress. Senate. *Congressional Globe.* 36th Cong., 2d sess. (See pp. 1447–51.)

———. *Congressional Globe.* 37th Cong., 1st sess. (See pp. 62–64.)

Mason, James M. *The Public Life and Diplomatic Correspondence of James M. Mason.* Roanoke, VA, 1903.

McPherson, James M. *Ordeal by Fire: The Civil War and Reconstruction.* New York, 1982.

Case 37

Waitman T. Willey and John S. Carlile

(1811–1900) (1817–1878)

Virginia

Election Case
July 13, 1861

Issues
Challenge to legislature's authority to elect

Result: Seated

Chronology:
Credentials presented: July 13, 1861
Senate vote: July 13, 1861

Background

The troubled status of the Civil War Senate failed to be resolved with the expulsion of senators from the seceding states. Virginia complicated matters when a portion of the state, strongly Unionist, refused to accept the secessionist moves of its government. This group formed a Unionist legislature at Wheeling in 1861 and replaced those expelled, Robert M. T. Hunter and James M. Mason, with two new senators, Waitman T. Willey (U) and John S. Carlile (U). Both forceful opponents of secession, these senators appeared with their credentials on July 13, 1861.

Statement of the Case

Andrew Johnson (D-TN) warmly introduced the senators and applauded "the return of the Old Dominion" to the Senate. Before the oaths could be administered, however, James A. Bayard, Jr. (D-DE) asked that the credentials be sent to the Committee on the Judiciary. To support his request, Bayard raised two issues about the validity of the credentials: he complained that, by accepting the new Virginia senators, the Senate would be recognizing an irregular state government, and he cautioned that the Senate had no authority to create a new state out of part of an existing state. In addition, he and others pointed out that on the previous day, July 12, the Senate had voted to expel Virginia Senators Robert M.T. Hunter and James M. Mason. Thus, at the time the Unionist legislature elected Carlile and Willey on July 9, there had in fact been no vacancies to fill, since the Senate had tacitly recognized Hunter and Mason as holding those seats until July 12. Based on these grave issues, Bayard thought a committee should investigate the matter before the oaths were administered.

Response of the Senate

The mood lingered from the previous day when the Senate had expelled ten southern senators. Opponents of the South, still exhilarated by the earlier expulsion events, refused to accept any delay and dismissed Bayard's concern that the Senate would be recognizing a state insurrection. John P. Hale (R-NH), viewing the events as the culmination of a struggle that had lasted many years, was anxious to recognize the credentials of these Virginians who had rallied to the beleaguered Union's cause. Hale urged the Senate not to search for precedents but rather to accept the present contest as a new challenge with new rules. Heeding his remarks, the Senate, by a vote of 5 yeas to 35 nays, rejected the motion to refer the credentials to committee and instead seated the new Virginia senators.

Conclusion

The acceptance of these credentials reflected the general war spirit of the nation. Yet the Senate's action did not follow either the letter or the spirit of constitutional law. If the Unionists denied the possibility of secession and contended that southern states had not separated from the Union, the Senate was bound to accept only credentials submitted by the duly elected governor of Virginia in accordance with the Constitution. The failure to do so, in addition to being a constitutional breach, placed the Unionists in a contradictory position. Andrew Johnson, for example, had welcomed back a state whose departure he supposedly did not recognize. Critics correctly accused the Unionists of assaulting their own doctrine and trampling on the Constitution. But July 1861 was not a time for measured arguments nor lengthy deliberations. The Senate, confused and apprehensive about the impact of secession, chose to respond to the cry of John Hale, "The day for compromise has gone by. . . we have lived on compromises. It was our daily food constantly. . . . I have no compromise to offer." In judging the qualifications of its members in this extraordinary case, the Senate chose to agree with Jacob Collamer (R-VT) that this was a "matter of political action and the political power is what settles it."

John Carlile, a forceful orator who vigorously opposed secession, served the nearly four years remaining in Hunter's term in the Senate. In 1865, he returned to West Virginia, the new state formed from the unionist portion of Virginia, where he resided until his death in 1878. Waitman Willey served the balance of Mason's term, which ended in March 1863 and, on August 4, 1863, became one of West Virginia's first two senators. He remained in the Senate until 1871. Willey distinguished himself as a Radical Republican who supported legislation to improve the status of recently freed blacks. He frequently gave public lectures and contributed to journals and reviews. He died in Morgantown, West Virginia, in 1900.

Sources

U.S. Congress. Senate. *Journal.* 37th Cong., 1st sess. (See pp. 39–40, Appendix, pp. 103–9.)

Ambler, Charles. *Waitman Thomas Willey: Orator, Churchman, Humanitarian.* Huntington, WV, 1954.

Belz, Herman. *Reconstructing the Union: Theory and Policy During the Civil War.* Ithaca, NY, 1969. (See pp. 31–32.)

Johnson, Allen, ed. *Dictionary of American Biography.* Vol. 4. New York, 1946; reprint of 1935 edition. (See p. 347.)

Malone, Dumas, ed. *Dictionary of American Biography.* Vol. 12. New York, 1946; reprint of 1935 edition. (See p. 455.)

John C. Breckinridge

(1821–1875)

Kentucky

Expulsion Case
December 4, 1861

Issues
Disloyalty to Union

Result: Expelled

Chronology:
Resolution introduced: Dec. 4, 1861
Senate vote: Dec. 4, 1861

Background

Among Kentucky's political leaders none enjoyed a more illustrious national career than John C. Breckinridge, who held the offices of representative, senator, and vice president. In the multi-candidate 1860 presidential race, he ran as the candidate of the Southern Democratic party. Breckinridge was then elected to the U.S. Senate for a term beginning on March 4, 1861, as Abraham Lincoln began his administration and after seven southern states had already seceded.

A defender of the South on the Senate floor, Breckinridge personally hoped that secession could be stopped. In August 1861, when it became apparent that the secession movement was a reality, Breckinridge devoted one of his final speeches in the Senate to urging an end to the war. "I would prefer to see these States all reunited upon true constitutional principles... But I infinitely prefer to see a peaceful separation of these States, than to see endless, aimless, devastating war, at the end of which I see the grave of public liberty and of personal freedom," he declared. He then returned to Kentucky, a border state torn by divided loyalties. Although sympathizing with the Confederacy, Breckinridge struggled to preserve peace and keep the state neutral, but in September the Kentucky legislature voted to side with the Union. Learning that he was about to be arrested and imprisoned, the senator hastily departed for Tennessee and soon after appeared in Richmond, the Confederate capital. There, Jefferson Davis appointed him a brigadier general in the Confederate army. Breckinridge, the champion of neutrality between the Union and the Confederacy, had finally been forced to choose.

Statement of the Case

Because he was versed in the protocol of the Senate from his service as vice president, Breckinridge, unlike many other senators who followed the Confederacy, sent a formal letter of resignation to the Senate in October. On December 4, 1861, Zachariah Chandler (R-MI) introduced a resolution of expulsion.

Response of the Senate

A brief discussion followed, in which Lyman Trumbull (R-IL) inquired of Breckinridge's Kentucky colleague, Democrat Lazarus Powell, whether it was true that Breckinridge had become a general in the Confederate army. After first trying to avoid a direct answer, Powell finally confirmed that Trumbull's information was correct. Because Breckinridge had accepted a prominent military position in the Confederacy, Trumbull asked that the resolution be amended to state:

> Whereas John C. Breckinridge, a member of this body from the State of Kentucky, has joined the enemies of his country, and is now in arms against the Government he had sworn to support: Therefore,
>
> *Resolved,* That the said John C. Breckinridge, the traitor, be, and he is hereby, expelled from the Senate.

That same day, the Senate voted 36 to 0 to pass the resolution as amended and expel Breckinridge.

Conclusion

In the earlier Civil War expulsion cases, friends of the South argued that the senators should not be penalized for the secessionist decisions of their state governments, but only for their own individual misconduct. As long as southerners did not take up arms against the United States government, their supporters maintained, they did not deserve the censure of their colleagues. In the case of John Breckinridge, with Kentucky a Union state and the senator an officer in the Confederate army, southern sympathizers were caught upon the horns of their own argument.

Promoted to major general, Breckinridge saw combat in several battles of the Civil War before Jefferson Davis appointed him secretary of war. Upon the collapse of the Confederacy, he fled to Cuba and then lived in England and Canada. Convinced by 1869 that he was finally safe from arrest, Breckinridge returned to Kentucky and quietly practiced law until his death in 1875.

Unlike the expulsions of senators from seceding states, which left those states unrepresented in the Senate, Breckinridge's departure left a vacancy that needed to be filled. On December 23, 1861, Garrett Davis, elected as a Unionist by the Kentucky legislature, arrived to take his seat in the Senate.

Sources

U.S. Congress. Senate. *Congressional Globe*. 37th Cong., 2d sess. (See pp. 9–10.)

Davis, William C. *Breckinridge: Statesman, Soldier, Symbol.* Baton Rouge, LA, 1974.

Heck, Frank H. *Proud Kentuckian: John C. Breckinridge, 1821–1875.* Lexington, KY, 1976.

Roller, David C. and Robert Twyman, eds. *Encyclopedia of Southern History.* Baton Rouge, LA, 1979.

Stillwell, Lucille. *Born to Be a Statesman.* Caldwell, ID, 1936.

Case 39

Waldo P. Johnson and Trusten Polk

(1817–1885) (1811–1876)

Missouri

Expulsion Case
December 10, 1861 to January 10, 1862

Issues
Disloyalty to Union

Result: Expelled

Chronology:
Resolutions introduced:
Dec. 10, Dec. 18,1861
Referred to committee:
Dec. 12, Dec. 18, 1861
Committee reports: Jan. 9, 1862
Senate votes: Jan. 10, 1862

Background

The political climate of Missouri grew increasingly tense as the nation moved toward Civil War in the early months of 1861. As a slave state with strong economic ties to the North, Missouri was torn by bitter fighting between secessionists and unionists. Ultimately, the state was forced to remain in the Union but at the cost of heavy casualties on both sides. During this struggle, both senators, Waldo P. Johnson (D) and Trusten Polk (D), angered their Senate colleagues by supporting the Missouri secessionists. Earlier in 1861, the Senate had penalized senators from the seceding states either by declaring their seats vacant and omitting their names from its roll call (See Case 34) or, once the war began, through the harsher move of expulsion (See Case 36). To many senators, the blatant support for the South voiced by these members from a Union state demanded an equally strong response.

Statement of the Case

On December 10, 1861, Solomon Foot (R-VT) asked that Waldo P. Johnson be expelled, based on the Missourian's sympathy for and participation in the rebellion. On December 18, Charles Sumner (R-MA) called for the expulsion of Trusten Polk as a traitor. Although the dates and the wording of the resolutions differed slightly, the Missouri situation essentially represented one case.

Response of the Senate

General floor discussion about the Missouri senators took place on December 12 and 18, 1861. In the debates earlier in the year, feelings had run so high that the expulsion question moved to a vote without first being referred to committee. By mid-December, however, senators had retreated to their traditional concern for evidence, form, and precedent. James McDougall (D-CA) and James A. Bayard, Jr. (D-DE) urged that correct procedures be followed. McDougall acknowledged that, while in the July cases he supported an immediate vote on the expulsions, in this case, there was no need for unseemly haste. He reminded the Senate that this was a serious matter, and their actions might be invoked as precedents in the future.

Senators who pressed for immediate action emphasized that neither Missouri senator had appeared at any time during the session to claim his seat or to answer the charges against him. Their failure to communicate with those in Washington lent credence to the unofficial information that Johnson held an officer's position in the Confederate army and that Polk wrote public letters urging Missouri to join the southern cause. The Senate, however, sent the complaints about both senators to the Judiciary Committee.

On January 9, 1862, the committee issued reports supporting the charges made against Johnson and Polk. Both were reported to have secretly crossed into rebel territory. Satisfied that neither demonstrated the slightest interest in answering the Senate charges and that both participated in secessionist war activities, the committee recommended expulsion. On January 10, 1862, the Senate expelled Waldo Johnson by a vote of 35 to 0 and Trusten Polk by a vote of 36 to 0.

Conclusion

In expelling Johnson and Polk the Senate continued the trend established in the John C. Breckinridge case (See Case 38) resolved in December 1861. The Senate could not tolerate a situation in which senators from a Union state gave open support to the enemy government.

Despite the insistence of their supporters that the charges against them were only rumor, Polk and Johnson belied this confidence by slipping back and forth into southern territory. Waldo Johnson, wounded at the Battle of Pea Ridge only two months after his expulsion, recruited and organized troops for the Confederate army, attaining the rank of lieutenant colonel. He served in the Confederate senate, lived briefly in Canada after the war, and returned to Missouri, where he served as president of the state's constitutional convention in 1875. He practiced law until his death in 1885. Trusten Polk accumulated a similar record of service for the Confederacy, first as a colonel in the Confederate army and later as a military judge in Mississippi. After the war he practiced law in St. Louis. He died in 1876.

As in the Breckinridge case, these expulsions left vacancies to be filled. On January 17, 1862, the governor appointed Unionists John B. Henderson and Robert Wilson as the new senators from Missouri.

Sources

U.S. Congress. Senate. *Congressional Globe.* 37th Cong., 2d sess. (See pp. 36, 70–71, 126, 263–64.)

———. Senate Report No. 4. 37th Cong., 2d sess., 1862.

———. Senate Report No. 5. 37th Cong., 2d sess., 1862.

Roller, David C., and Robert W. Twyman, eds. *The Encyclopedia of Southern History.* Baton Rouge, LA, 1979.

Case 40

Jesse D. Bright

(1812–1875)

Indiana

Expulsion Case
December 16, 1861 to February 5, 1862

Issues
Disloyalty to Union

Result: Expelled

Chronology:
Resolution introduced: Dec. 16, 1861
Referred to committee: Dec. 16, 1861
Committee report: Jan. 13, 1862
Senate vote: Feb. 5, 1862

Background

Among the forty-four senators who remained after the southern states seceded at the start of the Civil War, Jesse Bright of Indiana was the Senate's most senior Democrat. A senator since 1845, Bright was noted for his grasp of Senate rules and precedents and for his frank manner. He was willing to take firm positions on sensitive issues, regardless of the long-term consequences of his stands. Bright's colleagues regarded him as capable of unswerving friendship to those who shared his proslavery views and as "an enemy who knew how to inflict punishment" to those who did not. His principal Senate antagonists were abolitionists Charles Sumner (R-MA) and Morton Wilkinson (R-MN). In recognition of his seniority, Bright had served as the Senate's president pro tempore in 1854, 1856, and 1860. During his tenure in that position, Bright saw to it that Sumner received no committee assignments.

In mid-1861, the Democrats were a helpless minority in the Republican-controlled Senate. Shortly after the inglorious rout of Union troops at the first Battle of Bull Run, Thomas Lincoln, a Texas arms merchant, was captured by federal forces as he attempted to cross into Confederate territory. Lincoln's captors found among his possessions the following letter, dated March 1, 1861, from Jesse Bright to "His Excellency Jefferson Davis, President of the Confederation of States":

> My dear Sir:
>
> Allow me to introduce to your acquaintance my friend, Thomas B. Lincoln of Texas. He visits your capital mainly to dispose of what he regards a great improvement in fire-arms. I recommend him to your favorable consideration as a gentleman of the first respectability, and reliable in every respect.

In the following months before the Senate convened for the second session of the Thirty-seventh Congress, Washington was rife with speculation as to Bright's likely fate at the hands of his Republican Senate colleagues. Over the years, he had denounced those who equated abolitionism with loyalty to the Union. He believed that the rupture in the Union would be only temporary and that military force would have little effect in healing the break. Clearly, Bright was vulnerable in a Senate whose majority feared the influence of southern sympathizers in the national government.

Statement of the Case

On December 16, 1861, shortly after the Senate opened its new session, Morton Wilkinson introduced a resolution to expel Bright on the basis that the letter to Jefferson Davis was evidence of disloyalty. The Senate promptly referred the resolution to the Judiciary Committee, which then consisted of five Republican and two Democratic members.

In his own defense, Bright argued that, although he had written the letter, he did not specifically remember doing so because he frequently wrote such commendations on behalf of his friends and constituents. Early in his career, Bright had served as Thomas Lincoln's attorney and, in 1861, he felt it was only natural to introduce his friend to his former Senate colleague, Jefferson Davis. Bright contended that, in addressing his letter to "His Excellency, Jefferson Davis, President of the Confederation of States," he had simply followed the conventions of the day, using a polite form of address customary between two gentlemen and using the title Davis claimed at the time. At the heart of Bright's defense was the question of the state of relations between the Union and Confederacy on March 1, 1861, the date of the letter. He argued that no fighting had yet occurred and the break was then considered by no means irrevocable.

This was the weakest point in Bright's case. His opponents pictured Jefferson Davis as the archtraitor who, in March 1861, was busily assembling arms for his April attack on the federal garrison at Fort Sumter. For Bright to introduce an arms merchant to Davis was, in their view, clearly an act of treason. They also focused on the wording of his letter, underscoring its subservient tone with references to "His Excellency" and "your capital." Where Bright's defenders asserted that he was guilty only of bad timing and indiscretion, his opponents charged that he had violated his oath to defend the Constitution against foreign and domestic enemies.

Response of the Senate

The Judiciary Committee reported to the Senate on January 13, 1862, that it found the charges were not sufficient to justify expulsion. One committee member, Lafayette Foster (R-CT), subsequently changed his mind and supported expulsion. He explained that, in voting against expelling Bright for a letter written on March 1, 1861, he had followed the precedent set by the Senate when it failed on March 14 to expel Jefferson Davis and other senators from the seceding states and decided simply to declare their seats vacant, although he himself thought they should have been expelled.

Debate in the Senate began on January 20 and continued intermittently until February 5, 1862. The most dramatic and damaging speech was made by Charles Sumner, who demanded that the Senate purge itself of traitors. The decisive vote occurred on February 5, with members of both houses filling the chamber and the gallery overflowing with onlookers. During the proceedings, which lasted for five hours, Bright summarized his case. "From the hour this war actually commenced," he asserted, "I have had in view... one single object—the reunion of these States." Noting with resignation that the Republican caucus had undoubtedly already made the final decision, he declared that he was speaking only to set forth his case for posterity. Upon completing his address, Bright gathered his belongings from his desk and walked out of the chamber. Moments later, the Senate, by a vote of 32 to 14, expelled him. He thereby became the fourth nonsouthern senator, after Breckinridge, Johnson, and Polk (Cases 38 and 39), to be expelled during the war.

Conclusion

Bright returned to Indiana and sought reelection to the balance of his Senate term, but the state legislature, although under Democratic control, refused to return him to Washington. Bright then moved to Kentucky and was elected to that state's legislature. In 1874 he moved to Baltimore, where he died in 1875.

Sources

U.S. Congress. Senate. *Congressional Globe.* 37th Cong., 2d sess. (See pp. 89, 287, 391–98, 412–19, 431–35, 447–54, 470–71, 539–45, 559–64, 582–92, 622–29, 644–55, Appendix, pp. 37–42.)

Bright, Jesse D., papers. Indiana Historical Society, Indianapolis.

Johnson, Allen, ed. *Dictionary of American Biography.* Vol. 3. New York, 1946; reprint of 1935 edition. (See pp. 45–46.)

Murphy, Charles. "The Political Career of Jesse D. Bright." *Indiana Historical Society Publications* 10 (1931): 101–45.

Case 41

Benjamin Stark

(1820–1898)

Oregon

Election Case/Expulsion Case
(appointment) January 6, 1862 to June 6, 1862

Issues
Alleged disloyalty to Union

Result: Seated; Not expelled

Chronology:
Credentials presented: Jan. 6, 1862
Referred to committee: Jan. 10, 1862
Committee report: Feb. 7, 1862
Referred to select committee: March 18, 1862
Committee report: April 22, 1862
Senate vote: June 6, 1862

Background

Despite their distance from the battle zones, Oregon's political factions reflected the national divisiveness of the Civil War. Local party alliances shifted as Whigs converted to Republicans and as Democrats split into ardent Unionists or secessionists. Strongly committed to the Union cause, Oregon Senator Edward D. Baker joined both the Republican party and the Union army. Soon after Baker denied rumors that he planned to resign his Senate seat, through a communication to the Oregon legislature, he was killed at the Battle of Ball's Bluff in October 1861.

Governor John Whittaker, who was widely regarded as a secessionist, immediately appointed Benjamin Stark, a lawyer, land speculator, and former state legislator, to serve an interim Senate term until the next session of the legislature. Opposed to the abolitionist views of Republicans in the state, Stark, who began his career in the territory as a Whig, had bolted to the state Democratic organization. Oregon Democrats, however, considered Stark's defection to their party to be little more than political expediency. His appointment to fill Baker's seat elicited a storm of protest, both from Republicans grieving over the loss of their beloved Baker and from the divided Democrats.

Statement of the Case

On the day Stark left for Washington, a group of Oregon businessmen drew up a petition of charges against the new senator. Their strategy included sending a letter to Secretary of War William H. Seward, in which they accused Stark of disloyalty.

When Stark presented his credentials on January 6, 1862, William P. Fessenden (R-ME) led the opposition to seating him. Four days later, James A. Bayard, Jr. (D-DE), with whom Stark had conferred as soon as he learned of the petition, defended the constitutionality of the new senator's appointment. Bayard asserted that the candidate demonstrated all constitutional qualifications and that the Oregon governor had exercised legitimate authority when he named an interim appointee while the legislature was in recess. Therefore, he argued, Stark had a right to take his seat. If he were later found to be disloyal to the Union, the Senate could always expel him after a two-thirds vote. Bayard believed it was dangerous to set the precedent of excluding a qualified member on the basis of his views, because that action could be taken by a simple majority vote. Unconvinced, the Senate referred Stark's credentials to the Judiciary Committee for review.

Response of the Senate

On February 7, 1862, the committee issued a report favorable to Stark, despite some inflammatory testimony given by his Oregon foes. Among his public remarks in favor of secession, Stark was accused of saying, "The southern confederacy is the only legal government in existence; . . . Jeff. Davis is fighting in a good cause, and it will be impossible to defeat him." Although Stark's comments had been decidedly indiscreet, the Judiciary Committee appeared reluctant to bar him from the Senate and refused to rule on the charges. Radical Republicans quickly marshaled their forces to assail the committee's recommendations and tied their protests to a definition of the word "loyalty." During the course of the debate, Charles Sumner (R-MA) contended that loyalty should also be an added qualification for acceptance of a senator.

The tide turned on February 18 when Fessenden reversed his earlier stance. Since Stark's remarks had been made before he was elected senator and the committee had no way of knowing the circumstances, he stated that he had decided to vote in favor of seating Stark. On February 27, after days of wrangling, the Senate voted, 26 to 19, to seat Stark "without prejudice to any further proceedings in the case." Voting with the majority was his Oregon colleague James Nesmith (D) who, believing that Stark had an unshakable constitutional right to the seat, chose to ignore the damage an affirmative vote might do to his own reputation in Portland.

With the oath of office administered, the controversy would have ended had not Stark himself revived it. On February 28, Stark, stung by the fervor of the Republican opposition, asked the Judiciary Committee to review the matter and investigate the charges against him. The Senate delayed action on Stark's resolution until March 18, when it voted to establish a select committee to conclude the inquiry.

Relations between the select committee and Stark remained hostile. Stark wanted the committee to present specific charges. The committee, uninterested in sending an expensive investigating team to Oregon, wished the senator to produce new evidence of his innocence. In a long communication to the committee on April 10, Stark pointed out that he was being challenged simply for his opinions and renewed his request that the committee prepare charges. When the committee asked whether he wished to submit further testimony, Stark on April 15 responded, "I have nothing to add." With Stark steadfastly refusing to cooperate, the committee turned again to the original statements from Oregonians. It concluded that these affidavits, earlier judged to be the concoctions of political rivals, were, in fact, fair and unprejudiced. On April 22, the select committee reported to the Senate that Benjamin Stark was an advocate of rebellion, that he supported the Confederate constitution, and that he was disloyal to the United States government. Stark's failure to supply proof of his innocence, the committee asserted, left it no alternative but to believe the evidence placed before it.

Based on the committee's report, Charles Sumner, on May 7, 1862, introduced a resolution calling for the expulsion of Benjamin Stark, which the Senate defeated on June 6 by a vote of 21 to 16. Senators seemed not to consider the case as serious, since the Oregon legislature would meet in a few months to elect a senator to finish the term to which Stark had been appointed. The currents of political power in the state made it clear that the unpopular Stark would not be returned to his seat. Throughout the process, Stark made no replies in his own defense, and the Senate took no further action on the case.

Conclusion

In the midst of the angry turmoil associated with the Civil War, many senators believed that refusing to seat Stark would establish dangerous precedents. Exclusion of a duly appointed member would have been accomplished through a simple majority vote, rather than the two-thirds vote required for expulsion, thus opening the door to purely political vendettas. Moreover, the nature of the challenge threatened to add new qualifications—in this instance "loyalty"—to the existing constitutional requirements of age, citizenship, and residence. Fearing that adding one new qualification would make it hard to limit others in the future, the Senate opted not to tamper with the constitutional order.

Benjamin Stark's brief senatorial career, in which he served on no committees and remained an insignificant figure, concluded with the election of his successor in September 1862. Stark continued to be active in the Democratic party of Oregon and retained his business interests in the state when he later moved to Connecticut, where he resided until his death in 1898.

Sources

U.S. Congress. Senate. *Congressional Globe.* 37th Cong., 2d sess. (See pp. 183–85, 265–69, 696–97, 861–73, 925–29, 963–75, 988–94, 1011–14, 1261–66, 1983.)

———. Senate Report No. 11. 37th Cong., 2d sess. February 7, 1862.

———. Senate Report No. 38. 37th Cong., 2d sess., April 22, 1862.

Edwards, G. Thomas. "Benjamin Stark: The United States Senate, and 1862 Membership Issues." *Oregon Historical Quarterly* 72 (December 1971), 73 (March 1972).

Bogue, Allan G. *The Earnest Men: Republicans of the Civil War Senate.* Ithaca, NY, 1981.

Case 42

Lazarus W. Powell

(1812–1867)

Kentucky

Expulsion Case
February 20, 1862 to March 14, 1862

Issues
Alleged disloyalty to Union

Result: Not expelled

Chronology:
Resolution introduced: Feb. 20, 1862
Referred to committee: Feb. 20, 1862
Committee report: Mar. 12, 1862
Senate vote: Mar. 14, 1862

Background

At the onset of the Civil War, Peace Democrats, who advocated neutrality in the clash between the states, looked to Kentucky Senator John C. Breckinridge as their titular head. By the summer of 1861, however, Breckinridge had fled Washington to accept a position with the Confederacy. Left behind in the Senate was his Kentucky colleague and good friend, Lazarus Powell. A Democrat and a former governor of the state, Powell continued to insist that Peace Democrats were not merely Confederates in disguise, despite the actions of many who deserted to the South. As the war escalated and emotions heightened, Powell's position became increasingly awkward, especially among Unionists in Kentucky.

Statement of the Case

On February 20, 1862, Morton Wilkinson (R-MN) submitted a passionately worded resolution calling for Powell's expulsion. The resolution turned out to have been written by Powell's Kentucky colleague, Garrett Davis, who had been elected as a Unionist to fill Breckinridge's vacant seat. The lengthy list of charges concluded with the contention that "Under the false and delusive cry of neutrality and peace, . . . he has doubtless assisted to seduce hundreds and hundreds from loyalty and duty into rebellion and treason. He has not supported the Constitution of the United States, but he has sounded the charge to his recruits, and they have made the overt attack upon it." The Senate referred the matter to the Committee on the Judiciary.

Response of the Senate

On March 12, 1862, the committee, chaired by Republican Lyman Trumbull of Illinois, recommended that the resolution not pass. Although the committee disapproved of Powell's former activities aimed at keeping Kentucky neutral, it found no clear evidence that Powell favored the rebellion.

Garrett Davis took immediate exception to the recommendation. Announcing that he acted at the insistence of the Kentucky legislature, Davis bitterly assailed Powell for attending pro-Confederate political rallies in June and September of 1861. Davis, although gracious to Powell personally, told the senators that their colleague traveled to Henderson, Kentucky, where Powell presided over a states' rights convention that adopted resolutions encouraging Kentucky to resist troops from either army. A Republican senator charged: "This was long after the Battle of Bull Run. . . . It was when the Federal troops were marching upon Kentucky for the purpose of rescuing the State. . . . We had the solemn, stern, bloody fact of the existence of civil war; and even then we find a Senator counseling his people to resist the Government in crushing out that rebellion."

Republican Lyman Trumbull, however, eloquently defended the Democrat Powell. He reminded the Senate that, unlike Breckinridge and other secessionists who joined the Confederacy, Powell "came to the Government of the United States to discharge his duties here." "He does not agree with me in sentiment," Trumbull continued, "his opinions are not my opinions; I do not agree with the views that he has so often announced here; but he is entitled to his own opinions; and no man is to be expelled from this body because he disagrees with others in opinion."

Powell himself, however, stated his case most effectively. Although he had not intended to speak after the committee recommended in his favor, he decided that Davis' virulent assault required a response. Addressing the Senate on March 14, Powell admitted attending the Kentucky rallies, which were sponsored by long-time friends and political acquaintances. Regarding the Confederacy, he observed, "Breckinridge went there; I did not." He insisted that he had attempted to use his position in the Senate to resolve national difficulties through conciliation and compromise, rather than coercion. While acknowledging that his efforts had been doomed to failure, Powell defied the senators to find any speech in which he did not call for a constitutional Union. "If it comes to that, that a senator cannot speak and vote as he thinks proper and right without expulsion," he concluded, "then the majority are masters and the minority are slaves, and a seat in the American Senate would no longer be desired by an honest man or a patriot." Convinced of his innocence, the Senate on March 14 voted down the resolution, 11 yeas to 28 nays, and permitted Powell to retain his seat.

Conclusion

Amid the confusing currents of sectional and party factionalism that swirled about his case, Powell probably benefited most from the Senate's growing wariness about defining loyalty and treason. Even clearly drawn partisan lines could alter quickly; by 1864, for example, both Garrett Davis and the Kentucky legislature had shifted their political sympathies to the South. Powell remained in the Senate until 1865, when he returned to his law practice in Kentucky, reconciled with both Davis and the state assembly. He died in 1867.

Sources

U.S. Congress. Senate. *Congressional Globe.* 37th Cong., 2d sess. (See pp. 1112–13, 1208–16, 1230–34.)

———. *Journal.* 37th Cong., 2d sess. (See pp. 224–27, 292, 307.)

Bogue, Allan G. *The Earnest Men: Republicans of the Civil War Senate.* Ithaca, NY, 1981. (See pp. 90, 136.)

Dell, Christopher. *Lincoln and the War Democrats: The Grand Erosion of Conservative Tradition.* Cranbury, NJ, 1975.

General Assembly of Kentucky. *Biographical Sketch of the Hon. Lazarus W. Powell.* Frankfort, KY, 1868.

Johnson, Allen, and Dumas Malone, eds. *Dictionary of American Biography.* Vol. 5. New York, 1946; reprint of 1935 edition. See pp. 113–15, 148–49.)

Case 43

James F. Simmons

(1795–1864)

Rhode Island

Expulsion Case
July 2, 1862 to July 14, 1862

Issues
Corruption

Result: Not expelled
(resigned before Senate could act)

Chronology:
Resolution introduced: July 2, 1862
Referred to committee: July 8, 1862
Committee report: July 14, 1862
No Senate action

Background

Rhode Island industrialist James F. Simmons entered the Senate as a Whig in 1841. When he failed to capture a second term, Simmons returned to his manufacturing interests. His most successful ventures centered on the production of yarns, but his commercial contacts throughout the state were varied and far-reaching. In 1857 the Rhode Island legislature again sent Simmons to the Senate, this time as a Republican.

Statement of the Case

On July 2, 1862, Joseph A. Wright (U-IN) submitted a resolution that called for the expulsion of James Simmons. Acting upon information reported by Secretary of War Edwin M. Stanton, Wright charged that Simmons had blatantly misused his official influence to secure a war contract for two Rhode Island rifle manufacturers. In exchange for his lobbying efforts, Simmons was said to have received two promissory notes of $10,000 each, the first payments on a $50,000 share in the manufacturers' profits.

Response of the Senate

As early as 1853 widespread abuses of congressional influence had prompted the passage of a mildly worded law to check just such conduct as Simmons'. But the proliferation of wartime opportunities apparently proved too attractive, and the Senate again faced the need to curtail this questionable conduct. Congress responded to the charges against Simmons by quickly passing a law that prohibited members of Congress from accepting fees for services before agencies of the United States government.

A Republican-dominated Senate, already vexed by the prevalence of war lobbying, was embarrassed to have one of its own involved in a case so shockingly obvious. On July 8, the matter was referred to the Judiciary Committee, which reported within a week.

The committee ascertained that an agent of a Rhode Island business firm approached Simmons and requested aid in procuring a government contract for the manufacture of 50,000 breechloading rifles. Simmons corroborated the testimony of the agent, C. D. Schubarth, but insisted that the manufacturers' payments to him were not tied to a guarantee of government contracts. Simmons detailed the transaction with great frankness, expressing his complete astonishment at the charges and contending that he acted for the benefit of both his constituents and his government. Simmons cited the recent Union draft of 500,000 men, for whom the government had but 200,000 weapons. With such a critical shortage, Simmons assumed that prompt delivery from a responsible firm could only aid the war effort. The unabashed senator made no move to deny that he still held the promissory notes or that he expected them to be paid in full.

In its July 14 report, the committee set forth Simmons' case in the most deferential terms, citing his age and honorable life, but ultimately found the senator's behavior entirely inexcusable. Acknowledging that to penalize Simmons under the newly passed law would be unfair and would violate the constitutional prohibition against ex post facto laws, the committee reported back the expulsion resolution with the recommendation that the Senate take whatever action it thought appropriate. When the Senate adjourned three days later, it had taken no action in the Simmons case.

Conclusion

Rather than risk expulsion in the session scheduled to begin in December 1862, Simmons resigned from the Senate on August 15, 1862. He returned to his manufacturing interests in Rhode Island, where he died in 1864.

Sources

U.S. Congress. Senate. *Journal.* 37th Cong., 2d sess. (See pp. 739, 773, 831.)

———. Senate Report No. 69. 37th Cong., 2d sess., 1862.

Bogue, Allan G. *The Congressman's Civil War.* New York, 1989. (See pp. 104, 112.)

Case 44

William M. Fishback, Elisha Baxter, William D. Snow

(1831–1903) (1827–1899) (Dates unknown)

Arkansas

Election Case
May 21, 1864 to February 26, 1866

Issues
Reconstruction: challenge to legislature's authority to elect

Result: Not seated

Chronology:

Fishback and Baxter
Credentials presented: May 21, May 31, 1864
Referred to committee: June 13, 1864
Committee report: June 27, 1864
Senate vote: June 29, 1864

Baxter and Snow
Credentials presented: Mar. 7, 1865
Referred to committee: Mar. 8, 1865
Committee report: Mar. 9, 1865
Senate vote: Feb. 26, 1866

Background

In the closing months of the Civil War, a confused and divided Congress struggled to establish Reconstruction policies within a valid constitutional framework, while competing with the president for the right to define and control the program. On December 8, 1863, President Abraham Lincoln had issued a Proclamation of Amnesty and Reconstruction, pardoning citizens of the southern states who would take an oath of loyalty to the Union and accept the end of slavery. Residents of a state could set up a new state government once the number of those who took these actions equalled 10 percent of the voters the state had in 1860. Only the House and Senate, however, could decide whether to seat senators and representatives from the states that met these criteria.

In March 1864, Arkansas voters, representing nearly one-quarter of those who had voted in 1860, approved a revised state constitution that included the abolition of slavery. Election of a legislature, senators, and representatives followed. The U.S. House of Representatives and the Senate were then faced with the question of whether to seat the new members from Arkansas. In the House the three Arkansas representatives elected under the state's new government presented their credentials but, by the time their terms ended at the conclusion of the Thirty-eighth Congress in March 1865, the body had still not decided whether to seat them. The attempt to seat the two new senators elected to complete the unexpired terms of those expelled in 1861 proved to be a forerunner of the seating dilemmas caused by Reconstruction that were to torment the United States Congress until the 1870s.

Statement of the Case

On May 21, 1864, James H. Lane (R-KS) announced that forty-two of the fifty-four counties in Arkansas had voted to eliminate slavery by amending the state constitution. He recommended that the Senate should therefore accept the credentials of William M. Fishback, elected to fill the remainder of the term of expelled Senator William K. Sebastian that would expire in March 1865. Ten days later, on May 31, Solomon Foot (R-VT) asked the same recognition for Elisha Baxter, the replacement for Arkansas' expelled Charles B. Mitchel.

The presentation of these credentials stirred a storm of protest. Jacob Howard (R-MI), a constitutional expert, represented the basic congressional perspective when he demanded to know under what authority Arkansas, whose legislature had announced secession and sent delegates to the Confederate Congress, had restored itself to a legitimate position within the federal government. A state whose Unionism existed only by the force of a military presence should not be so easily readmitted.

Response of the Senate

On June 13, Lane tried a different approach, asking the Senate to consider a joint resolution recognizing the free state government in Arkansas. In the procedural debates that followed, senators agreed that discussion of the joint resolution would also include the Fishback and Baxter credentials. Charles Sumner (R-MA) questioned the right of Arkansas to participate in the national government while reconstruction policies were still being established. Sumner warned that every rebel state would note the Senate's decision in this case, which could set a precedent and unleash a flood of other requests for recognition.

Sumner dismissed Lincoln's reorganization plan as provisional and outlined several reasons Arkansas should not be readmitted to the Union. Since large portions of the state remained in rebel hands, the senators-elect could only represent a minority of the citizens, and the continuing military occupation there was inconsistent with the reordering of civil authority. He also made the practical point that an earlier proclamation issued by the president in 1861—which was still in effect—excluded Arkansas from commercial intercourse with the loyal states. It would therefore be absurdly inconsistent to grant the state full political representation.

William A. Richardson (D-IL), although disagreeing with Sumner's premise that the rebel states were divorced from the Union, condemned Fishback for his participation in secessionist activities. Fishback had offered a resolution stating that any attempt by the federal government to prevent the secession of Arkansas would be met by force within the state, and in May 1861 Fishback had voted for the ordinance of secession and then participated in the state convention's planning to raise troops.

Lane and other supporters defended Fishback, explaining that he had lived in Arkansas under suspicion of having abolitionist sympathies and, terrified by constant death threats, had simply voted for secession in order to save his life. On June 13, after some further discussion, the Senate decided to refer the matter to the Judiciary Committee.

The committee issued a brief report on June 27, 1864, focusing on the legality of the Arkansas government and ignoring the wartime activities of either claimant. Since this was the first of the postwar seating cases, the committee relied as precedent on the 1833 case of Asher Robbins and Elisha Potter (See Case 14), where two contestants had been elected by separate bodies, each claiming to be the legislature of Rhode Island. In that circumstance, the Senate had determined which was the legitimate legislature and therefore which candidate should be seated. As Committee Chairman Lyman Trumbull (R-IL) explained, the committee did not believe the legislature that "assumed to elect these gentlemen was a body of men selected by the loyal inhabitants of Arkansas entirely unrestrained by military authority." In the judgment of the Judiciary Committee, the circumstances described by Fishback and Baxter did not demonstrate that the Arkansas rebellion had been sufficiently suppressed or that the civil government could function without a military force in the state. Thus, the committee determined the Senate should not recognize the claims of the two.

Benjamin Wade (R-OH) urged the Senate to postpone action on the Arkansas senators until it had acted on a general Reconstruction bill already passed by the House. Sumner and others, however, insisted that the Arkansas matter needed to be dealt with promptly and the more general bill might require a lengthy debate. On June 29, the Senate agreed with the committee, voting 27 to 6 to approve a resolution stating that the two were not "entitled to seats as senators from the State of Arkansas."

The adverse votes on both the status of the free state government and the credentials of Fishback and Baxter did not conclude the problems of representation for Arkansas. On March 7, 1865, the credentials of William Snow were presented for the new term for the seat that William Fishback had claimed. The Senate on March 8 referred these credentials to the Judiciary Committee. Amid the turmoil of Reconstruction and with the status of Arkansas still unresolved, the committee the next day simply recommended postponing the subject until the next session of Congress, or until the situation in Arkansas was clarified.

On February 26, 1866, James Lane revived the question, asking that the credentials of Baxter and Snow be removed from the Senate files and referred to the Judiciary Committee. Lane stressed that the government established by the loyal citizens of Arkansas had now lasted for two years and deserved representation in the Senate. On behalf of the Judiciary Committee, however, Lyman Trumbull pointed out that in December 1865 the general question of recognizing the government of Arkansas had been referred to a joint House-Senate committee, known as the Joint Committee of Fifteen on Reconstruction. Until that question was settled, his committee considered it improper to take any action on seating these senators.

After a brief procedural debate, the Senate voted 29 to 17 to table Lane's motion; Baxter and Snow were not seated.

Conclusion

The credentials struggle of Fishback, Baxter, and Snow was only the first of many during the confused period of Reconstruction. The Joint Committee of Fifteen reported in June 1866 that the former Confederate states did not yet have a right to be represented in Congress. Not until March 1867 did Congress pass the First Reconstruction Act, setting forth the general criteria for readmission: new constitutional conventions must be held; the new state governments must guarantee suffrage for all, including blacks; and the states must ratify the Fourteenth Amendment. This act was followed later that year and in 1868 by supplementary acts setting specific steps to implement the process. Finally, in June 1868, Congress passed an Omnibus Act, readmitting Alabama, Arkansas, Florida, Georgia, Louisiana, North Carolina, and South Carolina. On June 23, 1868, two new Arkansas senators presented credentials and were seated.

A staunch Unionist who had been imprisoned by the Confederates before escaping to recruit and lead a Union regiment, Elisha Baxter became governor of Arkansas in the 1870s. In 1878, Baxter was defeated in another bid for the United States Senate and then retired to his farm, where he died in 1899.

William Fishback's erratic behavior during the war—voting for secession in 1861, then swearing support for the Union in 1862—antagonized both Unionists and Secessionists, but thirty years later, in 1892, he was elected governor of Arkansas as a Democrat. He died in 1903.

William Snow died in obscurity.

Sources

U.S. Congress. Senate. *Congressional Globe.* 38th Cong., 1st sess. (See pp. 2895–2907, 3360–68.)

———. *Congressional Globe.* 39th Cong., 1st sess. (See pp. 1025–27.)

———. Senate Report No. 94. 38th Cong., 1st sess., 1864.

———. Senate Report No. 1. 38th Cong., 2d sess., spec. sess., 1865.

Belz, Herman. *Reconstructing the Union.* Ithaca, NY, 1969.

Dell, Christopher. *Lincoln and the War Democrats.* Cranbury, NJ, 1975.

Foner, Eric. *Reconstruction: America's Unfinished Revolution, 1863–1877.* New York, 1988.

Johnson, Allen, and Dumas Malone, eds. *Dictionary of American Biography.* Vol. 5. New York, 1946; reprint of 1935 edition. (See p. 403.)

Case 45

R. King Cutler, Charles Smith, Michael Hahn

(dates unknown) (dates unknown) (1830–1886)

Louisiana

Election Case
December 7, 1864 to March 9, 1865

Issues
Reconstruction: challenge to legislature's authority to elect

Result: Not seated

Chronology:
Credentials presented: Dec. 7, 1864
Referred to committee: Dec. 8, 1864
Committee report: Jan. 11, 1865
Senate action postponed: Mar. 9, 1865

Background

As the Civil War wound to a close, Louisiana served as both a test case for the readmission of Confederate states into the Union and an arena for the clash between presidential and congressional Reconstruction. By 1864, Republican sentiment in Congress favored a vague schedule for granting rebel states full participation in the national government, as opposed to President Abraham Lincoln's desire for speedy reconciliation. As representatives of southern states occupied by Union forces presented their election credentials, Congress tackled the question of Reconstruction policies and oversight responsibilities.

Louisiana, which had adopted a new constitution in 1864 while it was under military occupation by Union forces, hoped to seat its congressional representatives promptly. Former Confederates feared the retaliatory spirit they sensed in Congress and hoped their representation there would dilute the power of the Radical Republicans. The latter, however, unwilling to share the decisions of government with politicians so recently disloyal, resisted seating representatives from former Confederate states, who they expected would block their Reconstruction policies.

Statement of the Case

On December 7, 1864, credentials were presented for R. King Cutler and Charles Smith, elected to fill the Louisiana seats of John Slidell and Judah P. Benjamin that had remained vacant since before the war. At the same time, the Senate received a memorial from citizens of Louisiana, urging that the two not be seated as senators. The Senate referred the matter to the Judiciary Committee on December 8.

Response of the Senate

The Judiciary Committee turned to Major General Nathaniel P. Banks, commander of the Department of the Gulf, for information about the civil condition of the state. He reported that properly elected delegates had met in New Orleans for a constitutional convention and adopted an acceptable state constitution. Banks expressed his satifaction with the organization of the state, asserting: "The sentiment of loyalty in Louisiana. . . . is based upon a thorough reform of all the elements of power . . . schools, churches, theatres, industry, commerce, financial establishments, the militia, fire departments, and society in general."

Although convinced by Banks that the election was valid, the committee reported on January 11, 1865, recommending that the Louisiana senators not be seated because of reports that significant insurrection continued throughout the state. The committee thought it inappropriate for senators to be admitted before the House and Senate jointly recognized the establishment of a legitimate state government, or while Louisiana remained excluded by statute from commercial transactions with the other states. The committee therefore proposed adoption of a resolution specifically recognizing the government of the state.

When the matter reached the Senate floor in February 1865, Banks' glowing accounts of Confederate conversions failed to convince many senators that the government of Louisiana genuinely represented the people of the state. Lazarus Powell (D-KY) charged Banks with being a usurper, asking, "Who clothed Nathaniel P. Banks, major general of the Army of the United States, with the power to amend the Constitution of the State of Louisiana?" From the other side, Republican Charles Sumner of Massachusetts challenged the validity of Louisiana's 1864 constitution as "a mere seven-months abortion, begotten by the bayonet in criminal conjunction with the spirit of caste, and born before its time, rickety, unformed, unfinished—whose continued existence will be a burden, a reproach, and a wrong." At the core of these attacks lay a power struggle between civilian and military institutions; the Senate adamantly refused to seat members who might have been picked by military overseers.

Subsequently, the debate shifted to an emotional exchange about black suffrage. Despite the late hour on a Saturday night, battle lines quickly formed and the debate raged, with Republicans on both sides of the issue. Democrat William Hendricks of Idaho charged that Sumner was determined that the rebellious states should never "be heard in the halls of Congress" until the men who spoke for them represented "the negroes as well as . . . the white men," adding that his party was united in opposing that view. Sumner, however, finally persuaded his colleagues not to seat the Louisiana claimants.

Since Smith's term ended in March 1865, the legislature elected Louisiana governor Michael Hahn to the new Senate term. His credentials, however, were no more welcome in the Senate than his predecessor's. On March 9, 1865, the Senate ordered that action on Hahn's credentials be postponed until the next session, but when Congress convened in December, it took no further action on the matter.

Conclusion

The case of Louisiana's senators remained unresolved. Not until 1868, the year the state was formally restored to the Union, was Louisiana again represented in the Senate.

Cutler and Smith have faded into historical obscurity. Michael Hahn, a native of Bavaria, was elected as a Unionist to the House of Representatives early in the war and later held a number of public offices in Louisiana. A newspaper publisher who opposed slavery, Hahn did not attempt to claim his Senate seat personally because he opposed President Andrew Johnson's Reconstruction policy. In addition to serving as governor, he was later speaker of the state legislature and a judge. Elected to the House of Representatives once more in 1884, he died in Washington two years later.

Sources

U.S. Congress. Senate. *Congressional Globe.* 38th Cong., 2d sess. (See pp. 1061–70, 1091–99, 1101–11.)

———. Senate Report No. 127. 38th Cong., 2d sess., 1865.

———. Senate Miscellaneous Documents Nos. 1, 2, and 9, 38th Cong., 2d sess., 1865.

Harrington, Fred H. *Fighting Politician: Major General N.P. Banks.* Philadelphia, 1948.

Merrill, Horace S. *Bourbon Democracy of the Middle West, 1865–1896.* Seattle, 1953.

Taylor, Joe Gray. *Louisiana Reconstructed, 1863–1877.* Baton Rouge, LA, 1974. (See pp. 17, 55.)

Case 46

Joseph E. Segar and John C. Underwood

(1804–1880) (dates unknown)

Virginia

Election Case
February 17, 1865 to March 9, 1865

Issues
Reconstruction: challenge to legislature's authority to elect

Result: Not seated

Chronology:
Credentials presented:
Feb. 17, Mar. 9, 1865
Senate action postponed: Mar. 9, 1865

Background

In contrast to the situation with the other seceding states, which remained unrepresented in Congress, Virginia had enough loyal citizens to form a government-in-exile, led by Governor Francis H. Pierpont and recognized by the Union. Originally situated in Wheeling, the government included most of the northwestern counties, which in 1863 formed the new state of West Virginia. The loyal Virginia legislature was crucial in the creation of the new state, since according to the U.S. Constitution no new state can be formed from the territory of an existing state without the permission of that state's legislature. Once the legislature gave its approval to the formation of West Virginia, the new state's legislature elected two U.S. senators. Meanwhile, the Unionist Virginia legislature—which had moved to Alexandria—also continued to be represented in the Senate by John S. Carlile and Lemuel J. Bowden. Bowden died on January 2, 1864, and Carlile's term expired on March 3, 1865, setting the stage for a battle over the seating of their successors. (In the Thirty-seventh Congress [1861–1863], the House of Representatives had seated some Virginia representatives while refusing to seat others because they had been elected by only a small number of voters and their districts were often still under rebel control. In the Thirty-eighth Congress [1863–1865] Virginia had no representatives in the House.)

Statement of the Case

The presentation of credentials on February 17, 1865, for Joseph Segar, elected to replace Bowden, brought objections from Senate Republicans who challenged the legitimacy of the Virginia state legislature. Jacob Howard (R-MI) told his colleagues the Senate should make a full inquiry into the status of Virginia. Howard wanted the credentials to go to the Judiciary Committee, because, he said, "If I understand it rightly, the constituency... is now in a state of insurrection and rebellion against the United States.... I am very much inclined to deny the right of that community to any representation upon this floor."

Response of the Senate

Charles Sumner (R-MA) supported the challenge to the credentials and spoke passionately about the importance of knowing for certain that Segar had been elected by a legitimate state legislature. Democrat Willard Saulsbury (DE) pounced on Sumner for political inconsistency. Recommending that Segar's credentials be referred to the Judiciary Committee, he reminded the Senate that in 1861 when Virginia Senators Waitman T. Willey (UU) and John T. Carlile (U) claimed the seats of the two expelled Virginians (See Case 37), some questioned the validity of their election. He noted, "a small corporal's guard objected (not on account of any personal dislike to those honorable members) to their being admitted . . . because we contended then the legislature of Virginia had not sent those men here." During that episode, Sumner had supported those who argued that, given the stress of war, the Unionist loyalty of Willey, Carlile, and the legislature that elected them superseded other procedural concerns. Yet, in this case, he was raising a challenge to a Virginia senator.

Waitman Willey, now a Republican senator from West Virginia, supported seating Segar, observing that it was inconsistent to object to admitting him when the state was already represented by Carlile, and Segar was simply replacing Bowden. In his view, it was a little late for the Senate to start objecting that the Virginia legislature was not legitimate.

The matter was postponed for several weeks until March 9, 1865, during a special session of the Senate, when credentials for Segar and John C. Underwood, who had been elected to replace Carlile, were again considered. As long as Virginia had been the only southern state seeking representation, the Senate had been glad to encourage the Unionist legislature. Now that other seceding states were beginning to apply for representation, the Senate began to rethink the principles at stake, particularly because President Abraham Lincoln had just vetoed the Wade-Davis bill that set forth the congressional plan for Reconstruction. That same day, the Senate had postponed considering the credentials of the two senators-elect from Arkansas (See Case 44). Apparently in the interests of consistency, it tabled the Virginia credentials, as well, until the next session of Congress in December 1865. At that time, Congress created the Joint Committee of Fifteen on Reconstruction to review the situation of all the former Confederate states, and no further action was taken on the credentials of Segar and Underwood.

Conclusion

Virginia remained unrepresented in the House and Senate until 1870, after the state's formal readmission to the Union.

Joseph Segar was no stranger to credential problems. Three times—in 1862, 1864, and 1869—his credentials for the House of Representatives were denied. In 1877 he became a member of the Spanish Claims Commission. In 1879 the Senate supported Segar's claim for expenses related to his 1865 case and paid him $5,000. Joseph Segar died in 1880. In 1886, the heirs of John Underwood, who had died years earlier, received the same amount.

Sources

U.S. Congress. Senate. *Congressional Globe.* 38th Cong., 2d sess. (See pp. 845–49, 1433–34.)

———. *Congressional Record.* 43d Cong., 1st sess. (See p. 1213.)

———. *Congressional Record.* 44th Cong., 2d sess. (See pp. 2195–96.)

———. *Congressional Record.* 45th Cong., 3d sess. (See pp. 1513–15.)

———. *Congressional Record.* 47th Cong., 1st sess. (See pp. 4616–18.) 2d sess. (See pp. 3697–3706.)

———. *Congressional Record.* 48th Cong., 1st sess. (See pp. 6067–70.)

———. Senate Report No. 509. 45th Cong., 2d sess., 1878.

———. Senate Report No. 656. 47th Cong., 1st sess., 1882.

———. Senate Report No. 748. 48th Cong., 1st sess., 1884.

Belz, Herman. *Reconstructing the Union: Theory and Policy During the Civil War.* Ithaca, NY, 1969. (See p. 47.)

Case 47

John P. Stockton

(1826–1900)

New Jersey

Election Case
December 4, 1865 to March 27, 1866

Issues
Conduct of election; whether senator could vote for himself on Senate floor in contested election case

Result: Unseated

Chronology:
Credentials presented: Dec. 4, 1865
Referred to committee: Jan. 8, 1866
Committee report: Jan. 30, 1866
Senate vote: Mar. 27, 1866

Background

John P. Stockton's family connections prepared him for political leadership in New Jersey, since both his father and grandfather had been United States senators. In 1858, President James Buchanan appointed Stockton, who was a lawyer, to be United States minister to Rome, where he served until 1861.

When Stockton, a Democrat, was elected to the Senate in 1865, the method of his election precipitated a major debate and ultimately passage of a law specifying procedures for state legislatures to follow in electing U.S. senators.

Statement of the Case

Stockton's credentials for the term to begin March 4, 1865, were presented on December 4, 1865, together with a memorial from a portion of the New Jersey legislature complaining that the election was invalid. Opponents in the legislature protested that Stockton had received only a plurality, rather than a majority, of the votes in the joint session. At the time of the election, the joint session of the legislature had voted, 41 to 40, to rescind the state requirement that a senator be elected by a majority of all the legislators and instead to permit election by a plurality of those present. The opponents contended that such a change would require a majority vote by each house and that a majority of the state assembly members had not voted for the resolution. The Senate, however, allowed Stockton to take his seat, while referring his credentials to the Judiciary Committee on January 8, 1866.

Response of the Senate

The Judiciary Committee, chaired by Lyman Trumbull (R-IL), reported on January 30 that Stockton's election had been valid. According to the committee, the New Jersey statute provided that a joint meeting of the senate and the general assembly would select the United States senators, but the law contained no stipulations regarding how the joint meeting would be organized and the election conducted. In fact, the committee noted that the New Jersey legislature's joint meetings had in the past operated under a variety of different rules, which were adopted at the beginning of the session, an arrangement apparently permitted by the state constitution.

On March 22, 1866, Daniel Clark (R-NH) initiated the Senate debate, challenging the recommendations of the Judiciary Committee. Clark argued that the Constitution remained silent on the subject of election by plurality or majority and that past custom represented the accepted common law for New Jersey. Additionally, Clark noted that when the New Jersey legislature had voted to change the traditional method of counting a victory, only one body, the state senate, had a majority present.

In defending the legislature's conduct, Stockton raised a point that was becoming increasingly apparent to the Senate. He said, "Senators are not always elected in New Jersey, or in any other State, I presume, in precisely the same way." "Since I have been in Washington," he complained, "the position I have occupied has been very unexpected.... It is a very unpleasant thing to have any one believe that a gentleman would claim a seat to which he was not clearly entitled."

Post-Civil War factional animosities continually surfaced during the complex legal arguments of the contending senators, adding considerable heat to the debate. On March 23 the Senate voted 22 to 21 to affirm the Judiciary Committee's recommendation but failed to end the controversy, since Stockton himself participated in the vote. Urged on by Radical Republicans William P. Fessenden (ME) and Charles Sumner (MA), Lot M. Morrill (R-ME), who had been paired with Stockton's absent New Jersey colleague, William Wright (D), insisted on voting against the resolution. He thus abandoned the pair arrangement—in which the vote of a senator who is present is neutralized by that of an absent senator on the opposite side of an issue. Contending that New Jersey was thus being denied a vote on an issue crucial to the state, Stockton then angrily demanded that his name be called, and he cast the deciding vote for the committee's resolution, although some senators objected that he could not properly vote in his own case. On Monday, March 26, Charles Sumner declared that the record in the Senate *Journal* showing Stockton voting on his own case reflected badly on the Senate. He therefore demanded that the *Journal* be amended to remove Stockton's name from the list of those voting. After considerable debate, Stockton offered to withdraw his vote, but the Senate finally decided that the proper approach was simply to reconsider its earlier action.

In the midst of the heated debate, Stockton asked the Senate not to act on the case until his ailing New Jersey colleague, Democrat William Wright, could return to Washington. The Senate, however, decided to move ahead the next day and take a new vote on the Judiciary Committee's resolutions, this time without Stockton's participation. On March 27, the Senate voted, 23 to 20, to deny the New Jersey senator his seat.

Conclusion

During the course of his defense, Stockton had prepared a detailed list of the procedures used by state legislatures across the country in electing their senators. This report dramatized the inconsistency in the way such elections were handled and led the Senate to take action. In response to this evidence, and to the burden of multiple election challenges resulting from extensive misconduct and corruption at the state level, Congress in July 1866 passed a law to regulate the time and procedure for the election of United States senators. This legislation represented the first major change in the selection process originally authorized by the Founding Fathers. It stipulated that, on the first Tuesday after a legislature met in a senatorial election year, the two houses would meet separately to each select a senator by voice vote. The next day, both houses would meet in joint session to report their individual selections. If both houses chose the same candidate, that candidate would be declared elected. If not, the law provided that "the joint assembly shall meet at twelve o'clock meridian, on each succeeding day of the legislature, and take at least one vote until a Senator shall be elected." The requirement that the two houses of a legislature meet together was designed to end the deadlocks in which each house of a legislature had ignored the other.

Although much of the extensive debate on this case dealt with the complexities of the New Jersey election, Radical Republican senators like Sumner and Fessenden had an additional agenda. The Senate had recently failed to override President Andrew Johnson's veto of the Freedmen's Bureau bill, and the president was also expected to veto the civil rights bill. They hoped that unseating Democrat Stockton would help them gain the necessary two-thirds vote to override that veto. As it happened, on April 6, 1866, the Senate succeeded in overriding the civil rights veto by a vote of 33 to 15, and in July the Senate overrode a veto of a second Freedmen's Bureau bill. Stockton's seat remained vacant until the following September when the legislature elected a Republican to serve out the remainder of the term.

In 1869, John Stockton was returned to the Senate, where he served until 1875. In 1877, he became attorney general of New Jersey, a position he held for fifteen years. Stockton died in 1900.

Sources

U.S. Congress. Senate. *Congressional Globe.* 39th Cong., 1st sess. (See pp. 1564–73, 1589–1602, 1635–48, 1666–79.)

———. Senate Report No. 4. 39th Cong., 1st sess., 1866.

Donald, David. *Charles Sumner and the Rights of Man.* New York, 1970. (See pp. 258–60.)

IV. Reconstruction: 1866–1877

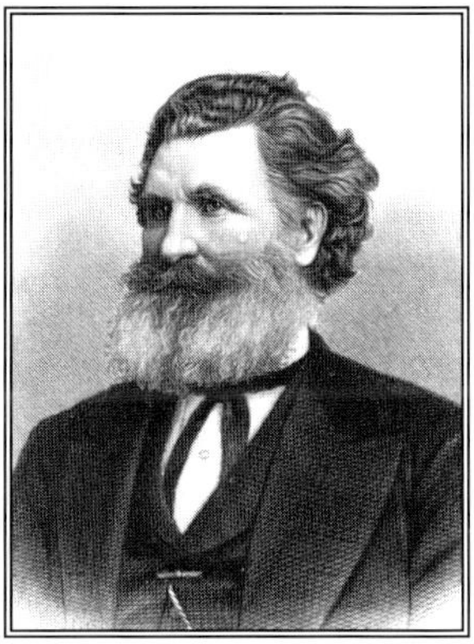

Joshua Hill
(Case 52)
Library of Congress

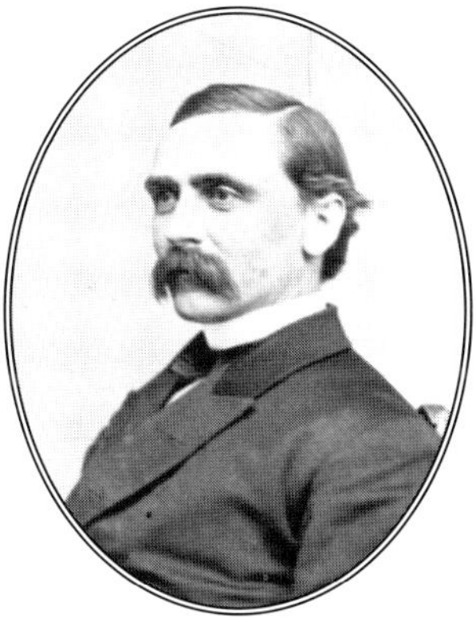

Adelbert Ames
(Case 53)
Library of Congress

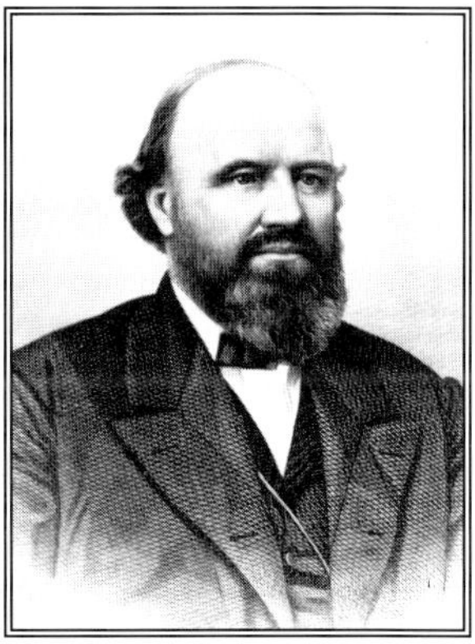

Samuel C. Pomeroy
(Case 61)
U.S. Senate Historical Office

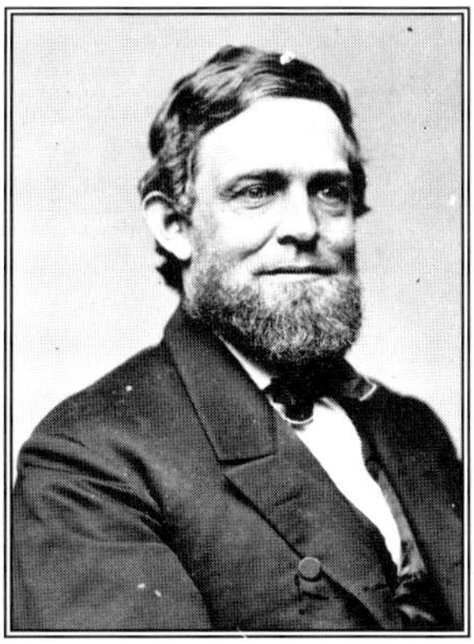

Vice President Schuyler Colfax
(Case 64)
Library of Congress

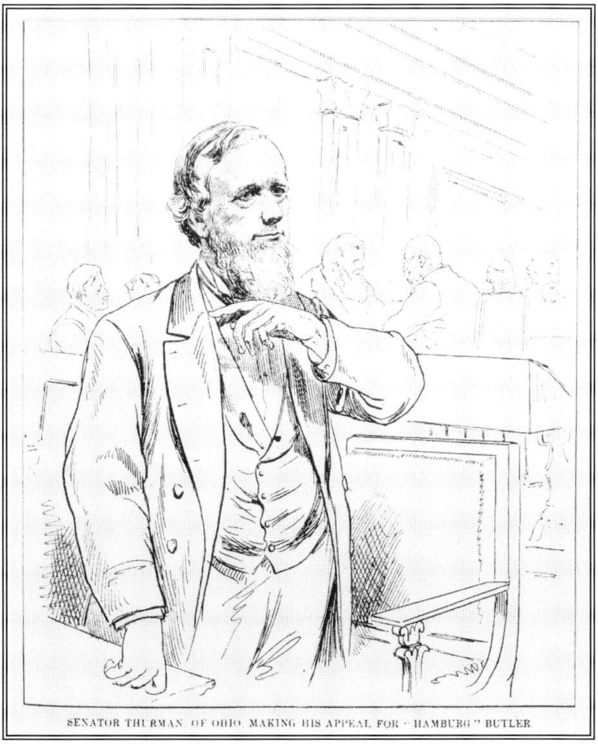

Allen G. Thurman *(Case 66)*
New York Daily Graphic, December 3, 1877

Case 48

David T. Patterson

(1818–1891)

Tennessee

Election Case
July 26, 1866 to July 28, 1866

Issues
Reconstruction: qualifications: ability to honestly swear to test oath

Result: Seated

Chronology:
Credentials presented: July 26, 1866
Referred to committee: July 26, 1866
Committee report: July 27, 1866
Senate vote: July 28, 1866

Background

Tennessee's desire to return to the Union following the Civil War caused great concern among Radical Republicans, who feared that the admission of that state's congressional representatives would establish precedents for other rebel states that would be difficult to check. On the other hand, the state had supported a large Unionist population throughout the war and was the home of President Andrew Johnson, who was certain to watch the proceedings in Congress with a keen eye. Once Tennessee ratified the Fourteenth Amendment and was readmitted to the Union on July 24, 1866, under an enabling act certifying that all necessary conditions had been fulfilled, Congress had little reason to refuse to seat the state's representatives.

Statement of the Case

On July 26, 1866, David T. Patterson (U), elected to complete the term that began on March 4, 1863, presented his credentials. Charles Sumner (R-MA) immediately asked that the certificates be sent to the Judiciary Committee. Sumner based his request on information from Tennessee that Patterson had taken an oath of allegiance to the rebel government and had served as a state judge during the war. Under the terms of Reconstruction, a person who acted as an official of a rebellious state was denied office in the national government.

Response of the Senate

Reverdy Johnson (D-MD) and James Grimes (R-IA) both objected to referring the matter to committee. They insisted that Patterson be seated at once to provide his state with Senate representation (his Tennessee colleague, Joseph Fowler, had been seated the previous day) while the Judiciary Committee examined the case. Edgar Cowan (R-PA) argued that the Senate could expel Patterson with a two-thirds vote after he was seated but that it was unwise to exclude him from his seat on a simple majority vote when he met all constitutional requirements. Others, however, believed the committee should review the case to determine whether Patterson, having served as a judge under the Confederacy, could properly take the "Ironclad Test Oath of Loyalty" required by the act of July 1862. Under that act, all future officials of the U.S. government must swear that they had not given aid or encouragement to the enemy nor exercised "the functions of any office" under an authority "in hostility to the United States." After considerable discussion, the Senate voted 26 to 14 to refer the matter to the Judiciary Committee.

On July 27, 1866, a divided Judiciary Committee reported back that it accepted the facts of Patterson's support for the Union, but members differed on whether he should be seated. James R. Doolittle (R-WI) had championed Patterson's loyalty, stating that it had not faltered in the face of constant harassment and repeated arrests by the Confederate army. Patterson held the judicial post when the war began and ran for reelection only because his east Tennessee Unionist friends greatly feared the other candidate, an aggressive Confederate. Although victorious, Patterson had difficulty pursuing his career as a judge, for he spent most of his days in hiding, unable to convene the court with regularity. Further, Doolittle added, "His house was the home of the fleeing men who sought their way through the mountains from North and South Carolina. His fortune was at their disposal. He organized a system by which the men of East Tennessee ran into Kentucky and flocked to our armies by thousands upon thousands." Patterson's personal suffering on behalf of the Union convinced the majority of the Judiciary Committee that he had subscribed to the Confederate oath simply as an expedient, in order to be in a position to help protect Union supporters in that part of Tennessee from civil disorder and violence by bands of armed rebels. Patterson had also been in touch with leaders of Union forces in the area, providing them with information on rebel movements. In light of his evident dedication to the Union, the panel recommended that Patterson be seated.

While Committee Chairman Lyman Trumbull (R-IL) concurred in these sentiments and sympathized with Patterson's plight, he maintained that Patterson could not honestly swear that he had never accepted any office in a government hostile to the United States. Trumbull objected to seating a member who knowingly swore a false oath, particularly since Republicans worried that many southern states were still trying to send to Congress known rebels who might not hesitate to swear that they had been loyal during the war. As a possible solution, Trumbull offered a joint resolution that would exempt Patterson from the troublesome portion of the oath. Other senators objected that the resolution would never pass the House, although they agreed that, if it did, President Johnson—who happened to be Patterson's father-in-law—could be depended upon not to veto it. The resolution, hastily drafted that day by Trumbull, passed the Senate 35 to 2.

The Senate remained in session until four in the morning of the next day, when the body again addressed the subject of David Patterson. Exhausted by the late hour and informed that the House—bowing to pressure from Republicans who objected to tampering with the oath in any way—had tabled the joint resolution, the Senate reverted to the original recommendation from the Judiciary Committee. Trumbull continued to insist that the only way to administer Patterson the oath was to exclude the portion that referred to the acceptance of a Confederate office. Benjamin Wade (R-OH) blamed Patterson for creating his own predicament: "No man can act as a judge under a rebel government and swear allegiance to it without committing an act of hostility and treason against his own Government.... If he is true to the confederacy he is a traitor to our Government. If he is true to our Government he is false to that to which he has voluntarily sworn." Faced with this impasse and unwilling to see the oath intended to exclude rebels and secessionists become a weapon against a vigorous Unionist, the Senate finally voted, 21 to 11, with 18 senators absent, to seat Patterson. He took his oath of office in the final hours of the congressional session on July 28.

Conclusion

Even after Patterson's seating, two concerns remained: he did, in fact, swear to the full oath, which his actions contradicted; and some senators could not shake the uneasy feeling that the oath itself represented an illegal addition to the constitutional qualifications for membership. Such dilemmas were to be repeated many times in the Senate throughout the troublesome era of Reconstruction.

David Patterson, who had risked his life in support of the Union in Tennessee, remained in the Senate until the end of his term in 1869, when he retired from public life. He died in Tennessee in 1891.

Sources

U.S. Congress. Senate. *Congressional Globe.* 39th Cong., 1st sess. (See pp. 4162–4169, 4213–4216, 4242–4245.)

Hyman, Harold M. *Era of the Oath: Northern Loyalty Tests During the Civil War and Reconstruction.* Philadelphia, 1954. (See pp. 91–94.)

Case 49

Phillip F. Thomas

(1810–1890)

Maryland

Election Case
March 18, 1867 to February 19, 1868

Issues
Reconstruction: qualifications: ability to honestly swear to test oath

Result: Not seated

Chronology:
Credentials presented: Mar. 18, 1867
Referred to committee: Mar. 19, 1867
Committee report: Dec. 18, 1867
Senate vote: Feb. 19, 1868

Background

Phillip Thomas, son of a prominent Maryland Whig family, abandoned his family's political affiliation and joined the Democratic party. A lawyer who was active in both state and national politics, Thomas served as governor of Maryland and in the United States House of Representatives. He was secretary of the treasury under President James Buchanan for one month before resigning in January 1861 at the outset of the Civil War. A Confederate sympathizer, he spent the war years in retirement at his farm on Maryland's Eastern Shore. Thomas was elected to the United States Senate for a term to begin March 4, 1867.

Statement of the Case

The presentation of Thomas' credentials on March 18, 1867, launched the Senate on a year-long controversy. Jacob Howard (R-MI) spearheaded the Republican attack, demanding that the Senate send Thomas' credentials to the Judiciary Committee before permitting him to take the oath of office. He feared that Thomas could not truthfully swear the so-called ironclad test oath, required by the act of 1862, that he had not provided "aid, countenance, counsel or encouragement" to the enemy during the war. Reverdy Johnson (D-MD), who was frequently at loggerheads with the Republicans on Reconstruction issues, denounced Howard's challenge to his Maryland colleague and long-time friend as incomprehensible. It could not, Johnson hoped, be because Republicans gave any credence to "unfounded rumors" that surrounded Thomas' tenure as secretary of the treasury.

Radicals, in a barrage of accusations, quickly made it clear that this was but one of the many charges they would level at Thomas. There were two principal allegations against the senator-elect: that he had resigned as a member of President Buchanan's cabinet because he opposed the reinforcement of

Fort Sumter; and that, as secretary of the treasury, he had transferred a substantial sum of federal money from New York to New Orleans once he knew rebels controlled the Louisiana bank and could easily seize the funds. Reverdy Johnson, defending his colleague, provided detailed information to refute this latter charge.

Unexpected support for Thomas came from Lyman Trumbull (R-IL), chairman of the Judiciary Committee, who argued that senators were bound by the Constitution to admit members who appeared with the correct qualifications. If the matter were referred to his committee, he inquired, "What is there for the committee to investigate?" He cited precedents in his own case (See Case 28) and that of James Harlan (See Case 29) that in such challenges, the senators were usually seated and then an investigation was conducted into the charges against them. Trumbull told his colleagues, "It will not do to assume the position that every person who disagrees with us politically is an enemy of his country." William P. Fessenden (R-ME) agreed with Trumbull and suggested that Thomas take his oath; then if the Senate had evidence that he committed perjury, he should be expelled through the traditional means. Fessenden recalled only two cases, both involving charges of disloyalty during the war (Cases 41 and 48), when he had urged investigating the serious allegations first.

The objections to Thomas intensified after John Sherman (R-OH) read aloud a newspaper account of a speech that Thomas made to the Maryland general assembly immediately after his senatorial nomination, in which he said, "The men now assembled at Washington, before the war occurred, were bent upon dissolving the Union . . . and were now bent upon the establishment of a military despotism." According to the report, he had declared that those in the Congress "are now and always were traitors to the Union." Democrats questioned the accuracy of the newspaper story, but the damaging impression remained. In response to these objections, the Senate sent Thomas' credentials to the Judiciary Committee on March 19, 1867.

Response of the Senate

On December 18, 1867, the committee returned a report without recommendation. After examining the evidence it had collected, the committee found no reason to prevent Thomas from taking his seat, with the possible exception of the fact that his son served in the Confederate army. For a judgment on whether that circumstance should disqualify him, the committee referred all the evidence to the full Senate.

On January 6, 1868, the Senate began debating the matter. Reverdy Johnson led the effort to seat Thomas, defending his Maryland colleague at length. Thomas, he said, had spent months unsuccessfully trying to dissuade his young son from joining the Confederate army. Once the young man was actually leaving to cross into southern territory, Thomas gave him $100 in case he was captured and needed money in prison. After the son left, the father refused to communicate with him again. Republican senators opposed to seating Thomas focused particularly on the $100 gift to the soldier-son as evidence that Thomas had given aid and comfort to the rebel cause.

Again, there was considerable procedural discussion over the recurring issue of whether the Senate should seat a challenged senator and then investigate the charges or should conduct the investigation first and, if appropriate, deny him his seat. If after a senator was sworn in an inquiry substantiated the charges, or the senator was found to have committed perjury when swearing the loyalty oath, the Senate could later expel him through a two-thirds vote. Judiciary Committee Chairman Trumbull, who—based on previous precedent—had urged seating Thomas when his credentials were first presented, changed his position and suggested that in the future it would be preferable for the Senate to conduct the investigation first, since there had been occasions in the past when a senator had been seated and served for a year or more before the Senate finally decided he was not entitled to a seat. In fact, he suggested adopting a Senate rule that "no person about whose right to a seat there is a question should be admitted to be sworn until that question is settled."

Charles Sumner (R-MA) expressed the continuing fear of many Republicans that the Senate was in danger of being overrun by former Confederates. "Everywhere in the rebel states," he said, "disloyal people are struggling for power; and now at the door of the Senate we witness a similar struggle.... Disloyalty must be met at the door and not allowed to enter in." Many of the Radical Republicans believed that Thomas' lack of active support for the Union was in itself evidence of disloyalty, but other senators considered that mere sympathy for the rebels should not be disqualifying as long as Thomas had taken no overt action on their behalf. Trumbull, for example, did not believe that Thomas' gift of $100 to his son constituted "encouragement" to the enemy in the meaning of the oath. He therefore concluded that Thomas should be seated.

After several more days of debate, the Senate on February 19 concurred with Sumner's view and voted, 27 to 20, to deny Thomas his seat. The resolution as adopted read that Thomas, "having voluntarily given aid, countenance, and encouragement to persons engaged in armed hostility to the United States," was not entitled to be seated as a senator.

Conclusion

The lengthy, heated debate in this case helped to weaken the unity among Senate Republicans. On the day of the final vote, Jacob Howard and Lyman Trumbull hurled at each other angry charges of "perverting the evidence." Trumbull, Fessenden, and several other Republicans broke with their colleagues and voted in favor of Thomas, a symptom of the deep-seated differences among Republican senators, some of whom could not shake the uneasy feeling that the required loyalty oath was an unconstitutional device, designed to limit political opposition.

Phillip Thomas was elected to the U.S. House of Representatives in 1875 and served one term. In 1878 he won a seat in the Maryland general assembly. Thomas died in Baltimore in 1890.

Sources

U.S. Congress. Senate. *Congressional Globe.* 40th Cong., 1st sess. (See pp. 171–180, 821–824.) 2d sess. (See pp. 320–30, 632–35, 653–62, 678–86, 1144–56, 1165–77, 1205–10, 1232–43, 1260–71.)

———. Senate Report No. 5. 40th Cong., 2d sess., 1867.

Hyman, Harold M. *Era of the Oath: Northern Loyalty Tests During the Civil War and Reconstruction.* Philadelphia, 1954. (See pp. 127–28.)

Malone, Dumas, ed. *Dictionary of American Biography.* Vol. 18. New York, 1946; reprint of 1935 edition. (See p. 443.)

Case 50

John T. Jones and Augustus H. Garland

(dates unknown) (1832–1899)

v.

Alexander McDonald and Benjamin F. Rice

(1832–1903) (1828–1905)

Arkansas

Election Case
June 23, 1868

Issues
Reconstruction: challenge to legislature's authority to elect

Result: McDonald and Rice Seated

Chronology:
Credentials presented: June 23, 1868
Senate vote: June 23, 1868

Background

Even after the unsuccessful Senate bids of William Fishback, Elisha Baxter, and William D. Snow in 1864 (See Case 44), Arkansas did not abandon efforts to have its representatives seated in the upper house. Undaunted by the Senate rebuff, the state legislature sent claimants in 1866 and 1867. In both cases the credentials—one set for John T. Jones and one for Augustus Garland (D)—were ordered to lie on the table.

Then, on June 22, 1868, after adopting a new constitution with the participation of black voters, Arkansas was readmitted to the Union under terms of the Reconstruction acts of 1867.

Statement of the Case

The next day, on June 23, 1868, the credentials of Republicans Alexander McDonald and Benjamin F. Rice, elected under the new constitution, were presented for the same terms claimed by Jones and Garland. A native of Pennsylvania who moved to Arkansas during the war, McDonald, a banker, was active in raising troops for the Union army. Rice, originally from New York, lived in Kentucky and Minnesota before settling in Arkansas after serving with Union forces in the war years.

Arkansas, having been unrepresented in the Senate since 1861, now had four sets of credentials under consideration. Neither of the earlier-elected senators had attempted to claim his seat: Garland did not appear, and Jones had died. Nonetheless, Garrett Davis (D-KY) requested that the earlier credentials be read and that all four sets be sent to the Judiciary Committee for a determination as to which senators should be seated.

Response of the Senate

Jacob Howard (R-MI) objected to Davis' strategy, pointing out that, in passing the 1867 Reconstruction acts, Congress had already refused to recognize the provisional state legislature of 1865 that was responsible for the first election attempts. The reorganized state government had elected McDonald and Rice under a constitution in accord with national Reconstruction policy.

As senators warmed to a debate on the fine points of procedure, Lyman Trumbull (R-IL), chairman of the Judiciary Committee, foresaw that his committee would be inundated with claimants to Senate seats from former Confederate states. With senatorial elections pending in North and South Carolina, Florida, Georgia, and Alabama, Trumbull recommended adoption of a rule to regulate the precise time when legislatures in the former rebel states were authorized to hold elections. By such a rule Trumbull hoped to deflect charges that state legislatures elected senators before Congress granted the proper authorization. Additionally, Trumbull rejected a suggestion that the Arkansas senators should be required to draw lots for the length of their terms, arguing that, even though the seats had been vacant for several years, the terms established when Arkansas entered the Union in 1836 had continued despite the secession period.

Garrett Davis insisted on the need to refer the matter to the Judiciary Committee, reiterating his own Reconstruction philosophy, which denied to either the president or Congress the power to prescribe the terms of readmission. Davis contended that, once a rebel state was defeated, "the Constitution restored them to the Union and enabled them to claim all their rights in the Government as States of the United States." Thus, he believed the Arkansas seats properly belonged to Jones and Garland rather than to the new arrivals.

Rejecting Davis' argument, the Senate, by voice vote, defeated the motion to refer the credentials to the Judiciary Committee. Alexander McDonald and Benjamin Rice then stepped forward to take the oath of office, and, for the first time in seven years, Arkansas had two senators.

Conclusion

Unlike the earlier claimants for Senate seats from the former Confederate states, there could be no question about the loyalty of McDonald and Rice, both of whom had served in the Union army during the war. The Reconstruction acts and the formal readmission of Arkansas to the Union had set the ground rules, and the Republican-dominated Senate took the next step by swearing in the senators elected under the state's new constitution.

McDonald failed to be reelected in 1870. A proponent of western railroad development, he died in 1903. Rice, an organizer of the Republican party in Arkansas, remained in the Senate until 1873, after which he practiced law until his death in 1905. More prominent was Augustus Garland, who, after his rejection by the Senate, was elected governor of Arkansas in 1874. Known for his affable style, Garland became a United States senator in 1876. From 1885 to 1889, he served as attorney general of the United States, after which he practiced law until his death in 1899.

Sources

U.S. Congress. Senate. *Congressional Globe.* 40th Cong., 2d sess. (See pp. 3384–89.)

Brock, W. R. *An American Crisis: Congress and Reconstruction, 1865–1867.* New York, 1963.

Johnson, Allen, and Dumas Malone, eds. *Dictionary of American Biography.* Vol. 7. New York, 1946; reprint of 1935 edition. (See pp. 150–51.)

Case 51

William Marvin v. Thomas W. Osborn

(1808–1902) (1833–1898)

Florida

Election Case
June 30, 1868

Issues
Reconstruction: challenge to legislature's authority to elect

Result: Osborn seated

Chronology:
Credentials presented: June 30, 1868
Senate vote: June 30, 1868

Background

In 1866, Florida's provisional state government elected two United States senators, but, believing the state had not taken sufficient steps to protect the rights of the freedmen, the Senate tabled their credentials and took no further action. Then, in 1868, under provisions of the Reconstruction acts of 1867, Florida adopted a new moderate constitution that enfranchised black voters. Having ratified the Thirteenth and Fourteenth Amendments, the newly constituted legislature elected two United States senators, former Freedmen's Bureau Commissioner Thomas W. Osborn (R) and Adonijah S. Welch (R). On June 25, the state was readmitted to the Union, together with North and South Carolina, Louisiana, Alabama, and Georgia.

Statement of the Case

Upon the presentation of Thomas Osborn's credentials on June 30, 1868, William P. Fessenden (R-ME), aware that well-publicized political discord and violence continued in Florida, inquired whether the state had met all requirements for representation in Congress. Osborn's supporter, Timothy Howe (R-WI), responded that the confirming evidence—the ordinance ratifying the two constitutional amendments—had just been laid on the table. Charles Drake (R-MO) nevertheless urged that the credentials be referred to committee.

Response of the Senate

Timothy Howe reminded his colleagues that the Senate had not referred the credentials of Arkansas' two senators to committee before swearing them in a week earlier under similar circumstances (See Case 50). Fessenden, however, reiterated his desire to know more about Florida's ratification of the Thirteenth and Fourteenth amendments, since even the 1868 legislature was dominated by those favoring white supremacy. Others agreed that a committee should review the matter. Jacob Howard (R-MI) and Charles Drake questioned the use of the word "adopted," rather than "ratified," by the Florida legislature in accepting the Thirteenth and Fourteenth amendments. They urged that the materials regarding ratification be referred to the Judiciary Committee, but the committee's chairman, Lyman Trumbull (R-IL), expressed little enthusiasm for the idea. "I have looked at these papers," he declared, "and I see no earthly object in referring them. We may as well act upon them now as tomorrow."

Conservative Republican James R. Doolittle (WI) added a twist to the proceedings by submitting the credentials of another Florida senator, William Marvin, elected by the provisional legislature in 1866 for the same term claimed by Osborn. The Wisconsin senator had first presented the credentials of the racially conservative Marvin, who had served as Florida's provisional governor, on January 19, 1866. At that time, they were tabled by the Senate. Doolittle now argued that Florida had never actually been out of the Union; since the war was over by 1866, the legislature therefore had had a right to elect U.S. senators. Marvin, he believed, had first claim upon the seat, and his credentials should be sent to the Judiciary Committee along with those of Osborn.

After extensive wrangling over whether Florida had properly ratified the two amendments and whether the question should be referred to committee, the Senate finally refused, by a vote of 13 to 31, to postpone the matter and then voted, 34 to 6, to seat Osborn. William Marvin's claim was disregarded because he had been elected before passage of the Reconstruction acts and by a Florida legislature that did not meet the stringent standards for renewal of representation in Congress. Osborn then came forward and took the oaths of office.

Conclusion

Resolving the controversy over Florida's readmission and the seating of one senator cleared the way for the state's second senator to take his place. On July 2, 1868, Adonijah Welch joined Osborn in the chamber and took his oaths of office. Welch, a Michigan educator who moved to Florida after the war, served only until the end of his brief term in March 1869.

Thomas Osborn, a native of New Jersey who parlayed his service in the Union army during the Civil War into a powerful Florida political career, retired from the Senate in March 1873 at the completion of his term. He returned to Florida to practice law, and in later years moved to New York City. He died in New York in 1898.

William Marvin later returned to his native New York, where he remained until his death in 1902.

Sources

U.S. Congress. Senate. *Congressional Globe.* 40th Cong., 2d sess. (See pp. 3598–3607.)

Shofner, Jerrell H. *Nor Is It Over Yet: Florida in the Era of Reconstruction, 1863–1877.* Gainesville, FL, 1974.

Case 52

Richard H. Whiteley and Henry P. Farrow

(1830–1890) (dates unknown)

v.

Joshua Hill and H. V. M. Miller

(1812–1891) (1814–1896)

Georgia

Election Case
December 7, 1868 to February 1, 1871

Issues
Reconstruction: challenge to legislature's authority to elect; qualifications: ability to honestly swear to test oath

Result: Hill and Miller Seated

Chronology:
Credentials presented: Dec. 7, 1868
Referred to committee: Dec. 10, 1868
Committee reports:
Jan. 25, Feb. 17, 1869
Credentials presented: July 15, 1870
Referred to committee: Dec. 13, 1870
Committee report: Jan. 23, 1871
Senate vote: Feb. 1, 1871

Background

Resistance to granting blacks political equality in some southern states created a basic tension with the Radical Republican Congress in the late 1860s. This attitude, coupled with factionalism within the states and a suspicious and divided Congress, kept several southern Senate election cases in uncertainty for inordinately long periods. Such political conflicts blocked the seating of Georgia's senators for over two years.

By June of 1868, Georgia had adopted a new constitution conforming to the Reconstruction acts of 1867 and elected a legislature that ratified the Thirteenth and Fourteenth amendments. Since the state had met the necessary criteria, Congress on June 25 passed a law restoring Georgia to representation in Congress, along with North and South Carolina, Alabama, Louisiana, and Florida. A month later, the five Georgia members were seated in the House of Representatives, and, on July 28, the state legislature elected to the state's two Senate seats Republican Joshua Hill, who had served in the U.S. House of Representatives before the war, and Democrat Homer V.M. Miller, a physician who had participated in the new Georgia constitutional convention. But then, in September, the situation changed dramatically when the white members of the Georgia legislature expelled twenty-eight black representatives and senators, in effect returning the legislature to rebel control. As a result, when Hill's credentials were presented to the U.S. Senate on December 7, 1868, at the beginning of the third session of the Fortieth Congress, the scene was set for a fight.

Statement of the Case

Even though Joshua Hill was known to have remained a loyal unionist throughout the war, Charles Drake (R-MO) registered a protest upon the presentation of his credentials. Informing his colleagues that the white Georgia legislators had banded together and expelled all the black members, Drake asked the Judiciary Committee to investigate Hill's credentials. Drake's fellow-Republican, John Sherman (OH), disagreed. Sherman maintained that Georgia had complied with all conditions imposed by Congress, the state had been readmitted to representation, and the governor inaugurated on July 18, 1868. Ten days later, the legislature had elected Hill by a large majority, because the Democrats were so anxious to defeat his principal opponent, whom they violently disliked, that they unenthusiastically joined with Georgia Republicans to vote for him. The expulsion of the black Republican legislators after the election, Sherman declared, "is as much disapproved by the senator-elect as by any one of us. It was a gross outrage; a violation of the constitutional amendment, and a violation of the reconstruction acts." Sherman concluded, however, that the Senate should not penalize Hill, a faithful unionist who decried the behavior of the state legislature.

Drake refused to abandon his opposition, stressing his belief that Congress retained its power over the reconstructed states even after a state government was reorganized and recognized. Claiming to have no objection to Hill personally, he stated: "I wish this matter to be investigated. I wish the facts to go before the country."

In October 1868, a convention representing the black population of Georgia had sent to Congress a memorial describing the situation there. It set forth the circumstances under which the black legislators had originally been elected and noted that the white members had encouraged them to ratify the constitutional amendments. Then, once the state was safely restored to the Union, the white legislators declared that the black members were actually ineligible to serve and voted to expel them in a body after "the Speaker ruled that none of the persons involved in the charge had the right to vote upon the question." The memorialists asked for redress from Congress to uphold their rights as citizens.

According to John Thayer (R-NE), the rebellion in the Georgia legislature occurred because the body had been "composed in part of men who had been expressly disqualified" from holding public office under terms of the Fourteenth Amendment's prohibition on service by anyone who had previously served in a federal or state government office and later "engaged in insurrection or rebellion against" the United States. Contending that the illegal inclusion in the state legislature of these members undermined the legitimacy of the reorganized Georgia government, the Nebraska Republican dismissed concerns that sending the credentials to committee would place Hill in a state of suspense. After all, Thayer said, "civil order is in suspense in Georgia; loyalty is in suspense in Georgia; human liberty is in suspense in Georgia."

On December 10, 1868, the Senate decided to refer the credentials of Joshua Hill to the Judiciary Committee, together with the memorial of the black voters and a letter on the matter from the governor of Georgia. A month later, the Senate also sent to committee the credentials of the senator-elect for the second Georgia vacancy, Homer V.M. Miller.

Response of the Senate

On January 25, 1869, the Judiciary Committee returned majority and minority reports on the credentials of Joshua Hill. Most committee members agreed with Roscoe Conkling (R-NY) that Congress could not overlook outrageous irregularities in the organization of the Georgia legislature or the expulsion of its black members. According to the committee, an essentially rebel legislature controlled the civil government, and widespread persecution, assault, and murder were being perpetrated against black Georgians and others loyal to the national government. Concerned about these conditions in the state, Conkling and his associates decided that Hill should not be seated.

The minority view, espoused by Judiciary Committee Chairman Lyman Trumbull (R-IL), accepted a statement by Georgia's provisional governor that no ineligible members sat in the legislature; it therefore recommended that the loyal unionist Hill should be seated. Trumbull believed that time and the influence of a new state administration would "soon correct whatever of lawlessness and disorder now remain in the State," of which there had been conflicting reports.

Before the Senate took further action on either senator-elect, the National Union Republican Association of Georgia submitted resolutions to the Senate condemning the expulsion of the black legislators and urging that Joshua Hill and H.V.M. Miller not be seated. These resolutions were referred to the Judiciary Committee, which recommended on February 17, 1869, that Miller not be seated. Shortly thereafter, Congress adjourned.

Lyman Trumbull promptly reactivated the Hill and Miller case when the Forty-first Congress convened several weeks later in early March, but the Senate failed to take action during this brief first session, and reports of disorder in the state continued. In December 1869, at the start of the second session, Congress responded by passing an act setting additional requirements for Georgia's reconstruction, including reorganization of the state legislature. After complying with these provisions and ratifying the Fifteenth Amendment, the state was again formally admitted to representation in Congress on July 15, 1870. That same day, credentials were presented to the Senate for two new senators—Richard H. Whiteley (R) and Henry P. Farrow—chosen by the reorganized legislature. In the early days of the third session of the Forty-first Congress, on December 13, 1870, the Senate referred these credentials to the Judiciary Committee.

Once again, the committee was divided, issuing majority and minority reports in January 1871. On January 23, the majority report recommended that Joshua Hill be seated but that H.V.M. Miller, who had acted as a surgeon in the Confederate army, should be denied his seat, because he could not swear the required ironclad test oath of loyalty that he had not given aid to the enemy. In presenting the report, Lyman Trumbull expressed the view that the Senate was not in a position to investigate the eligibility of individual members of a legislature that elected U.S. senators. "All that the Senate of the United States can do," he asserted, "is to ascertain whether there was a Legislature duly organized with a constitutional quorum in each of its branches which has sent the member here." He reiterated that, at the time Hill and Miller were elected, the Georgia legislature had been recognized by Congress, along with those from the other states readmitted to representation in June 1868. The problem, he explained, had arisen from the subsequent action of that legislature in expelling the black members and replacing them with white men who had not been properly elected.

On January 30, 1871, William M. Stewart (R-NV) presented the minority report, expressing his opposition to seating Hill and Miller in extensive floor remarks. The two claimants elected before the December 1869 law was enacted, he believed, were not entitled to their seats, and Whiteley and Farrow, having been elected by a duly recognized legislature, should be sworn in. By a vote of 19 to 36, the Senate defeated Stewart's motion to seat Farrow and Whiteley, but Stewart continued to press his position. He contended that, in passing the December 1869 act, Congress had repudiated the 1868 legislature as illegally constituted and thus not empowered to elect U.S. senators. A majority of the Senate, however, rejected this view, believing that the legislature had elected Hill and Miller in conformity with the law. On February 1, 1871, senators anxious to settle the case voted to seat Joshua Hill, and he came forward to take the oaths of office.

Debate on Miller's credentials followed. Allen Thurman (D-OH) introduced a joint resolution providing that Miller need not take the ironclad oath regarding his past actions and instead could simply swear future loyalty to the United States. Thurman argued that, since other southerners who aided the rebellion both militarily and politically had had their disabilities removed, it seemed illogical to turn away Miller, who as a Confederate surgeon had been a noncombatant charged with saving lives. The Senate referred the joint resolution to the Judiciary Committee, and it was subsequently passed by both houses of Congress and signed by the president. On February 24, 1871, Miller took the oath prescribed by the resolution and was seated. His term of office expired less than two weeks later.

Conclusion

The questions raised by the stormy history of the 1868 Georgia legislature were not yet finally settled. Throughout 1871, the Senate also wrestled with the case of Foster Blodgett, elected to succeed Miller by the same reorganized legislature that selected Whiteley and Farrow (See Case 57).

On February 27, the Senate voted compensation to Henry P. Farrow and Richard H. Whiteley for the eleven months they waited for a decision in the case.

Both Joshua Hill and Homer Miller returned to Georgia on the completion of their terms, Hill in 1873 and Miller in 1871. Hill participated in Georgia's constitutional convention of 1877, after which he returned to private life. He died in 1891, and Miller died in 1896.

Sources

U.S. Congress. Senate. *Congressional Globe.* 40th Cong., 3d sess. (See pp. 1–5.)

———. *Congressional Globe.* 41st Cong., 1st sess. (See p. 102.) 3d sess. (See pp. 816–30, 848–51, 871–74.)

———. Senate Report No. 192. 40th Cong., 3d sess., 1869.

———. Senate Report No. 58. 41st Cong., 2d sess., 1870.

———. Senate Report No. 308. 41st Cong., 3d sess., 1871.

Malone, Dumas, ed. *Dictionary of American Biography.* Vol. 9. New York, 1946; reprint of 1935 edition. (See pp. 42–43.)

Seip, Terry L. *The South Returns to Congress: Men, Economic Measures, and Intersectional Relationships, 1868–1879.* Baton Rouge, LA, 1983.

Case 53

Adelbert Ames

(1835–1933)

Mississippi

Election Case
February 25, 1870 to April 1, 1870

Issues
Reconstruction: qualifications: residency

Result: Seated

Chronology:
Credentials presented: Feb. 15, 1870
Referred to committee: Feb. 25, 1870
Committee report: Mar. 18, 1870
Senate vote: April 1, 1870

Background

In 1867 Congress passed the first of the Reconstruction acts returning the former Confederate states, including Mississippi, to military rule. President Ulysses S. Grant in 1869 selected Adelbert Ames as provisional governor and military commander of the district. A Maine native and West Point graduate, who had been awarded the Congressional Medal of Honor for his valor during the Civil War, Ames proved an articulate and dedicated spokesman for the policies of radical Republicanism, as befitted the future son-in-law of Radical Republican Representative Benjamin F. Butler. Concerned about the violence against African Americans that he saw in Mississippi and elsewhere in the South, Ames joined the Republican party and championed the rights of Mississippi blacks.

Despite bitter infighting that split the state's Republican party into two factions, Mississippi succeeded in establishing a state constitution in January 1870, and, on February 23 of that year, the state was readmitted to representation in Congress. When the Republicans who dominated the legislature elected the thirty-four-year-old Ames to the United States Senate, he resigned from the army to take the post. As his colleague, the legislature chose Hiram Revels, the first black to serve in the Senate (See Case 54).

Statement of the Case

When the credentials of Adelbert Ames were presented to the Senate on February 25, 1870, Democrats questioned his qualifications, and the matter was referred to the Committee on the Judiciary. His opponents charged that, at the time of his election, Ames held two military posts: he was commander of the military district of the Mississippi as well as the provisional governor of the same jurisdiction. Some senators therefore questioned whether Ames, who as provisional governor had signed both his own credentials and those of Revels, was in fact a legal resident of Mississippi.

Response of the Senate

On March 18, Roscoe Conkling (R-NY) submitted the report of the Judiciary Committee, with a resolution unfavorable to Ames. The report included Ames' statement to the committee, explaining that, when he decided to leave army life, he made a public declaration of his intentions, began negotiations to purchase property in the state, and resigned his military office before the readmission of Mississippi to the Union. The committee, however, did not consider these actions sufficient and recommended that Ames not be seated, because it believed the Constitution required a senator-elect to be an inhabitant of the state at the time of election and not merely upon the convening of the Senate. The committee maintained that Ames did not resign his military commission and announce his intention to remain permanently in Mississippi until after his election.

Conkling spoke at length in support of the committee's interpretation of the constitutional wording. He began his remarks by praising the personal worth, military courage, and obvious integrity of the senator-elect. He hoped to see Ames in the Senate but not on the basis of the election that had been held in January. Conkling was sure that, once the Senate rejected these credentials, the Mississippi legislature would promptly reelect Ames, who was now clearly eligible for the seat, and he could then be seated. Based purely on the technical facts of the case, the committee believed that Ames did not meet the legal requirement for residency at the time of the election. In support of this assertion, Conkling explained that one could not become a resident of a state by "mere locality of existence" but must move there voluntarily and demonstrate a firm intention to remain there. Because Ames had gone to Mississippi in compliance with military orders and would have to leave if ordered elsewhere, he could not be said to have moved there voluntarily or to be in a position to plan to remain there permanently. The Judiciary Committee therefore ruled that he could not legally claim to have been an inhabitant of Mississippi at the time of his election.

Senate Republicans, however, were not united on the issue, for most believed that Ames should be seated. Committee member Benjamin F. Rice (R-AR) disagreed with the committee's recommendation. He contended that the intention to remain in Mississippi was enough to make Ames an inhabitant, an intention Ames had formed at the time he was elected. An extensive debate ensued, continuing on March 23 and 31 and April 1, with supporters and opponents of Ames citing various legal authorities to support their positions that Ames should or should not be considered an inhabitant of Mississippi in the constitutional meaning of the term.

A more severe view was expressed by several Democratic senators, who questioned the validity of the election itself. Garrett Davis (KY) charged that, since Ames as military governor had overseen the election of the legislators who later elected him senator, "that Legislature, the men who composed it, . . . were . . . the creatures of General Ames." "Will the Senate," he asked, "enact the solemn farce . . . of admitting here a man thus appointed by his own military chieftain, and sent here by a Legislature selected by himself, and whose action in the election of Senator was controlled by himself?"

When word of the Senate's wrangling reached Mississippi, the legislature adopted a resolution—which arrived in Washington on March 31—assuring the Senate that the election of Ames had been legal and urging that he be seated immediately.

Perhaps convinced by this message, the Senate finally acted on April 1. It first voted 40 to 12 to amend the Judiciary Committee's resolution, striking the word "not," and then voted to seat Ames. He immediately came forward and took the oaths of office.

Conclusion

Differences among Republicans over Reconstruction continued to plague the party at both the state and national levels. In the Senate, five Republicans, including Conkling and Judiciary Committee Chairman Trumbull, cast their votes against Ames, thus reflecting the widening breach among party members over Reconstruction policies.

Adelbert Ames served until 1874, when he resigned from the Senate and returned to Mississippi to become governor. There his efforts to guarantee civil rights for all citizens met with tragic defeat. In 1875, a rejuvenated Democratic party in the state used terror and violence to recapture the legislature. Threatened with impeachment by the hostile legislators, Ames resigned, left the state, and retired from politics. Returning to New York and Massachusetts, he accumulated great personal wealth yet seemed always haunted by his experiences in Mississippi. Ames lived until 1933.

Sources

U.S. Congress. Senate. *Congressional Globe.* 41st Cong., 2d sess. (See pp. 2087–88, 2122–23, 2125–35, 2156–69, 2303–16, 2335–49.)

———. Senate Report, No. 75. 41st Cong., 2d sess., 1870.

Ames, B. A. *Adelbert Ames, 1835–1933: General, Senator, Governor.* New York, 1964.

Current, Richard N. *Three Carpetbag Governors.* Baton Rouge, LA, 1967.

Harris, William C., ed. *The Facts of Reconstruction: John R. Lynch.* Indianapolis, 1970.

McFeely, William S. *Grant: A Biography.* New York, 1982. (See pp. 359–60, 419–25.)

Roller, David, and Robert Twyman, eds. *The Encyclopedia of Southern History.* Baton Rouge, LA, 1979. (See p. 42.)

Case 54

Hiram R. Revels

(1827–1901)

Mississippi

Election Case
February 23, 1870 to February 25, 1870

Chronology:
Credentials presented: Feb. 23, 1870
Senate vote: Feb. 25, 1870

Issues
Reconstruction: qualifications: citizenship

Result: Seated

Background

When the credentials of Hiram Revels (R) of Mississippi were presented to the Senate on February 23, 1870, the occasion marked the first time that a black American entered the chamber to serve as a United States senator.

In earlier years, Revels, an ordained minister in the A.M.E. Church, distinguished himself with his educational work among slaves. Born into a free black family in North Carolina, Revels traveled widely as a teacher and chaplain in a variety of states. At the close of the Civil War, Revels moved to Mississippi, where he became active in Republican politics in 1868, serving in local government and then in the state legislature. In preparation for the state's readmission to the Union, which occurred on February 23, 1870, the Mississippi legislature elected Revels to a brief unexpired term ending on March 3, 1871. For the other Senate seat, the legislature chose Adelbert Ames (R), who had been serving as the state's military governor. His credentials, too, were challenged (See Case 53).

Statement of the Case

Revels' arrival in the Senate precipitated intense responses from two political camps. Radical Republicans, led by Henry Wilson and Charles Sumner of Massachusetts, warmly welcomed Revels. A second group, led by Democratic Senators Willard Saulsbury of Delaware, Garrett Davis of Kentucky, and John Stockton of New Jersey, launched a bitter attack upon Revels' credentials.

Response of the Senate

At the outset, the debate was cloaked in technical arguments. The challengers charged that Adelbert Ames, the provisional governor of Mississippi who had signed Revels' credentials, could not legitimately certify an election. This claim was quickly answered by senators pointing out that such provisional governors had signed election certificates for senators from a number of the recently reconstructed states. Opponents also contended that, since the Supreme Court's 1857 Dred Scott decision ruled that those of African blood were not U.S. citizens, Revels had only become a citizen upon ratification of the Fourteenth Amendment in 1868; thus he had not held citizenship for the nine years required for a Senate seat. Revels' supporters countered that both the Civil Rights Act of 1866 and the Fourteenth Amendment stated that "all persons born . . . in the United States . . . are citizens." In addition, Henry Wilson pointed out that "as a citizen of Ohio, more than twenty years ago, [Revels] was a voter and voted in that state."

The nature of the discussion quickly shifted from these technicalities to the subject of Revels' race. Senators exchanged stinging rounds of racial insults and inflammatory rhetoric, stretching over two days of debate. Although badly outnumbered in the Senate, the small band of Democrats argued fiercely against seating the Mississippi senator. Finally, on February 25, 1870, the Senate voted not to refer the matter to the Judiciary Committee and, by a second party-line vote of 48 to 8, accepted the credentials of Hiram Revels. He then came forward to take the oaths of office and took his seat as the first black member of the United States Senate.

Conclusion

Hiram Revels made his initial Senate speech less than a month later, on March 16, 1870, in opposition to a bill readmitting Georgia without sufficient protection for the rights of black citizens. The galleries overflowed with black people who came to hear the historic, first oration of the Mississippi senator. For the rest of his term, Revels was a quiet worker on the committees on Education and Labor and the District of Columbia, supporting such issues as integration of the D.C. public schools. When his term expired in March 1871, Revels returned to Mississippi to become president of Alcorn University. He died in 1901.

Sources

U.S. Congress. Senate. *Congressional Globe.* 41st Cong., 2d sess. (See pp. 1503–14, 1542–44, 1557–68, Appendix, pp. 125–30.)

Libby, Billy W. "Senator Hiram Revels of Mississippi Takes His Seat, January–February 1870." *The Journal of Mississippi History* 37 (November 1975).

Roller, David, and Robert W. Twyman, eds. *The Encyclopedia of Southern History.* Baton Rouge, LA, 1979. (See p. 1052.)

Singer, Donald L. "For Whites Only: The Seating of Hiram Revels in The United States Senate." *Negro History Bulletin* 35 (March 1972).

Thompson, Julius Eric. *Hiram R. Revels: 1828–1901, A Biography.* New York, 1982.

Case 55

Ossian B. Hart v. Abijah Gilbert

(1821–1874) (1806–1881)

Florida

Election Case
April 1, 1870 to April 28, 1870

Issues
Reconstruction: challenge to legislature's authority to elect; right of a challenger in contested election to address the Senate

Result: Gilbert retained seat

Chronology:
Credentials presented: April 1, 1870
Referred to committee: April 1, 1870
Committee report: April 13, 1870
Senate vote: April 28, 1870

Background

Successful maneuvers in 1868 to seat Florida's first two post-Civil War senators did not end the controversy over that state's representation in Congress. Shortly after selecting Adonijah Welch and Thomas Osborn (See Case 51), the Florida legislature picked Abijah Gilbert (R) for the full term beginning in March 1869. He would succeed Welch, whose term was to expire seven months after he arrived in Washington. Gilbert was a New York businessman and committed abolitionist, who moved to Florida after the Civil War because of poor health. There, he participated actively in Reconstruction efforts. The Senate therefore seated him without incident in March 1869.

All three Florida Senate elections took place after the passage of the Reconstruction acts of 1867 but before adoption of the June 1868 act declaring Florida entitled to representation in Congress. Political opponents took advantage of this latter fact to challenge the validity of Gilbert's election. In January 1870, the legislature, splintered by political factionalism, decided to vote again for the term that had begun in March 1869. This time, it bypassed the main contenders and elected Florida supreme court justice Ossian B. Hart (R), a native Floridian who, although a former slaveholder, was a staunch advocate of black suffrage. An opponent of secession, Hart had suffered persecution for his views.

Statement of the Case

On April 1, 1870, Florida Senator Thomas Osborn presented the credentials of Ossian B. Hart for the seat already held by Abijah Gilbert. In his remarks, Osborn indicated that, while he believed Gilbert had been elected legally to the Senate, some Florida officials expressed doubts about that 1868 election. Hart and his supporters based their protest upon alleged irregularities in the observance of the 1866 law regulating senatorial elections. The Senate referred the challenge to the Judiciary Committee.

Response of the Senate

On April 13, 1870, the Judiciary Committee returned a report favorable to Abijah Gilbert. The committee ruled that, when Congress recognized the Florida state government, it validated any actions that government had taken since the time of its organization. In electing Gilbert, the committee determined, the legislature had acted in conformity with the procedures established by Congress in the 1866 act "regulating the times and manner of holding elections for Senators in Congress."

This report failed to resolve the matter. On April 15, Judiciary Committee Chairman Lyman Trumbull (R-IL), presented a petition from Ossian Hart, contending that the Judiciary Committee's report did not correctly present the facts and requesting an opportunity to appear before the Senate to plead his case. Although he submitted the petition as a favor to Hart, Trumbull declined to participate further in the matter because he disapproved of the precedent set in an 1851 election challenge from Florida, when the claimant, David Yulee, was granted two hours to address the Senate (See Case 24).

The question of a claimant's right to speak on the Senate floor generated a brief debate about the difference between the Senate and the House of Representatives, which permitted claimants to address the members. Because representatives were chosen by popular vote, cases there were often more complicated and the contestants needed a chance to explain. In the case of Senate elections, the necessary information was usually incorporated in the documentation of the state legislature's action. At the conclusion of the discussion, the Senate took no further action until April 28, 1870. On that day, Trumbull again read the report of the Judiciary Committee. Deciding that the Florida problems were caused by ambiguities in the law and by the confusion of Reconstruction, the Senate permitted Abijah Gilbert to retain his seat. Ossian Hart received mileage and the pay of a senator for one month.

Conclusion

Abijah Gilbert served until the end of his term in 1875. He then returned to his birthplace in New York, where he died in 1881.

Ossian Hart retained his seat on the Florida supreme bench. In 1872 Hart, who managed to establish good relations with both black Republicans and white conservatives in Florida, was elected governor. Having injured his health during the campaign, however, he died in 1874.

Sources

U.S. Congress. Senate. *Congressional Globe.* 41st Cong., 2d sess. (See pp. 2330–31, 2705–06, 3053–54.)

———. Senate Report No. 101. 41st Cong., 2d sess., 1870.

———. Senate Miscellaneous Document No. 102. 41st Cong., 2d sess., 1870.

Shofner, Jerrell H. *Nor Is It Over Yet: Florida in the Era of Reconstruction: 1863–1877.* Gainesville, FL, 1974.

Case 56

George Goldthwaite

(1809–1879)

Alabama

Election Case
February 6, 1871 to January 9, 1872

Issues
Reconstruction: challenge to legislature's authority to elect

Result: Seated

Chronology:
Credentials presented: Feb. 6, 1871
Referred to committee: Mar. 13, 1871
Committee report: Mar. 20, 1871
Senate vote: Jan. 9, 1872

Background

The rancor and mistrust that divided Congress during the Reconstruction period gathered force as the years passed, and many senators greeted with suspicion and hostility those arriving with credentials from former Confederate states.

Boston-born George Goldthwaite moved to Alabama as a young man and built a career there as a lawyer. During the Civil War, he served as the state's adjutant-general. In 1870 the legislature elected him as a Democrat to the United States Senate.

Statement of the Case

George Goldthwaite's credentials were presented on February 6, 1871, for the term to begin March 4. Before he could be seated, however, members of the Alabama legislature submitted a protest charging that the legislators voting for Goldthwaite included some who had been fraudulently elected, one who had no certificate of election, and several who were still under political disabilities. On March 13, 1871, the Senate sent the credentials, with the petition of protest, to the newly established Committee on Privileges and Elections, which also received contests from Georgia, Texas, and North Carolina that same day (Cases 57, 58, 59).

Response of the Senate

Convinced that the circumstances surrounding the contested election in Alabama were identical to the case of Georgia's Foster Blodgett (See Case 57), and acutely conscious of the workload of cases it faced, the committee on March 20 reported jointly on the two cases. Explaining that there was not sufficient time remaining in the brief congressional session that would end on April 20 to conduct a proper investigation into the charges, the committee recommended that both Goldthwaite and Blodgett be permitted to take their seats while the investigation continued, since they presented proper credentials and were not under any disability for prewar and wartime activities.

This proposal prompted a lengthy and convoluted debate, as senators spoke about both the Goldthwaite and the Blodgett elections. Committee member Allen Thurman (D-OH), who wanted the cases considered separately, argued for seating Goldthwaite. He complained that the state legislators appeared to have extended their challenge beyond the election of George Goldthwaite to contest the election of every member of the Alabama legislature. The questions they raised regarding procedural legalities, election conduct, and qualifying certificates threatened to embrace the entire voting population of Alabama and delay a decision in the case for the next six years. Thurman stressed the longstanding precedent that "where a member of this body is elected by a Legislature competent to elect him" and presents proper credentials, the Senate would accept this as prima facie evidence of his right to a seat, seating the claimant so that the state would not be deprived of representation. The investigation could then be pursued afterwards. Thurman believed that the Democrat, Goldthwaite, was clearly elected by the appropriate body and thus should be allowed to take his seat. At the same time, he argued that Georgia's Blodgett, a Republican, had not been elected by a legislature with the power to elect for that term and thus should not be admitted.

Republican senators, however, expressed concern about the political conditions in Alabama portrayed in the legislators' protest. John Sherman (R-OH) cited the allegation that "by organized force and violence, extending over large regions of the State of Alabama, the local authority was subverted, and that no elections were held in certain counties." On April 11 the Senate tabled the matter until the next session.

When Congress reconvened in December 1871, the arrival of a properly elected senator from Georgia paved the way for the Senate to refuse to seat Foster Blodgett. With that case eliminated, the Senate was able to move ahead on the credentials of George Goldthwaite. On January 9, 1872, the Senate agreed to accept Goldthwaite's credentials while the committee continued its investigation, and he took his seat on January 15, 1872. The committee made no subsequent report on the matter, and the Senate took no further action.

Conclusion

The attempt to consolidate challenged elections from different states proved a failure in the cases of George Goldthwaite and Foster Blodgett. With the Senate already confused and divided, combining the cases only complicated the floor debates. Not until it disposed of the Blodgett credentials by seating a different claimant, could the Senate resolve the Alabama case. George Goldthwaite served in the Senate until 1877 and died two years later.

Sources

U.S. Congress. Senate. *Congressional Globe.* 42d Cong., 1st sess. (See pp. 1–4, 218–19, 271–74, 494–98, 504–58.) 2d sess. (See pp. 261–62, 319–20.)

———. Senate Report No. 3. 42d Cong., 1st sess., 1871.

Johnson, Allen, and Dumas Malone, eds. *Dictionary of American Biography.* Vol. 7. New York, 1946; reprint of 1935 edition. (See pp. 368–69.)

Case 57

Thomas M. Norwood v. Foster Blodgett, Jr.

(1830–1913) (1826–1877)

Georgia

Election Case
March 2, 1871 to December 19, 1871

Issues
Reconstruction: challenge to legislature's authority to elect; qualifications: corruption

Result: Norwood Seated

Chronology:
Petition received: Mar. 2, 1871
Referred to committee: Mar. 13, 1871
Committee report: Mar. 20, 1871
Credentials presented (Norwood): Dec. 4, 1871
Referred to committee: Dec. 11, 1871
Committee report: Dec. 18, 1871
Senate vote: Dec. 19, 1871

Background

As governance of the South under Reconstruction became mired in factionalism and political and economic corruption, emotional charges and countercharges often overwhelmed the legal issues. The Senate, splintered by disagreements about Reconstruction policies, found the disputes surrounding senatorial elections both tedious and frustrating. In one effort to expedite matters, a Senate committee in 1871 decided to link debate about two election cases, one from Georgia and one from Alabama. Rather than ensuring a speedy resolution, however, this approach simply confused the proceedings.

Statement of the Case

On January 20, 1871, the credentials of Georgian Foster Blodgett, Jr. (R) were presented for a term to begin March 4, 1871. In late February, Homer V.M. Miller (D), who had defeated Blodgett in the 1868 election, was seated, after two years of delay, for the few days remaining in the term that ended on March 3. Thus, the discussions in the Blodgett case followed soon after those in the long-running Georgia case of Miller and Joshua Hill (R), who finally took his oath for the other Georgia seat on February 1 (See Case 52).

In response to a March 2 petition from members of the Georgia legislature, protesting Blodgett's claim, he was not sworn in, and his credentials were ordered to lie on the table. The petition cited three formal grievances against Blodgett: that he was chosen by a legislature not competent to elect, that he was elected at a time not in accord with the legal elections schedule, and that there was no quorum present in the state house of representatives at the time of the voting. On March 13, shortly after the new Congress convened, the Senate sent the credentials and the protest to the Committee on Privileges and Elections, which had been established three days earlier to relieve the Judiciary Committee of the growing burden of reviewing such contests, four of which were referred to committee on this same day (See Cases 56, 58, 59).

Response of the Senate

One week later, on March 20, the committee, concerned about the volume of cases and pleading lack of time to conduct a full investigation, issued a report recommending that both Foster Blodgett and George Goldthwaite of Alabama (See Case 56) be seated while the investigations continued, since their credentials were in proper form. Combining the two cases, however, only complicated the debate, when committee members Joshua Hill, the other Georgia senator, and Allen Thurman (D-OH) urged separate consideration of the two claims, because they supported seating Goldthwaite but not Blodgett. Thurman argued that Blodgett had not been elected by the legislature closest to the time of the vacancy.

Hill spoke at length in opposition to seating Blodgett. He charged that the legislature elected in 1868 had deliberately usurped authority that should belong to the one elected in December 1870 by postponing the convening of the new legislature from January until November 1871. The delay was designed to prevent election of a U.S. senator for the term beginning in March 1871, thus allowing Blodgett, the candidate chosen by the old legislature, to be seated. Hill considered this an outrageous power grab against the incoming legislature, which he noted had been chosen in a peaceful election. Blodgett had been elected by the same 1868 legislature, as reorganized in January 1870, that had also sent Richard Whiteley and Henry Farrow to the Senate as unsuccessful claimants for the seats of Miller and Hill in the earlier Georgia case (Case 52).

Joshua Hill then submitted a series of documents from Georgia challenging Blodgett's fitness to serve in the Senate. It was charged that, when the 1868 legislature reorganized as required by the December 1869 federal law, Blodgett had manipulated the process to block the seating of those unlikely to vote for him as U.S. senator and to replace them with others favorable to him. The documents also attacked the Georgia Republican's record during and after the Civil War. They claimed that Blodgett, the mayor of Augusta in the early 1860s, had served voluntarily as a captain in the Confederate army, then, in 1865, he had secured the office of postmaster by swearing the required postwar test oath that he had never borne arms against the United States. When Blodgett was indicted for perjury, he denied having taken the oath, and his lawyers managed to have the indictment quashed for lack of evidence by postponing the trial until after the death of the official who had administered the oath. Blodgett explained that he had actually been able to obtain the post without swearing, because federal authorities, confused by the name similarity, had administered the oath to his son, E.F. Blodgett. Blodgett's detractors further insisted that $940,000 of state funds had disappeared during his administration of a state-owned railroad and that he had bribed legislators to vote for him in the Senate election.

Calling the charges "the most extraordinary attack I have ever heard made on any individual in this body before," William Stewart (R-NV) countered that they were simply political fabrications, invented by Blodgett's enemies because he had boldly supported the unpopular Republican Reconstruction policies throughout Georgia. Many senators were clearly uncomfortable with having such defamatory remarks aired on the Senate floor and quickly reverted to discussing the legality of the election. On April 20, the short, first session of the Forty-second Congress ended, and the Blodgett affair was tabled until the next session.

When Congress reconvened on December 4, 1871, the controversy intensified with the presentation of credentials for Thomas M. Norwood (D). The Georgia legislature that was elected in 1870 had finally convened in November 1871 and had elected him to the same Senate term claimed by Blodgett. A Georgia native, Norwood was a lawyer and state legislator. On December 11, the Senate referred the new credentials to the Committee on Privileges and Elections, which returned its report a week later. Avoiding the allegations lodged against Blodgett personally, the committee focused on the clearcut issue of the legality of the election. The election law passed by Congress in 1866 stated that a U.S. senator should be elected by the state legislature that was "chosen next preceding the expiration" of the previous senator's term. Foster Blodgett was elected on February 15, 1870, by a legislature that had been elected in April 1868. A new legislature was elected in December 1870, prior to the March 1871 expiration of the previous Senate term, making it the legislature with the legal right to choose the new senator. This legislature had elected Thomas Norwood, and the committee therefore recommended that Norwood be seated. The Senate agreed, and Thomas Norwood took the oaths of office on December 19, 1871.

Conclusion

Because the Senate had been reluctant to reject Blodgett and leave the state with a vacant seat, it had become enmeshed in endless legal arguments about the validity of the legislature that elected him. The arrival of a new claimant clearly chosen in conformity with the letter of the 1866 election law provided a noncontroversial escape from the dilemma. It also relieved the Senate of the need to consider the charges against Blodgett's character.

On January 9, 1872, the Senate agreed to pay Foster Blodgett the per diem and mileage of a senator for the nine months he waited for a decision. Blodgett, who had managed a political metamorphosis from Confederate officer to Radical Republican, became an outcast when the Democrats returned to power in Georgia. In 1876 he was arrested for embezzlement tied to his administration of the state railroad. He died in 1877.

Thomas Norwood served in the Senate until 1877, and in 1885 he was elected to the House of Representatives. An advocate of rebuilding the economy of the South through industrial growth, Norwood led the movement for the construction of the Southern Pacific Railroad. He died in 1913.

Sources

U.S. Congress. Senate. *Congressional Globe.* 42d Cong., 1st sess. (See pp. 4–5, 218–19, 271–74, 494–98, 506–7, 540–58.)

———. Senate Report No.3. 42d Cong., 1st sess., 1871.

———. Senate Miscellaneous Documents No. 24 and 30. 42d Cong., 1st sess., 1871.

———. Senate Report No. 10, 42d Cong., 2d sess., 1871.

Chapman, Kenneth, and Charles S. Gurr. *Dictionary of Georgia Biography.* Athens, GA, 1983. (See pp. 91–93.)

Case 58

Joseph J. Reynolds v. Morgan C. Hamilton

(1822–1899) (1809–1893)

Texas

Election Case
March 3, 1871 to March 18, 1871

Issues
Reconstruction: challenge to legislature's authority to elect

Result: Hamilton seated

Chronology:
Credentials presented: Mar. 3, 1871
Referred to committee: Mar. 13, 1871
Committee report: Mar. 18, 1871
Senate vote: Mar. 18, 1871

Background

In November 1869, Texas ratified a new state constitution that permitted blacks to vote, and on March 30, 1870, Congress readmitted the state to representation for the first time since 1861. The next day, credentials were presented for Morgan C. Hamilton (R), elected to fill the vacancy in the term ending on March 3, 1871. Hamilton, whose brother Andrew Jackson Hamilton had served as provisional governor until the election of 1870, was sworn in without incident for the brief term. His Texas colleague, James W. Flanagan (R), was also seated. On the same day it conducted the two Senate elections, the legislature also elected Hamilton to the full Senate term beginning March 4, 1871.

Statement of the Case

When Morgan Hamilton's credentials for the new term were presented on July 13, 1870, the Senate tabled them until the beginning of the next Congress. On March 3, 1871, the day before Hamilton's new term began, the credentials of Joseph J. Reynolds were presented for the same seat. The legislature had elected him at its second session in January 1871. Reynolds, who as military commander of Texas had manipulated the 1870 gubernatorial election to ensure the defeat of A. J. Hamilton by the Radical Republican candidate, claimed that the legislature elected Morgan Hamilton before the passage of the act declaring Texas entitled to representation, thus making the selection illegal. On March 13, the Senate sent both sets of credentials to the Committee on Privileges and Elections, along with contests from Georgia, Alabama, and North Carolina (Cases 56, 57, 59).

Response of the Senate

Unlike some other contested Reconstruction elections, the Texas dispute came to a speedy conclusion. On March 18, the Committee on Privileges and

Elections returned a report favorable to Hamilton. The committee dismissed Reynolds' argument that his later election by the state assembly superseded Hamilton's, basing its conclusion upon the precedent set in the similar case of Florida Senator Abijah Gilbert (See Case 55). In that instance, the Senate had determined that the act admitting the state to representation ratified the actions previously taken by the legislature it approved.

A relieved Senate quickly accepted the Florida precedent and adopted the committee's recommendation by voice vote without debate. Hamilton took the prescribed oaths and was seated on March 20, 1871.

Conclusion

Morgan C. Hamilton served only one term in the Senate. After traveling extensively, he settled in Brooklyn, New York. He died in 1893.

Sources

U.S. Congress. Senate. Senate Report No. 2. 42d Cong., 1st sess., 1871.

Malone, Dumas, ed. *Dictionary of American Biography.* Vol. 15. New York, 1946: reprint of 1935 edition. (See pp. 521–22.)

Roller, David C., and Robert W. Twyman, eds. *The Enclopedia of Southern History.* Baton Rouge, LA, 1979. (See p. 1217.)

Joseph C. Abbott
(1825–1881)

v.

Zebulon B. Vance and Matt W. Ransom
(1830–1894) (1826–1904)

North Carolina

Election Case
March 7, 1871 to April 24, 1872

Issues
Reconstruction: qualifications: disability under 14th Amendment; challenge to legislature's authority to elect; Senate refused to seat losing candidate if winner disqualified

Chronology:
Abbott v. Vance
Memorial presented: Mar. 7, 1871
Referred to committee: Mar. 13, 1871
Committee report: Feb. 28, 1872
Senate vote: April 23, 1872
Result: Not seated

Ransom
Credentials presented: Feb. 5, 1872
Referred to committee: Feb. 5, 1872
Committee report: April 24, 1872
Senate vote: April 24, 1872
Result: Seated

Background

As the Reconstruction era waned and the dominance of the Radicals declined, Senate Republicans began increasingly to splinter over the treatment of senators elected from the former Confederate states. This factionalism became particularly apparent during Senate consideration of a contested North Carolina election.

New Hampshire native Joseph C. Abbott, a former brigadier general in the Union army and steadfast Republican, settled in North Carolina after the war. When the state first returned to Congress in 1868, he was elected to the United States Senate. A hard-working advocate for North Carolina, particularly for the Wilmington harbor area, Abbott nonetheless had political strength only among the state's black voters. By 1870, white supremacy groups had so far suppressed black suffrage that the state legislature easily chose Zebulon B. Vance (D), who had been the state's governor during the Civil War, over Abbott for the Senate term beginning in March 1871.

Statement of the Case

Abbott immediately challenged the results of the election, pointing out that Vance was still hampered by political disabilities imposed under the

Fourteenth Amendment to the Constitution because of his support for the Confederacy. Abbott maintained that, if the electors knew that the winning candidate was disqualified from serving in the Senate, then those votes should be voided and the election granted to the person with the next highest count.

No credentials were presented for Vance, a North Carolinian who had served in the U.S. House of Representatives from 1858 to 1861 and then fought for the Confederacy before being elected governor of the state in 1862. Vance had received a pardon in 1867 under President Andrew Johnson's amnesty program, but the Fourteenth Amendment adopted in 1868 prohibited service in Congress by anyone who had been a member of Congress and then engaged in rebellion against the United States. Vance had not been relieved of this disability at the time of his election.

On March 13, 1871, the Senate referred Abbott's complaint to the Committee on Privileges and Elections, together with contests from three other states (Cases 56, 57, 58).

Response of the Senate

Nearly a year later, on February 28, 1872, a divided committee returned a report recommending that Abbott was not entitled to a seat in the Senate since he had received only a small minority of the votes cast in the state legislature. In the meantime, apparently convinced that Congress would not remove his political disability, Vance had submitted his resignation from the Senate on January 20, 1872.

Abbott and his supporters had drawn upon examples in English law applicable to contested elections, in which the votes for an ineligible candidate were not counted and the candidate with the next highest number of votes was declared elected. The committee pointed out, however, that the practice in the United States was to declare such an election void, rather than to grant the seat to a competitor. In addition, the Fourteenth Amendment gave Congress the power to remove the disabilities from an individual elected to office and thus permit him to take his seat.

As precedents, the majority report cited such previous Senate qualifications cases as those of Albert Gallatin (Case 1) and James Shields (Case 32) to show that, when the Senate ruled the claimants ineligible, it called for a new election rather than giving the election to the defeated candidate. Committee member John A. Logan (R-IL) noted that, even in the case of David Yulee (Case 24) where Yulee received half the votes of the Florida legislature and the other half were blank, the Senate refused to seat Yulee and called for a new election. Yulee had claimed victory because he had a majority of the nonblank votes, but under a rule of the Florida legislature a majority of all the votes was required to elect. Logan also pointed out that, even if the North Carolina legislators voting for Vance knew he was disqualified, they also knew that Congress had removed the disabilities from the state's governor and several other officials after they were elected, and they could therefore reasonably assume it would do the same for Vance. Even John Pool (R), the other North Carolina senator, was under the impression that Congress would remove Vance's disabilities.

According to Logan, under the 1866 election law, a candidate must receive a majority of all the votes cast in each house of the legislature, even if some votes were for an ineligible person. Abbott, he declared, had received less than one-third of the votes in the North Carolina house and less than one-fourth of the votes in the senate, and thus clearly had not been elected by the North Carolina legislature.

Abbott supporters Matthew R. Carpenter (R-WI) and Benjamin F. Rice (R-AR) submitted a minority report, asserting that under federal election law a candidate needed only to receive a majority of the votes cast in each house of the legislature rather than the votes of a majority of the legislators present. Thus, if the votes for Vance were disqualified, Abbott, having received a majority of the remaining votes cast in each house, should be considered elected, even without receiving the votes of a majority of the full legislature as required by the 1866 election law. The minority report dismissed as irrelevant the previous qualification cases cited by the majority, because in the Gallatin and Shields cases the legislators voted for the candidates in the belief that they were eligible. The legislators voting for Vance, however, knew that he was ineligible and thus were deliberately throwing away their votes. The minority report therefore recommended that Abbott be seated.

The debate continued for several days in April, as complex discussions about the meaning of majority and minority candidates, equal suffrage, blank votes, and voided votes frayed senatorial tempers and further divided the Republicans. Underlying the legal arguments was the strong suspicion by some Republican senators, as George F. Edmunds of Vermont complained, that "the Legislature of North Carolina intended to pronounce an insult upon the people of the United States who did not agree with them in politics by electing the particular person the majority voted for." In fact, Matthew Carpenter cited affidavits stating that North Carolina legislators had heard Democratic and Conservative members declare, "We vote for Vance because his disabilities have not been removed; we have eaten dirt long enough." North Carolina Republican John Pool reinforced this view, reporting that "members were allowed seats in the [legislature] who were notoriously and confessedly under the disability imposed by the fourteenth amendment." Many citizens of the state, he believed, would be delighted to have Abbott seated as a rebuke to the legislature, and a number of Senate Republicans agreed.

On April 23, 1872, the Senate finally accepted the committee report, agreeing that, as Joseph Abbott did not have a majority of the votes cast in the North Carolina assembly, he could not claim the seat. The Senate did, however, vote him compensation and mileage for the year he had waited for a decision.

Conclusion

In denying the seat to Abbott, the Senate accepted the premise that, if it chose, it could have removed the disabilities of Zebulon Vance after his election, a procedure that had been followed for officials elected by several other southern states.

On February 5, 1872, while the Senate was still wrestling with the dilemma of turning out the well-liked and effective Abbott, Matt W. Ransom (D) had appeared with credentials for the disputed seat, having been elected to replace Vance. Unlike Vance, Ransom, a former brigadier general in the Confederate army, had not served in Congress before the war and thus was not hampered by the same disability. The Senate referred his credentials to the Committee on Privileges and Elections. On April 24, 1872, the committee reported that Ransom's credentials were in order. He was immediately seated and granted his pay from the beginning of the term in March 1871.

All three of the North Carolina politicians in this case continued to serve in public life. Joseph Abbott, who earlier demonstrated his concern for the harbor at Wilmington, accepted an appointment as inspector of ports under President Rutherford B. Hayes. Abbott died in 1882. Zebulon Vance eventually came to the Senate in 1879 and served until his death in 1894. Matt Ransom remained in the Senate until 1895 and died in 1904.

Sources

U.S. Congress. Senate. *Congressional Globe.* 42d Cong., 2d sess. (See pp. 2387–90, 2431–34, 2639, 2676, Appendix, pp. 219–29, 234–57, 272–79, 328–34.)

———. Senate Report No. 58. 42d Cong., 2d sess., 1872.

Blaine, James G. *Twenty Years of Congress.* Vol. 2. Norwich, CT, 1886.

Johnson, Allen, ed. *Dictionary of American Biography*. New York, 1946; reprint of 1935 edition. Vol. 1. (See pp. 23–24.)

Malone, Dumas, ed. *Dictionary of American Biography.* New York, 1946; reprint of 1935 edition. Vol. 15. (See p. 379.) Vol. 19. (See pp. 158–61.)

Case 60

Powell Clayton

(1833–1914)

Arkansas

Censure Case
January 9, 1872 to March 25, 1873

Issues
Charges of corruption prior to member's Senate term

Result: Not censured

Chronology:
Referred to committee: Jan. 9, 1872
Committee report: Feb. 26, 1872
Senate vote: Mar. 25, 1873

Background

Arkansas had elected Pennsylvania native and former Union officer Powell Clayton as governor under the new constitution a few months before the state reentered the Union in 1868. After first using the militia to restore order in the state, Clayton over the next three years built a record of achievement. His administration funded the state debt, expanded the railroads, and overhauled the public school system, incorporating special provisions for deaf and blind students. He was also, however, a highly partisan and controversial politician. During Clayton's Reconstruction governorship, the Arkansas Republican party splintered into at least three factions: the dominant Radical carpetbaggers of his regime, a dissident faction of reformers, and the native unionists known as Liberal Republicans. When Clayton was elected to the United States Senate in 1871, the bitterness engendered by this local factionalism followed him to Washington.

Statement of the Case

Powell Clayton (R) began his Senate service on March 4, 1871. The following January the Joint Select Committee to Inquire into the Condition of the Late Insurrectionary States notified the Senate that it had heard testimony raising questions about Clayton's behavior and integrity as governor. The committee judged the issue to be beyond the scope of its jurisdiction and turned the matter over to the Senate for disposition.

A former United States district attorney had testified to the joint select committee that, in April 1871 after Clayton became a U. S. senator, a grand jury had indicted him. The charge was that as governor Clayton had issued fraudulent election credentials for the U. S. House of Representatives to John Edwards (LR), whose opponent had allegedly received the most votes. Since Clayton and Edwards supported opposing factions in the Republican-dominated legislature, the district attorney speculated that Governor

Clayton had traded political favors in return for votes from his opponents in the election for U. S. senator.

In response to these allegations, Clayton contended that in eight precincts there had been two separate sets of polls, one set overseen by authorized judges and the other under the unauthorized auspices of the reform faction. The state supreme court, made up of Clayton supporters, had ruled that the legal election had been conducted at the authorized polling places and that the returns from the others were fraudulent. As governor, Clayton had then discarded the returns from the bogus election and certified the candidate who won with the genuine votes. (The opposing candidate, Thomas Boles (R), successfully contested the election, however, and on February 9, 1872, he replaced Edwards in the House.)

Response of the Senate

At Clayton's request, the Senate on January 9, 1872, appointed a special three-member committee to investigate the events in Arkansas. On June 10, after taking testimony for five months, questioning thirty-eight witnesses, and generating five thousand pages of transcript, the committee issued a partial report, asserting that fairness to Clayton demanded that a response be given before the session closed. The committee indicated that the testimony received appeared not to sustain the charges against Clayton but that the committee members would need to review the testimony more thoroughly and issue a final report in the next session. According to the committee report, the charges came from Clayton's bitter political opponents. The committee noted that the indictment against Clayton had subsequently been dropped for lack of evidence.

After the preliminary report, the committee continued its investigation and, on February 26, 1873, issued a final report declaring that the testimony failed to sustain the charges against Powell Clayton. There was no evidence that Clayton had any fraudulent intent in certifying the election of Edwards as directed by the state supreme court. Another allegation had declared that, when Clayton was first elected to the Senate in January 1871, he had declined to serve because he would have been succeeded as governor by James M. Johnson, the lieutenant governor, who was a political opponent. After failing to oust Johnson from his post, Clayton, it was charged, then arranged for the secretary of state of Arkansas to resign, so that Johnson could be appointed secretary of state, a more lucrative position. Thus, when Clayton was again elected to the Senate in March 1871 and stepped down as governor, he was succeeded by the Republican president pro tempore of the state senate, one of his supporters, rather than by the former lieutenant governor. According to the committee majority, this arrangement to keep the governorship in politically friendly hands was neither criminal nor corrupt. The committee also reported that the evidence reviewed did not establish any conspiracy regarding Clayton's election to the Senate.

Thomas Norwood (D-GA) submitted a lengthy minority report, setting forth in detail the background of the charges against Clayton. Norwood contended the evidence showed that Clayton had, in fact, secured votes from legislators by giving them "lucrative offices" and that he had paid the secretary of state to resign in order to make possible the appointment of Johnson.

The Senate took up the report on March 24, 1873, voting down a Democratic effort to delay consideration until the next session because of the massive volume of evidence. During the special session of the Forty-third Congress, the Senate had already been occupied with a lengthy case of electoral misconduct (Case 61) that had left little time for other matters.

On March 25, Thomas Norwood took the floor to reiterate his concerns, especially about the payment made to the secretary of state after he resigned. George G. Wright (R-IA), the chairman of the special committee, responded that Clayton's supporters held a large majority in the legislature, making bribery or official influence unnecessary to secure his election. He also noted that the secretary of state received nothing from Clayton in return for resigning. The charge had arisen because Clayton had passed along to the former secretary funds raised by others to compensate him for financial losses incurred when he alienated some business associates in the course of his official duties. Convinced by Wright and by Clayton's own testimony, the Senate voted 33 to 6 to accept the committee's resolution that the charges "affecting the official character and conduct" of Powell Clayton were not sustained. Nine senators—most of them Democrats—announced that they would abstain from voting because they had been given insufficient time to review all the testimony.

Conclusion

The crumbling of the Arkansas Republican party enabled the state's Democratic conservatives in 1874 to gain sufficient power to prepare and have ratified a more conservative state constitution. When Democratic representatives elected under the new constitution arrived in Washington, Powell Clayton demanded an investigation in an unsuccessful effort to prevent their seating. Clayton completed his Senate service in 1877 and returned to Arkansas. From 1897 to 1905, he served as U. S. ambassador to Mexico. He died in Washington, D.C., in 1914 and is buried in Arlington National Cemetery.

Sources

U.S. Congress. Senate. *Congressional Globe.* 42d Cong., 2d sess. (See pp. 311–18.)

———. *Congressional Record.* 43d Cong., spec. sess. (See pp. 165–73, 184–92.)

———. Senate Reports No. 15 and 232. 42d Cong., 2d sess., 1872.

———. Senate Report No. 512. 42d Cong., 3d sess., 1873.

Driggs, Orval T., Jr. "The Issues of the Powell Clayton Regime, 1868–1871." *Arkansas Historical Quarterly* 8 (Spring 1949).

Johnson, Allen, ed. *Dictionary of American Biography.* Vol. 3. New York, 1946; reprint of 1935 edition. (See pp. 187–88.)

Roller, David, and Robert Twyman, editions. *The Encyclopedia of Southern History.* Baton Rouge, LA, 1979.

Swinney, Everette. "United States v. Powell Clayton: Use of the Federal Enforcement Acts in Arkansas." *Arkansas Historical Quarterly* 26 (Summer 1967).

Case 61

Samuel C. Pomeroy and Alexander Caldwell

(1816–1891) (1830–1917)

Kansas

Election Case/Expulsion Case
March 5, 1872 to March 24, 1873

Issues
Electoral misconduct:
bribery and corruption

Chronology:
Pomeroy
Resolution submitted: Mar. 5, 1872
Referred to committee: April 8, 1872
Committee report: June 3, 1872
Referred to committee: Feb. 10, 1873
Committee report: Mar. 3, 1873
Result: Not expelled;
Pomeroy's term ended

Caldwell
Referred to committee: May 11, 1872
Committee report: Feb. 17, 1873
Resignation: Mar. 24, 1873
Result: Not expelled;
Caldwell resigned

Background

In Kansas during the 1860s and 1870s, commercial and political interests remained closely entwined, as they had been in the territorial period. The free-wheeling style of Kansas politics affected the United States Senate, as rumors of bribes and corruption marred the senatorial elections of Samuel C. Pomeroy (R) in 1867 and Alexander Caldwell (R) in 1871. Pomeroy, who had been born and educated in Massachusetts, settled in Kansas in the 1850s. A powerful Radical Republican and a friend to railroad interests, he had represented the state in the U. S. Senate since its admission to the Union in 1861. Caldwell was a wealthy railroad entrepreneur and a political novice at the time of his election.

Statement of the Case

In 1872, Samuel Pomeroy became aware that within a few weeks the Kansas legislature planned to submit to the Senate its findings in an investigation of his 1867 election. On March 5, he moved that all such communications be forwarded to the Committee on Privileges and Elections. On April 8, the anticipated documents relating to his election in 1867 and Caldwell's in 1871 arrived and were sent to the committee. The charges were essentially the same against both Pomeroy and Caldwell. Witnesses accused each of using money to secure votes. Pomeroy's opponents maintained that he paid members of the state legislature to vote for him, while Caldwell's detractors declared that he both bought votes and paid other candidates to remove themselves from the contest. On May 11, 1872, the Senate authorized the committee to investigate the charges and to call the necessary witnesses.

Response of the Senate

On May 21 the committee convened to begin its hearings, but before they could start, Alexander Caldwell appeared and requested an early disposition of his case. Pleading insufficient time remaining in the congressional session to investigate both cases, the committee, however, chose to deal first with the charges against Pomeroy.

Pomeroy

On June 3, the Committee on Privileges and Elections reported in favor of Samuel Pomeroy. It found no evidence to support the allegations and asked to be discharged from further inquiries into Pomeroy's election conduct. The session of Congress concluded on June 10 with no consideration of the Caldwell case.

The cloud of scandal still hung over Pomeroy, however. When he unsuccessfully sought reelection in January 1873, he faced renewed allegations of bribery and corruption from both houses of the Kansas legislature and was actually arrested for bribery. When Pomeroy returned to Washington in February 1873, having had his trial postponed, he publicly denied any wrongdoing. At his request, the Senate on February 10 established a special five-member committee to investigate the new charges against him.

The committee conducted a week of public hearings, calling a parade of witnesses from Kansas. The testimony received related a melodramatic tale of a midnight rendezvous in Pomeroy's private suite at a Topeka hotel, attended by the senator and state legislator Alexander M. York; a $2,000 downpayment for York's vote; a locked valise stuffed with a $5,000 post-vote installment; and an emotional anti-Pomeroy speech delivered by York as he displayed the cash to members of the state convention during the senatorial election. York testified that he had conspired with four colleagues to defeat Pomeroy by accepting a bribe from the senator and then exposing the action to the legislature just prior to the vote for U.S. senator. The plot had succeeded, for the legislators responded by changing their votes and electing another candidate.

Pomeroy did not deny giving the money to the legislator but claimed that York, a longtime political opponent, was going to deliver it to a mutual friend who was establishing a bank at Independence, Kansas. As the inquiry progressed, testimony from both the defendant and his accusers became shrouded in contradictions, evasions, and faulty memories; the only clear fact to emerge was that the 1873 Kansas elections had been conducted under unsavory circumstances. Newspapers across the country covered the story in all its lurid detail, fueling the public's perception that Congress was rife with corruption.

With all the witnesses tainted, the special committee remained uncertain about its verdict. When it issued its report on March 3 at the conclusion of the Forty-second Congress, the three Republican committee members, Frederick Frelinghuysen (NJ), William Buckingham (CT), and James L. Alcorn (MS), dismissed the entire transaction as a concerted and successful plot to defeat Pomeroy. Democrat George Vickers (MD) did not find Pomeroy to be "guilty beyond a reasonable doubt." He argued that the charges against Pomeroy should not be sustained because the accuser's deceit cast doubt on the accuracy of his testimony. Only Allen Thurman (D-OH) submitted a brief minority report pronouncing Pomeroy guilty of making corrupt offers to secure votes. Thurman declined to elaborate, noting that the report was being issued on Pomeroy's final day in office. His defeat in the election saved him from discipline by his colleagues, and the Senate took no action on the committee's report.

Caldwell

No brighter picture of Kansas election procedures greeted the Senate when it turned its attention to the report of the Committee on Privileges and Elections in the case of Alexander Caldwell. The most damaging testimony came from Sidney Clarke, Caldwell's personal and professional foe. Prior to the election, Clarke had been informed by Caldwell's associates that the candidate was determined to have the seat and was prepared to pay $250,000 for it. The only other serious candidate, Thomas Carney, a former governor of Kansas, admitted to the committee that he had accepted $15,000 to leave the race and assist in Caldwell's election. Even Caldwell's friends and political cronies acknowledged that after the election the senator-elect told them the contest had cost him over $60,000.

Caldwell did not enhance his position when he adopted an arrogant attitude toward the committee. Caldwell insisted that the charges were made by disappointed and ambitious politicians who were maliciously seeking his downfall. He then imprudently asked under what authority the Senate presumed to investigate him, to which the committee responded by returning a report that condemned the fraudulent manner in which Caldwell captured his seat. On February 17, 1873, the committee submitted a well-documented report unanimously concluding that Caldwell had bribed legislators to vote for him. After debating whether Caldwell's crimes warranted expulsion or a declaration of a voided election, the committee opted for the latter. It declared that Caldwell had not been "duly and legally elected" to the Senate.

The many issues involved in the case—election procedures, party factionalism, expulsion—guaranteed a vigorous and lengthy floor debate when the special session of the new Senate convened on March 4. Ultimately, it was Oliver H.P.T. Morton (R-IN) who destroyed Caldwell's already shaky defense. Morton pointed out four flaws in Caldwell's excuses: he had called his bribe to an opponent a private arrangement of no concern to the Senate; he claimed that bribery of state legislators was not a criminal offense; he doubted the Senate's right to make the inquiry; and he denied that the Senate could expel a member for actions taken before he entered that body. Morton's summary indicated how poorly Caldwell understood the Senate; he had sealed his doom by challenging the right of the Senate to govern its own affairs. He had apparently misjudged the situation from the outset. As the committee report noted in explaining, though not condoning, his actions, "He was a novice in politics and evidently in the hands of men who encouraged him in the belief that Senatorial elections in Kansas were carried by the use of money."

The focus of the debates shifted to the two options available to the Senate—expulsion or invalidation. Allen Thurman explained his view of the dilemma: "I believe that this election is an invalid election; but, sir, my believing that does not preclude my voting to expel upon the same facts, because . . . the turpitude of the member is equal in either case, and the expulsion will be for good cause, and will be in the exercise of the legal discretion of the Senate." Alexander Caldwell belatedly appeared to understand the power of the United States Senate; on March 24, 1873, before a vote could be taken, he resigned his seat.

Conclusion

The two cases illustrate the type of corruption much of the country believed to be widespread in the Reconstruction Congress. The Pomeroy case in particular was so dramatic that it even found its way into fiction, when Mark Twain and Charles Dudley Warner included a thinly disguised version of the story in their novel *The Gilded Age,* published in December 1873.

Samuel Pomeroy's Kansas trial for bribery was postponed several times, until the prosecution finally dropped the case in 1875. Pomeroy remained in Washington for several years before returning to Massachusetts, where he died in 1891. Alexander Caldwell returned to his substantial business interests in Kansas. He became president of the First National Bank of Leavenworth in 1897 and died in 1917.

Sources

U.S. Congress. Senate. *Congressional Globe.* 42d Cong., 2d sess. (See pp. 1410–11, 3316–17.) 3d sess. (See pp. 1448–54.)

———. *Congressional Record.* 43d Cong., spec. sess. (See pp. 30–38, 41–62, 66–77, 80–102, 104–13, 118–34, 137–65.)

———. Senate Report No. 224. 42d Cong., 2d sess., 1872.

———. Senate Reports No. 451 and 523. 42d Cong., 3d sess., 1873.

Johnson, Allen, ed. *Dictionary of American Biography.* Vol. 3. New York, 1946; reprint of 1935 edition. (See pp. 405–6.)

Kitzhaber, Albert R. "Götterdämmerung in Topeka: The Downfall of Senator Pomeroy." *Kansas Historical Quarterly* 18 (1950): 243–78.

Malone, Dumas, ed. *Dictionary of American Biography.* Vol. 15. New York, 1946; reprint of 1935 edition. (See pp. 54–55.)

Francis W. Sykes v. George E. Spencer

(1816–1883) (1836–1893)

Alabama

Election Case
December 13, 1872 to May 20, 1876

Issues
Reconstruction: challenge to legislature's authority to elect (rival legislatures)

Result: Spencer retained seat

Chronology:
Credentials presented: Dec. 13, 1872
Referred to committee: Dec. 8, 1873
Committee report: April 20, 1874
Senate vote: May 28, 1874
Referred to committee: Dec. 16, 1875
Committee report: May 20, 1876
No Senate action

Background

In 1872 intense political fights in Alabama produced two separate bodies claiming to be the proper legislature, each of which elected a United States senator. One group, called the "statehouse legislature" because it met in the state capitol, elected Democrat Francis W. Sykes, a physician. The action of this legislature was recognized by the outgoing Democratic governor, Robert B. Lindsay, although he did not sign any credentials. The second group, the "courthouse legislature," elected Republican George E. Spencer, a native of New York and a former Union army officer who had been serving in the Senate since 1868. This latter election was recognized by the incoming Republican governor, David P. Lewis, who signed the credentials for Spencer. Once again, intrastate discord in the wake of Reconstruction set the stage for dissension in the United States Senate.

Statement of the Case

At the special session of the Senate in March 1873, George Spencer and Francis Sykes claimed the same senatorial seat. When Spencer stepped forward to be sworn in on March 6, James A. Bayard, Jr. (D-DE) objected, asking that both sets of credentials be sent to the Committee on Privileges and Elections. Republican Roscoe Conkling of New York, however, urged the Senate to continue its usual practice of seating a senator who presented credentials that were on their face valid and then allow the Committee on Privileges and Elections to conduct an investigation. Bayard insisted that the credentials for Sykes should be read to the Senate, along with those of Spencer, even though they were not in the proper form and not signed by the governor. Not all Democrats agreed, however, for others urged that Spencer be seated while the committee carried out its investigation, so that Alabama would not be deprived of her right to representation upon the floor of the Senate. They felt particularly strongly in light of the recent case of Alabama's other senator, George

Goldthwaite (D), who had waited almost a year before finally being seated (See Case 56). Precedents were cited by senators to support each approach.

After considerable debate, the Senate agreed to have the clerk read the credentials of Sykes, which were in the form of a memorial signed by the president of the senate and speaker of the house of the legislature that elected him. During the debate, information arrived from Alabama that the state supreme court had recognized as the legitimate legislature the courthouse general assembly that elected Spencer.

On March 7, after further discussion, the Senate rejected two motions by Bayard that consideration of the case be postponed for another day or that both sets of credentials be referred to a special five-member committee. George Goldthwaite, still smarting from the months he had been forced to wait before being sworn, supported the claim of Francis Sykes, urging that at the very least the two sets of credentials should be referred to a committee. The Senate, however, ignored his plea, and George Spencer came forward to take the oath of office.

But the controversy continued. When the Forty-third Congress convened in December 1873, John Gordon (D-GA) requested that the memorial of Francis Sykes and the appropriate documents be referred to the Committee on Privileges and Elections. Aware of continuing discord in Alabama, the Senate agreed.

Response of the Senate

On April 20, 1874, a divided committee submitted majority and minority reports. The committee had attempted to identify which of the two Alabama legislatures was the legitimate one, so that the seat could go to the senator it had selected. The statehouse body included a number of Democratic members who had election certificates, even though they had not been elected, while the courthouse group included the Republicans who had in fact been elected to those seats but had no certificates. Without the questionable members, the statehouse legislature would have had no quorum, and with those actually elected who had no certificates, the courthouse legislature did have a quorum. Subsequently, a compromise had been reached under the auspices of the U.S. attorney general, in which the conflicting legislatures were merged and the Republican legislators from the contested counties seated. According to the majority report supported by all the Republicans on the committee, "Were the Senate to hold Sykes's election to be valid, it would follow that erroneous certificates, delivered to men conceded not to be elected, had enabled persons who in fact ought not to vote for a Senator to elect a Senator to misrepresent the State for six years." The situation thus required them "to choose between the form and the substance." Arguing that the incoming legitimate governor, Lewis, recognized only the courthouse legislature, the majority of the committee upheld the right of George Spencer to his place in the Senate.

The two committee Democrats, Eli Saulsbury (DE) and William T. Hamilton (MD), protested vehemently, asserting that without the necessary qualifying certificates, the courthouse legislature constituted nothing more than an illegal gathering. They pointed out that, although the two competing legislatures had subsequently been merged, that action had occurred a week or more after the elections for U.S. senator were completed and should have no bearing on the validity of those elections. They also stressed the failure of those without certificates to take the appropriate steps to contest the election of those in the statehouse legislature. If the Senate granted the seat to Spencer, they hinted, it would raise suspicions of partisanship.

During the ensuing debate, the background on the dual legislatures emerged. Oliver H.P.T. Morton (R-IN), the chairman of the Privileges and Elections Committee, charged that there had been a conspiracy to obtain a Democratic majority in the legislature. Among the details: an official in one county had issued an injunction against counting the votes for legislative candidates from that county. The uncounted votes were sufficient to have elected Republican candidates from that area, and the lack of those votes led to the election of their Democratic opponents. The secretary of state promptly issued certificates of election to these Democratic legislators. Two days later, the injunction against counting the ballots was lifted, and county officials reported the Republican candidates as elected, but the secretary of state refused to correct the certificates. There were allegations in other counties that large numbers of Republican votes had been illegally thrown out.

After considerable emotional debate, the Senate acted on May 28, 1874. After defeating, by a vote of 11 to 33, an amendment declaring that George Spencer had not been elected, the Senate by voice vote agreed with the majority report and permitted Spencer to retain his seat. But Spencer's troubles with his Senate seat did not end there. On December 16, 1875, Spencer asked the Senate to investigate charges made by a new and hostile Alabama legislature that he had secured his seat through corrupt means, and the Senate referred the matter to committee. On May 20, 1876, the Privileges and Elections Committee dismissed as worthless hearsay the allegations that Spencer offered money or any object of value in return for votes in the legislature. The committee asserted that those who claimed to have received money for their votes did not appear before it and the admission of the second-hand testimony could only contribute to scandal while proving nothing. Although complaints of Republican malfeasance in the southern states multiplied during the Reconstruction years, in this instance the committee did not consider them sufficiently substantiated to act upon.

Conclusion

In March 1876, at the recommendation of the Committee on Privileges and Elections, the Senate granted Francis Sykes the compensation of a senator from March 1873 to May 1874 while the case had been under consideration. That decision had been delayed for two years because some senators objected to the existing precedent that those unsuccessfully contesting a senatorial election should receive compensation, fearing it might encourage frivolous election challenges. Some also believed that Spencer and other senators who successfully defended their seats deserved to have their expenses paid as well, although such payments had never been made in the past. Sykes continued to live in Alabama until his death in 1883.

In 1885, George Spencer sought and received more than $7,000 from the Senate as compensation for his expenses incurred during the corruption investigation. Spencer remained in the Senate until 1879, after which he became commissioner of the Union Pacific Railroad. Later involved with ranching and mining in Nevada, Spencer died in 1893 in Washington, D.C.

Sources

U.S. Congress. Senate. *Congressional Record.* 43d Cong., spec. sess. (See pp. 3–29.) 1st sess. (See pp. 4287–90, 4325–30, 4596–98, 4798–4800, 4850–52, Appendix, pp. 323–31.)

———. *Congressional Record.* 44th Cong., 1st sess. (See pp. 232–33.)

———. Senate Report No. 291. 43d Cong., 1st sess., 1874.

———. Senate Reports No. 135 and 331. 44th Cong., 1st sess., 1876.

Owen, Thomas M. *History of Alabama and Dictionary of Alabama Biography* 4 (Chicago, 1921).

John Ray v. William L. McMillen
(1816–1888) (dates unknown)

William L. McMillen, James B. Eustis
(dates unknown) (1834–1899)

Robert H. Marr
(1819–1892)

v.

P.B.S. Pinchback
(1837–1921)

Henry M. Spofford, Thomas C. Manning
(1821–1880) (1825–1887)

v.

William P. Kellogg
(1830–1918)

Election Cases
January 22, 1873, to December 7, 1880

Issues
Reconstruction: challenge to legislature's authority to elect; challenge to governor's authority to appoint; (rival legislatures)

Chronology:
Ray v. McMillen
Credentials presented: Jan. 11, 1873
Referred to committee: Jan. 22, 1873
Committee report: Feb. 20, 1873
No Senate action
Result: Not seated

McMillen, Eustis, Marr v. Pinchback
Credentials presented: Jan. 21, 1873
Referred to committee: Dec. 4, 1873
Committee report: Feb. 8, 1875
Senate vote: Dec. 10, 1877
Result: Eustis seated

Spofford, Manning v. Kellogg
Credentials presented: Jan. 20, 1877
Referred to committee: Mar. 7, 1877
Committee report: Nov. 26, 1877
Senate vote: Nov. 30, 1877
Result: Kellogg seated

Complaint of corruption: May 7, 1879
Referred to committee: May 7, 1879
Committee report: Mar. 22, 1880
Senate vote to postpone: June 11, 1880
Credentials presented (Manning): Dec. 7, 1880
Result: Kellogg retained seat

Background

Reconstruction politics battered Louisiana as furiously as any natural hurricane had ever done. Improper election conduct, corruption, blatant disregard for legal procedures, and open violence by members of both parties left the state government in shreds. This turbulence even reached the United States Senate when, between 1873 and 1880, eight different men claimed the right to be seated for Louisiana.

The resignation on November 1, 1872, of Radical Republican William P. Kellogg, who had represented Louisiana in the Senate since the state's readmission to the Union in 1868, launched three separate election challenges, leading to several Senate investigations and intense floor debates on the subject of Reconstruction. Senate concern in each case focused on the persistence of severe domestic disorder in Louisiana, culminating in the establishment of two legislatures led by rival governors.

Statement of the Case

Ray v. McMillen

On January 22, 1873, soon after Kellogg's resignation to run for governor, two claimants, John Ray (R) and William L. McMillen (D), appeared with certificates of election for the unexpired six weeks of Kellogg's term. Ray was elected by one legislature, with credentials signed by Kellogg as governor, while McMillen, chosen by the rival legislature, was certified by Acting Governor P.B.S. Pinchback. The Senate quickly referred the matter to its Committee on Privileges and Elections.

Response of the Senate

The committee heard a confusing chronicle of abuses, among them that, during the election for state assembly members, ten thousand Louisiana blacks had been denied the right to register, while an additional three thousand had been turned away at the polls. In addition, the committee learned that the two rival legislatures came into existence because, after the election and before the ballots were counted, the governor at the time, H.C. Warmoth, dissolved the existing election board responsible for counting ballots. A former Radical Republican who supported the Democratic gubernatorial candidate, Warmoth approved a new state law governing election procedures and appointed a new board. Meanwhile, the original board went ahead and counted the ballots, announcing the election of a Republican legislature and Kellogg as governor. The new board, for its part, declared that a Democratic legislature had been elected with John McEnery as governor. Then, ruling in a suit between the two parties, a federal judge ordered the U.S. marshal to take possession of the statehouse to "prevent all unlawful assemblage" there of the Democratic legislature, which he considered to be fraudulently elected. Under the judge's order, carried out with the aid of federal troops, the Republican-dominated legislature was declared elected and permitted to assemble, with Kellogg as the future governor. This legislature promptly voted to impeach Governor Warmoth for dissolving the original elections board and creating a new one. During Warmoth's trial, the Republican lieutenant governor, P.B.S. Pinchback, served as acting governor, thus becoming the first black governor of any state.

When the Senate committee reported on February 20, 1873, the majority of its members recommended that Congress order a new election in Louisiana. They also proposed that the Senate adopt two resolutions, declaring that "there is no State government at present existing in the State of Louisiana" and that "neither John Ray nor W.L. McMillen is entitled to a seat in the Senate, neither having been elected by the legislature of the State of Louisiana." The senators reached this conclusion even though they strongly disapproved of the judge's action as "inexcusable" and overstepping the powers of the federal government. Three members of the committee filed minority reports: Joshua Hill (R-GA) and Lyman Trumbull (R-IL) supported McMillen's claim, while committee chairman Oliver H.P.T. Morton (R-IN) expressed concern at the idea of overturning the state government.

With less than a month remaining in Kellogg's term, the Senate rejected the committee's proposal to call a new election. It took no further action on the committee's report, and neither candidate was seated. Five years later, in 1878, the Senate voted to pay $1,000 each to Ray and McMillen in compensation for their expenses during Senate consideration of their claims.

Pinchback v. McMillen/Marr/Eustis

Since the two competing legislatures still existed in Louisiana, both assemblies returned new claimants to the vacant seat for the term beginning on March 4, 1873. Almost three years passed before the Senate untangled the dilemma; in the meantime, four different men presented credentials signed by various Louisiana governors.

The first to arrive, on January 21, 1873, was Pinckney B.S. Pinchback, who had been Louisiana's acting governor. Elected by the Republican legislature to the new Senate term, he presented credentials signed by Governor Kellogg. Soon after, William McMillen appeared to claim the same seat, with credentials signed by Governor McEnery. In May 1873, President Ulysses S. Grant had recognized Kellogg as the legitimate governor. Still, on December 4, 1873, an uneasy Senate sent the credentials of both Pinchback, a black Republican, and McMillen, a white Democrat, to the Committee on Privileges and Elections. After attempting vainly to reach a resolution, the committee reported on December 15, 1873, that it was evenly divided on the question and referred the matter back to the full Senate. The Senate, in turn, after considerable debate, returned the credentials to the committee, and on February 8, 1875, the committee submitted a new report. The Republican majority, led by committee chairman Oliver Morton, argued that Pinchback's claim was valid and he should be sworn in. The two Democratic committee members objected, however, and denounced the entire 1872 election in Louisiana as "a crime against our civilization and a blot upon our free institutions."

The Senate still took no action, continuing to waver on the issue until December 9, 1875, when a weary William McMillen withdrew his claim. The McMillen faction in Louisiana promptly replaced him with a new candidate, Robert H. Marr. A month later, on January 18, 1876, the papers of James B. Eustis, a Democrat, were presented for the same seat, thus replacing Marr as the Democratic claimant. The Senate referred Eustis' credentials to the Privileges and Elections Committee. Within ten days, the harried committee reported that no vacancy existed, since Pinchback had been elected to that seat. It therefore recommended that Eustis' papers be laid on the table. The Senate then, on March 8, 1876, voted 32 to 29 not to seat Pinchback, although it later did grant him salary and mileage for the three years of the dispute.

A year later, at the request of Ohio Democrat Allen G. Thurman, the Senate in March 1877 agreed to reconsider the claim of J.B. Eustis and referred the matter to the Committee on Privileges and Elections. The committee submitted its report on December 1, 1877. Reflecting the Senate's confusion and embarrassment over the lengthy dispute, the report asserted that Eustis had been legally elected by the "lawful Legislature" of Louisiana, although the election took place at a time when Pinchback was already claiming the same seat. The committee argued that the Senate's 1876 action in refusing to seat Pinchback should be considered the final ruling in that case. In order to end the long vacancy, it recommended that Eustis be seated, even though it acknowledged an apparent conflict with an 1834 Senate decision. In that case, the Senate had determined that the Rhode Island legislature had unlawfully elected Elisha R. Potter to the seat of Asher Robbins when no vacancy existed (See Case 14). The committee explained that Pinchback's case differed from the earlier one in that Robbins had already been seated at the time he was challenged.

On December 10, 1877, the Senate voted, 49 to 8, to seat J.B. Eustis, and he took the oath of office. Still, some senators continued to be troubled by the decision to turn away Pinchback when he almost certainly had a prima facie claim to the seat.

Kellogg v. Spofford/Manning

In 1877 a controversy was also raging over the other Louisiana Senate seat for the term to begin March 4, 1877. P.B.S. Pinchback, who had endured public racial abuse throughout his long struggle to secure his seat, anticipated that Louisiana would elect him to this new Senate term. Once again, he faced disappointment, as his former ally William Kellogg, reportedly through the use of lavish bribes, secured the certificate of election. When Kellogg arrived to take the oath of office, however, objection was raised to seating him, and the Senate on March 7, 1877, referred his credentials to the Privileges and Elections Committee. In fact, the election of 1876 in Louisiana created even greater controversy than the previous ones. Not only did conflicting claims over the state's electoral votes complicate the presidential race between Republican Rutherford B. Hayes and Democrat Samuel J. Tilden, but the state again found itself with two governors and two rival legislatures. This situation, in turn, meant two claimants for the Senate seat, as Henry M. Spofford arrived in October 1877 to challenge Kellogg. His credentials, too, were sent to the Privileges and Elections Committee. On November 26, the committee's Republican majority reported in favor of Kellogg. The committee found that, because Democrats had used violence and intimidation to prevent blacks from voting in some legislative districts, election officials had thrown out the results and declared the Republican candidates elected from those districts. The resulting Republican-dominated legislature had elected Kellogg. The three committee Democrats filed a minority report, complaining that the committee had refused to receive evidence gathered by Spofford and failed adequately to investigate the Louisiana election. They pointed out that, as part of the agreement that resolved his disputed election, even Republican President Hayes had recognized the legitimacy of the Democratic legislature. His withdrawal of the federal troops that had been keeping the peace in Louisiana had led to the collapse of the Republican legislature, so that by April 1877 when Spofford was elected, only the Democratic legislature remained. On November 30, 1877, the Senate, still narrowly under Republican control, voted 30 to 28 to seat Kellogg.

Spofford, undaunted, continued to press his claim in the next Congress, since Democrats had become the majority party in the Senate. On May 7, 1879, the Senate voted 26 to 17 to direct the Committee on Privileges and Elections to investigate the reports of corruption in the 1876 Louisiana elections. On March 22, 1880, after holding extensive hearings both in Washington and in Louisiana, questioning nearly 150 witnesses, and gathering 1,200 pages of testimony, the committee reported that it had learned of fraudulent and corrupt practices by Kellogg in the election. It accused him of deliberately misleading the committee in its earlier investigation, so that his seating was based on false information. The committee majority therefore recommended that Kellogg be unseated and replaced by Spofford. The three Republican committee members charged that no new evidence had been obtained and that the only change since the earlier investigation was the change in party control of the Senate, placing the Democrats in a position to oust Kellogg. Debate on the proposal moved slowly until Congress adjourned in mid-June. Then, in August of that year, Spofford died. Thomas C. Manning (D), who had been a justice on the state supreme court, appeared as a replacement on December 7, 1880, but he had no success in supplanting Kellogg, who served out his term.

Conclusion

These election cases demonstrate the extent to which postwar disorder in Louisiana, exacerbated by local factionalism, federal mismanagement, personal dishonesty, and deep-seated racial biases, had an impact on the U.S. Senate.

P.B.S. Pinchback, although prevented from becoming the second black United States senator, lived out his life in affluence. He remained in Louisiana for many years but eventually retired to Washington, D.C., where he died in 1921.

In 1882, the Senate agreed to reimburse William Kellogg more than $9,000 for the expenses incurred in defending his seat. He remained in the Senate until 1883 and then served one term in the U.S. House of Representatives before retiring in Washington, D.C., where he lived until his death in 1918.

The Louisiana legislature did not reelect James Eustis at the conclusion of his term in 1879 but did return him to the Senate again in 1885. He served until 1891, became ambassador to France in 1893, and died in 1899.

Robert Marr served on the Louisiana supreme court from 1877 to 1880. Thomas Manning also served on that court during the same period and again from 1882 to 1886, when he was appointed U.S. minister to Mexico. The Senate in 1882 granted Manning $1,000 to cover his expenses in claiming the seat.

Henry Spofford's heirs also received compensation from the Senate for the three years he had spent in contesting the Louisiana election.

Sources

U.S. Congress. Senate. *Congressional Globe.* 42d Cong., 3d sess. (See p. 2147.)

———. *Congressional Record.* 43d Cong., 1st sess. (See pp. 220–28, 913–21, 1036–58, 1109–11, Appendix. pp. 41–48.) 2d sess. (See pp. 647, 1063, 1277–89, 1306–10, 1327–53, 1358–82.)

———. *Congressional Record.* 44th Cong., spec. sess. (See pp. 3–7, 9–25, 32–53, 55–91, 190.) 1st sess. (See pp. 200–204, 451–55, 886–89, 907–13, 1382–92, 1436–44, 1511–16, 1545–58, 4319–23, 4368–72, 4382–4400.)

———. *Congressional Record.* 45th Cong, spec. sess. (See pp. 1–2, 15–23.) 1st sess. (See pp. 78–83, 99–115, 730–64, 767–97.) 2d sess.(See pp. 82–87, 2053–56, 2147.)

———. *Congressional Record.* 46th Cong., 1st sess. (See pp. 468–69, 1022–24, 1071–87, 1099–1123.) 2d sess. (See pp. 833–35, 1758–68, 1985–88, 2676–83, 2735–54, 2909–11, 2952–60, 2972–82, 3108–16, 3161–66, 3232–40, 3270–77, 3313–22, 3362–67, 3456–62, 3511–15, 3551–65, 4238–44, 4414–31.) 3d sess. (See pp. 1911–12.)

———. Senate Report No. 457. 42d Cong., 3d sess., 1873.

———. Senate Report No. 476. 43d Cong., 1st sess., 1874.

———. Senate Report No. 626. 43d Cong., 2d sess., 1875.

———. Senate Report No. 274. 44th Cong., 1st sess., 1876.

Background

Rumors of financial scandal clouded the national celebrations over completion of the transcontinental railroad in 1869. Three years later, these suspicions were confirmed when a select committee of the House of Representatives uncovered a fraudulent relationship between the Union Pacific Railroad and the Crédit Mobilier of America Corporation, which had been formed to supervise the contracts to build the Union Pacific. A common group of stockholders secretly managed both companies, a scheme that permitted the construction firm to charge the railroad (and ultimately the government) two million dollars more than the actual building expenses. The major sensation of the exposé proved to be that many of the Crédit Mobilier stockholders were highly respected Republican members of Congress. The revelation shocked the nation and significantly weakened the Republican party's leadership.

Statement of the Case

The House investigation focused on the conduct of Representative Oakes Ames (R-MA), for many years an ardent spokesman for the railroad industry. In 1865 Ames permitted himself to be drawn into the machinations of the Crédit Mobilier. Since the secret organization of one group of stockholders under two different titles was questionable at best and since the government had initially granted the railroad exceedingly generous land and loan privileges, Thomas C. Durant, former president of the Crédit Mobilier and mastermind of the scheme, persuaded Ames to dispense company shares to his congressional associates, in order to deter any formal investigations into the shady dealings.

In September 1872 a New York newspaper, acting upon a tip from a disgruntled Ames crony, published the names of congressmen reported to have profited from the company's largesse. Unable to ignore the rising furor, the House of Representatives assembled a committee of inquiry chaired by Representative (and former Senator) Luke P. Poland (R-VT). By December of that year, the stunned Poland committee had received allegations against almost every important committee chairman of the House of Representatives, several senators, and Vice President Schuyler Colfax. Oakes Ames, the source of these charges, added to the confusion by rambling, erratic testimony that relied upon a complicated set of records kept on scraps of paper or in inscrutable ledgers. Nor were matters helped by Ames' repeated assertion that he was never good at remembering dates.

By February 1873, the House had become convinced that the Senate should be presented with the information. The House offered no recommendations to the Senate but simply made available all the testimony it had gathered. In this manner, the names of Senators William B. Allison (R-IA), James A. Bayard, Jr. (D-DE), George S. Boutwell (R-MA), Roscoe Conkling (R-NY), James Harlan (R-IA), John A. Logan (R-IL), James W. Patterson

(R-NH), Henry Wilson (R-MA), and Vice President Schuyler Colfax (R-IN) formally came to the attention of the Senate.

Response of the Senate

On February 4, 1873, James Patterson asked the Senate to appoint a select committee to investigate the charges. When Vice President Colfax excused himself from appointing the committee, the task fell to Henry B. Anthony (R-RI), who chose Lot M. Morrill (R-ME) to chair the group of five. Two Democratic committee members, John P. Stockton (NJ) and John W. Stevenson (KY), promptly asked to be replaced, claiming that they were already excessively burdened by their other Senate obligations, but their colleagues refused to excuse them from serving.

In its preliminary meeting on February 8, 1873, the Morrill committee tried to limit the scope of the investigation to ensure that the report would be completed before the close of the Forty-second Congress on March 3. Since less than a month remained for the committee to review all the evidence from the Poland Committee, interview witnesses, and hold public hearings, the thoroughness of the inquiry came into question from the outset.

William B. Allison, who had served in the House until 1871 and entered the Senate in 1873, described his financial association with Oakes Ames as a casual one, which he terminated by returning the Crédit Mobilier certificates when his Iowa constituents severely criticized him for holding any type of railroad stock. The Morrill committee made no mention of Allison in its final report. He continued to serve in the Senate and was chairman of the Appropriations Committee when he died in 1908.

James A. Bayard, Jr., who had left the Senate in 1869, submitted a letter disavowing knowledge of the nature of the corporation or personal acquaintance with Ames. As the seventy-four-year-old Bayard no longer served in the Senate, the Morrill committee gave only scant attention to the charges against him. His name was not included in the final report, and the elderly senator lived quietly until his death in 1880.

George S. Boutwell, one of the original founders of the Republican party and secretary of the treasury under President Ulysses S. Grant, also received little notice from the Morrill committee, which did not mention him in its report. Boutwell's connection to Ames stemmed from their joint service in the House of Representatives in the late 1860s, a tie that all witnesses agreed was tenuous. Boutwell did not actually enter the Senate until March 1873, after the investigation was completed. He served only one term and later was appointed to codify the Statutes at Large. Active in the field of international law, Boutwell died in 1905.

Roscoe Conkling also escaped the scandal unscathed. Conkling, a former member of the House of Representatives and a senator since 1867, had been alluded to briefly during the House hearings. Based on Conkling's testimony and that of other witnesses, the Morrill committee report specifically dismissed all charges against him as entirely unfounded. An aggressive and powerful senator, Conkling remained an influential member until his dramatic resignation from the Senate in 1881 in a dispute with President James A. Garfield over patronage. He died seven years later.

James Harlan, an outspoken supporter of railroad construction throughout the West, fared less well, even though he had a prestigious reputation, having served in the Senate before and during the Civil War and as Andrew Johnson's secretary of the interior. The Morrill committee was concerned to discover that in 1865, while he was secretary of the interior, Harlan had accepted a $10,000 contribution toward a future campaign for the Senate from Thomas Durant, the notorious former president of Crédit Mobilier, who was at the time a vice president of Union Pacific. Declaring that "the use of large sums of money to influence either popular or legislative elections strikes directly at the fundamental principle of a Republican government," the committee suggested that such action deserved censure, although it found no evidence that Harlan had permitted the money to influence his behavior as a senator. Time saved Harlan from the possibility of formal censure, for his term expired on March 3, 1873, before further action could be taken. Harlan's subsequent campaigns for senator and governor proved unsuccessful. He died in 1899.

John Logan, who had served in the House before and after the Civil War and entered the Senate in 1871, was completely exonerated by the committee report. In a straightforward account of his dealings with Ames, Logan explained that he refused Ames' original offer but that a few months later the Massachusetts congressman presented him with a $329 check for his dividends. A reluctant Logan accepted the check, cashed it at the sergeant at arms' office, held the money for two days, and then returned it to Ames with $2 interest. Logan's detailed testimony convinced the committee that the episode, which occurred while Logan served in the House, required no further action by the Senate. Logan's long public service was interrupted briefly when he was not reelected at the conclusion of his term, but in 1879 Illinois again sent him to the Senate, where he remained until his death in 1886. In 1884 he was the Republican nominee for vice president on the ticket with James G. Blaine.

A more serious case was that of James Patterson, who had served in the Senate since 1867. He testified that, on separate occasions, he had given Ames $3,000 and $4,000 to invest for him. The $4,000 was invested in Union Pacific and the $3,000 in Crédit Mobilier. Patterson had told the House committee that, since Ames gave him no receipt in writing, he was unaware that he owned the Crédit Mobilier stock. Ames, however, contradicted Patterson on this point, producing a receipt signed by the senator that specified the stock as Crédit Mobilier. Patterson attributed the contradictions between his testimony and that of Ames to a faulty memory and his ignorance of financial matters. He also asserted strongly that there was no reason he should not own stock in that corporation. The Senate committee, however, concluded that Patterson, as a U.S. senator, knowingly arranged with Representative Ames "for the purchase of thirty shares in the stock of the Crédit Mobilier of America at rates greatly below its esteemed value," obtained the stock, received the dividends on it, and later bought and sold Union Pacific stock, knowing about the relations between the two companies and about Ames' involvement in them. He also knew that Ames' goal was to influence his actions as a senator in relation to the two companies. The committee therefore charged in its February 27, 1873, report to the Senate that Patterson gave false testimony to both the House and Senate committees. It unanimously recommended that he be expelled.

On March 3, the day his term expired, Patterson asked the Senate to take up the committee's resolution, so that there would be a full discussion of the case. The Senate, however, pleading the press of end-of-session business, decided not to consider the recommendation until the next session of Congress. On March 14, 1873, during the special session of the new Senate, Henry B. Anthony submitted a resolution declaring that inaction on the committee's resolution should be interpreted neither as approval nor disapproval. The resolution would also have permitted Patterson to submit a statement to be published in the *Congressional Record,* which just days earlier had begun publication as the official proceedings of Congress and the successor to the privately produced *Congressional Globe.* After a lengthy discussion, the Senate on March 26 amended the resolution to state only that a pamphlet prepared by Patterson in his defense would be printed, bound, and distributed with the report of the committee. The Senate adopted the amended resolution, believing that this would be the fairest way to give Patterson a chance to state his defense, since he had had no opportunity to defend himself on the Senate floor. At the same time, this approach avoided setting the dangerous precedent of permitting someone who was no longer a member of the body to place a statement in the official *Congressional Record.*

The unrepentant Patterson, whose friends felt he deserved expulsion no more than several other members, returned to New Hampshire, where he served in the state legislature and later as state superintendent of public instruction. He died in 1893.

Henry Wilson offered the committee the most original explanation for his connection with Ames. He related that in 1865 his wife had received a monetary gift of $3,800, $1,000 of which she then lost through an unfortunate investment Wilson recommended. Wilson reimbursed her for this loss from his own money, then, anxious to provide his wife with a successful investment, he turned to the Crédit Mobilier Corporation. He had learned about the company from dinner-table conversation with Ames at their Washington boardinghouse. Mrs. Wilson, placing undeserved trust in her husband's financial skills, did purchase the stocks, although she never received the certificates. Wilson later had second thoughts about the propriety of the business deal and asked Ames to refund his wife's money, which Wilson returned to her. Out of his own pocket, he added the $814 that Ames told him would have been the profit on the transaction. Thus, Wilson told the committee, he was "and ever shall be, $1,814 poorer than I should have been had . . . the investment with Mr. Ames not been made." The Morrill committee agreed that these actions in no way benefitted or tainted Wilson, who in March 1873 had become vice president of the United States after the political ruin of Schuyler Colfax through his part in the Crédit Mobilier scandal. The Morrill committee report did, however, mildly reprimand Wilson for insisting vehemently and erroneously during his election campaign that he had never known anything of the infamous company or any person connected with it. Wilson, who—unlike many of his colleagues—was a poor man, having been a shoemaker before entering politics, died in office in 1875.

Schuyler Colfax, the bright and popular vice president under Grant, had previously served in the House for fourteen years, six of them as Speaker. He contributed to his own downfall by delivering an impassioned speech asserting his innocence in the scandal shortly before the House convened the Poland committee. The resulting testimony implicated Colfax so clearly that his political credibility never recovered. Colfax tried to cloak each new revelation with respectability, but he could not explain away a $1,200 canceled check in his name that Ames held. Colfax's status as president of the Senate made his position slightly different from that of the charged senators. Neither the Poland committee nor the Morrill committee reports discussed the allegations against him. On February 20, 1873, a resolution introduced in the House called for the impeachment of Colfax, but four days later the House Judiciary Committee rejected the measure. Again, time aided the accused. Before further action could be taken in either the House or the Senate, Congress adjourned and the term ended for Colfax, who had failed to be renominated for vice president. No formal adjudication resolved the Colfax scandal. Although he remained active in politics and gave many speeches, his brilliant career was destroyed. Colfax died in 1885.

Conclusion

The Morrill committee completed its work in less than three weeks. Given the complexity and the seriousness of the charges, many believed the investigations in both the House and the Senate had been little more than cosmetic cover-ups. Political observers wondered how many other politicians had escaped undetected. Still, the reputations of several leading Republicans, and indeed of the entire party, suffered from the scandal. In spite of efforts to limit the damage, it became clear that the Crédit Mobilier affair had seriously undermined the Republican party.

Sources

U.S. Congress. Senate. *Congressional Globe.* 42d Cong., 3d sess. (See pp. 1065, 1076, 1099, 1136–37, 1605, 1873, 2068–69, 2184–85.)

———. *Congressional Record.* 43d Cong., spec. sess. (See pp. 193–97, 204.)

———. Senate Report No. 519 (Morrill Committee). 42d Cong., 3d sess., 1873.

U.S. Congress. House. House Report No. 77 (Poland Committee). 42d Cong., 3d sess., 1872.

———. House Report No. 78 (Wilson Committee). 42d Cong., 3d sess., 1872.

Crawford, J. B. *The Credit Mobilier of America: Its Origin and History.* New York, 1961; reprint of 1880 edition.

Johnson, Allen, ed. *Dictionary of American Biography.* New York, 1946; reprint of 1935 edition. Vol. 1. (See pp. 489–90) Vol. 3. (See pp. 297–98, 346–47.)

Johnson, Allen, and Dumas Malone, eds. *Dictionary of American Biography.* Vol. 7. New York, 1946; reprint of 1935 edition. (See pp. 268–69.)

Malone, Dumas, ed. *Dictionary of American Biography.* New York, 1946; reprint of 1935 edition. Vol. 11. (See pp. 363–65.) Vol. 13. (See pp. 303–4.)

New York Times, June 14, 1872; February 3, 1873.

Smith, Willard H. *Schuyler Colfax: The Changing Fortunes of a Political Idol.* Indianapolis, 1952.

Summers, Mark Wahlgren. *The Era of Good Stealings.* New York, 1993. (See pp. 50–54, 226–27, 231–37.)

Case 65

Lewis V. Bogy

(1813–1877)

Missouri

Election Case
March 17, 1873 to March 25, 1873

Issues
Electoral misconduct:
allegations of bribery and corruption

Result: Retained seat

Chronology:
Memorial received: Mar. 17, 1873
Referred to committee: Mar. 17, 1873
Committee report: Mar. 25, 1873
Senate vote: Mar. 25, 1873

Background

Caught between the pull of southern cultural traditions and the attraction of frontier opportunity, post-Civil War Missouri opted for the wealth promised by commercial development. Thus, Reconstruction politics brought only a mild stir to Missouri as the state concentrated on the industrial growth encouraged by a new constitution friendly to corporate ventures. When the Missouri legislature elected Lewis V. Bogy, Democratic president of the St. Louis city council, to the United States Senate in 1873, the dispute over that election proved mild in comparison to the violent contests that characterized the states of the deep South.

Statement of the Case

On March 4, 1873, Lewis Bogy took his seat in the Senate. On March 17, the Senate received, and referred to the Committee on Privileges and Elections, a memorial from several members of the Missouri legislature charging that Bogy had secured his seat through bribery and corruption.

The following day, Bogy demanded that the Senate move promptly to investigate the matter. "It is true," he said, "our contests in the West for this distinguished position, as is known to western Senators upon this floor, are always attended by heat and animation, and success is no easy matter." He insisted, however, that an inquiry by the state legislature had already exonerated him from any wrongdoing, although it had uncovered some attempts at bribery by another candidate. Bogy contended that the memorial sent to the Senate by his political opponents offered no new evidence but simply complained that the investigation by the Democratic legislature had been hasty and incomplete. He requested speedy action by the Committee on Privileges and Elections, pointing out that he did not consider it appropriate for him to vote on any of the other election cases pending before the Senate while he himself was under investigation.

Response of the Senate

A week later, on March 25, 1873, the Committee on Privileges and Elections reported that the evidence in the Missouri memorial was vague and unworthy of further Senate consideration. The Missouri complainants had not presented sufficient information to convince the committee that the Senate should launch its own investigation.

That same day, the members agreed without debate and discharged the committee from further consideration of the subject. Bogy thus retained his seat.

Conclusion

The Senate was glad to dispose quickly of one contested election in an era when an abundance of other challenges required its attention. Once his case was resolved, Bogy took an active part in the debates over the Louisiana elections (See Case 63) as a critic of the Republican governor's tactics. Bogy remained in the Senate until his death in 1877.

Sources

U.S. Congress. Senate. *Congressional Record.* 43d Cong., spec. sess. (See pp. 102–3, 182.)

———. Senate Report No. 1. 43d Cong., spec. sess., 1873.

Johnson, Allen, ed. *Dictionary of American Biography.* Vol. 1. New York, 1946; reprint of 1935 edition. (See pp. 410–11.)

Roller, David C., and Robert W. Twyman, eds. *The Encyclopedia of Southern History.* Baton Rouge, LA, 1979.

Case 66

David T. Corbin v. Matthew C. Butler

(1833–1905) (1836–1909)

South Carolina

Election Case
February 13, 1877 to February 25, 1879

Issues
Reconstruction: challenge to legislature's authority to elect (rival legislatures); allegations of electoral misconduct: intimidation of voters

Chronology #1:
Credentials presented: Feb. 13, 1877
Referred to committee: Mar. 7, 1877
Senate vote: Nov. 30, 1877
Result: Butler seated

Chronology #2:
Petition presented: Dec. 13, 1877
Referred to committee: Mar. 26, 1878
Committee report: Feb. 4, 1879
Senate vote: Feb. 25, 1879
Result: Butler retained seat

Background

South Carolina did not escape the heated dissension that marked Reconstruction politics throughout the South. Manipulation of voting districts, establishment of inaccessible polling places, and violent disruption of political gatherings typified the conduct of resurgent Democrats seeking to regain political control of the state from the Radical Republicans. At the same time, the composition of the United States Senate was also changing, as an influx of new Democratic members at the beginning of the Forty-fifth Congress in 1877 reduced the margin of Republican control to a slim 38 to 34 (with one Independent who generally voted with the Democrats). The closeness of the party division also contributed to the intensity of the struggle over these election cases.

Statement of the Case

After the November 1876 election, the upheaval in South Carolina led to the formation of two rival legislatures. One faction organized itself into a body called the Wallace house of representatives, which acted alone as a legislature without any state senate, while the other legislature consisted of a state senate and a house of representatives known as the Mackey house. Each claimed to be the lawful body and promptly elected a United States senator for the term beginning March 4, 1877. The Mackey house, dominated by Republicans, elected David T. Corbin, whose election was certified by the outgoing Republican governor, D.H. Chamberlain, while the Wallace house named Matthew C. Butler (D), whose credentials were signed by the incoming Democratic governor, Wade Hampton. A native South Carolinian,

Butler was an attorney and had served as a general in the Confederate army. Corbin was the Republican U.S. attorney in South Carolina.

All too familiar with the convoluted, time-consuming arguments associated with contests between dual state legislatures, the Senate on March 7, 1877, sent the credentials of both David Corbin and M. C. Butler to the Committee on Privileges and Elections.

Response of the Senate

On November 20, 1877, Allen Thurman (D-OH) asked that the committee be discharged from further consideration of Butler's credentials. He pointed out that five weeks after the Senate had reconvened in mid-October the committee had still not reported, leaving South Carolina without full representation in the Senate. Thurman questioned the value of waiting for a committee report, since the facts were all on the record, both candidates had submitted statements, and neither wished to call witnesses. Because the full Senate would want to discuss the case anyway, he thought the debate should start as soon as possible. He chided his colleagues for their failure to work diligently to find solutions to the three contested elections facing the Senate at that time. The new chairman of the Privileges and Elections Committee, Bainbridge Wadleigh (R-NH), responded that, although the full Senate had been holding brief daily sessions, the committee had been putting in long hours on two election cases from Louisiana (See Case 63), which had been referred to it before the Butler-Corbin case. He suggested that Thurman's eagerness to remove the South Carolina case from the committee might indicate that there was "something in the case which will not bear the scrutiny of the committee." Wadleigh, who had succeeded to the chairmanship after the death of Oliver Morton (R-IN) on November 1, observed that he and the other Senate Republicans had not yet had a chance to study the issues involved, in order to make an informed decision between the two claimants.

On November 26, committee chairman Wadleigh, having in the interim looked into the Corbin-Butler case, reminded the Senate that a special committee sent to South Carolina to investigate the 1876 election was due to produce a report very soon. The evidence collected by that committee, Wadleigh declared, supported Republican Corbin's position and implicated Democrat Butler in some of the violence and intimidation, so that "his path to this Chamber is slippery with blood." Thus, he contended, there was ample reason for the Privileges and Elections Committee to review the case.

Wadleigh then insisted on having the clerk read to the Senate excerpts from the evidence gathered by the committee investigating the situation in South Carolina, particularly portions regarding a massacre of black militiamen that occurred in the town of Hamburg in July 1876. Some testimony regarding the incident at Hamburg indicated that M.C. Butler had been a leader of the white mob that fired on the town armory where members of the black militia were taking shelter and later murdered a number of militiamen when they tried to escape. Black witnesses were convinced that the idea was to kill the principal black men of the area and intimidate enough black voters to enable the Democrats to carry the election. According to Wadleigh, "Mr. Corbin contends that in two counties in South Carolina at the last election there was such an enormous amount of violence, intimidation, and crime from the date of this Hamburgh [sic] massacre . . . up to . . . the time of the election, that nobody who wished to vote the republican ticket could feel safe in so doing." This intimidation of black voters led the Republican legislature to invalidate the election in two South Carolina counties. Without the representatives who claimed election from those counties, the Wallace house that elected Butler would have had no quorum.

In a lengthy session that continued all night and into the next day, November 27, Democratic senators countered by demanding that Butler's testimony to the special committee be read as well. Butler had told the committee that he saw no evidence of violence during the election campaign, as the Democratic candidates sought the support of black voters. He did, however, acknowledge that at his precinct in one of the disputed counties five or six hundred black citizens were prevented from voting. Regarding the Hamburg massacre, Butler complained that he had been unfairly treated in Governor Chamberlain's report on the incident. He had been in the town when the riot began but soon saw that he could not control the white mob and therefore left before the murders took place.

Finally, a closely divided Senate voted 29 to 27 in favor of Thurman's motion and discharged the Privileges and Elections Committee from further consideration of the credentials. Although the vote was generally along party lines, two Republicans—John J. Patterson of South Carolina and Simon B. Conover of Florida—joined the Democrats in voting for the discharge. Both offered lengthy explanations of their action, in response to charges from their party colleagues regarding possible "corrupt bargains" for their vote. Patterson, known as "Honest John," had been charged in South Carolina with bribing legislators in his 1872 election. Rumor and a newspaper story claimed that, in return for Patterson's support, Butler had promised the senator would not be prosecuted. Patterson, however, assured the Senate that he was simply representing his constituents, since both Democrats and Republicans in South Carolina now wanted Butler to be seated.

On November 30, 1877, the Senate voted 29 to 28 to seat M. C. Butler, but that action did not conclude the controversy. On December 13, Angus Cameron (R-WI) presented David Corbin's petition for a review of his right to the seat, which was eventually referred to the Privileges and Elections Committee on March 26, 1878. After taking nearly a year to review the complicated South Carolina election, the committee issued a majority and a minority report on February 4, 1879. The committee's Republican majority determined that in the November 1876 election the members of the state senate were duly elected and that body legally organized. The report also found that, on December 12 and 13, 1876, the senate and the Mackey house (consisting of 59 Republicans) voted for U.S. senator and elected David T. Corbin. Governor Chamberlain signed Corbin's credentials before leaving office on December 14. On December 19, the Wallace house (composed of 57 Democratic representatives plus 8 from the two counties where the election was invalidated because of violence) elected M.C. Butler as U.S. senator. The state senate as a body never participated in this latter election, although eleven of its members did.

The committee majority noted that the Wallace house appeared to recognize that it had no legal standing, for it never attempted to pass any legislation or take official action other than electing a U.S. senator. In addition, the majority declared that, since Corbin was elected on December 12, there was no vacancy in the office of U.S. senator when Butler was elected on December 19; the Butler election was completely invalid because the state senate did not participate; and the Wallace house had no quorum when it held the election for Butler. The Mackey house, on the other hand, had had a quorum of the 116 house members certified as elected, even if not of the 124 members authorized by the state constitution. Citing numerous precedents for accepting this approach, the committee majority therefore concluded that Corbin had been duly elected.

In a minority report, the three committee Democrats argued that the matter had been finally settled by the Senate's decision in November 1877 to seat Butler, since the body had also reviewed information from Corbin at that time. Since then, Corbin had presented no new facts, and there were thus no grounds for reopening the inquiry. They stressed as crucial the point that the Mackey house did not have a quorum of all 124 house members when it elected Corbin.

Having been in the Senate for more than a year, Butler had accumulated sufficient support among his colleagues that, on February 25, 1879, a resolution to consider the report of the committee failed on a vote of 25 to 36, and he retained his seat.

Conclusion

Corbin's claim suffered not only from the narrowness of the Republican margin in the Senate but also from the backlog of cases that prevented the Privileges and Elections Committee from moving promptly to investigate the election, thus providing the opportunity for Butler's supporters to discharge the matter from committee and press for an immediate Senate vote. The Senate debate then focused on Butler's fitness to serve, depending on what his role had been in the Hamburg massacre, rather than directly on the election. Only when Corbin subsequently insisted, did the committee carefully examine the events of the election. By the time the committee majority decided that Corbin had in fact been elected, the Senate was unwilling to reopen the matter.

On February 28, 1879, David Corbin withdrew his claim to the seat, and on March 3 he was reimbursed $10,000 for his expenses in contesting the election. In 1882, the Senate granted M.C. Butler $3,500 to cover the costs of his defense. Butler served in the Senate until 1895. Upon completion of his senatorial career, he practiced law in Washington, D.C. and then participated in the Spanish American War. Butler died in Washington in 1909.

Sources

U.S. Congress. Senate. *Congressional Record.* 45th Cong., 1st sess. (See pp. 556–59, 571–81, 603–05, 638–714, 730–40.) 2d sess. (See pp. 235–36.)

———. Senate Report No. 707. 45th Cong., 3d sess., 1879.

Coté, Richard N. ed. *Dictionary of South Carolina Biography.* Vol. 1. Easley, S.C., 1985. (See p. 72.)

Foner, Eric. *Reconstruction: America's Unfinished Revolution, 1863–1877.* New York, 1988. (See pp. 570–72.)

Johnson, Allen, ed. *Dictionary of American Biography.* Vol. 3. New York, 1946; reprint of 1935 edition. (See pp. 363–64.)

Case 67

L. Q. C. Lamar

(1825–1893)

Mississippi

Election Case
March 5, 1877 to March 6, 1877

Issues
Reconstruction: challenge to legislature's authority to elect; electoral misconduct: voter intimidation

Result: Seated

Chronology:
Resolution submitted: Mar. 5, 1877
Senate vote: Mar. 6, 1877

Background

In 1862, L.Q.C. Lamar withdrew from the United States House of Representatives to serve as a colonel and diplomat for the Confederacy. In 1873, his political disabilities removed, Lamar returned to the House. There, on the death of Charles Sumner in 1874, Lamar delivered a brilliant eulogy honoring the late Radical Republican that did much to heal sectional wounds. On the other hand, Lamar was also a leader in the 1875 Mississippi campaign in which the Democrats, by both wooing and intimidating black voters, succeeded in regaining control of the state. This "Mississippi plan" of carefully orchestrated violence and fear served as a model for the next year's winning Democratic campaign in South Carolina (See Case 66). In 1876, Lamar was easily elected to a United States Senate seat as a Democrat.

Statement of the Case

Even though the Civil War had been over for a dozen years by March 1877, no former high-level official of the Confederacy had yet been admitted to the U.S. Senate. When L.Q.C. Lamar arrived to take his seat, George Spencer (R-AL) sought to prevent his admission. To demonstrate that Lamar drew his credentials from an illegal legislature, Spencer proposed to read the report of a select committee from the previous Congress regarding "force, fraud, and intimidation" in the 1875 Mississippi election. The spontaneous response of "Oh, no!" from his colleagues made clear the waning congressional interest in the progress of Reconstruction.

Response of the Senate

When Allen G. Thurman (D-OH) urged that Lamar should be seated, since his credentials were in order, Oliver H.P.T. Morton (R-IN), chairman of the Privileges and Elections Committee, balked. He recalled that, in identical circumstances the previous year, Thurman had insisted that Louisiana's black Republican senator-elect, Pinckney B. S. Pinchback, not be seated until his credentials had been reviewed by the committee (See Case 63). Thurman objected that there was a major difference between the two cases: "the defect in Pinchback's case was that, according to the testimony . . . that body which elected Pinchback was not the Legislature of Louisiana." Countering that "the Legislature that chose Mr. Lamar was not a lawful Legislature," Morton charged that "from my knowledge of what took place in Mississippi in 1875 it presented a field of carnage; that that election was a fraud from beginning to end, the most monstrous fraud that was ever practiced in this country."

Spencer prevailed in his proposal, and the clerk began to read descriptions of the 1875 campaign to terrorize black voters in Mississippi. The few senators remaining in the chamber heard the testimony that had been received from several black women about the whippings and murders of their husbands. At one point, John Gordon (D-GA) interrupted the litany of fear and intimidation to point out that no one was listening, but Spencer insisted that the reading continue. When the clerk finished, the Senate debated the matter briefly before voting 57 to 1, with 12 members absent, to seat L.Q.C. Lamar. Among those voting to seat Lamar was his Mississippi colleague, Blanche K. Bruce, a black Republican, whose support proved influential with many Republicans. Even Oliver Morton voted with the majority, once he had made the point that Democrats had acted from partisanship rather than principle in the Pinchback case.

Conclusion

At the beginning of the Forty-fifth Congress, the Senate was confronted with a number of other electoral challenges (See Cases 63, 66, 68, and 69) related to the end of Reconstruction. The perfunctory attention given to the Lamar case, even in the face of outrages committed in Mississippi, demonstrated the Senate's weariness with the entire question of violence and disorder in the former Confederate states.

A talented and skillful politician, Lamar served in the Senate until 1885, when he resigned to become secretary of the interior for President Grover Cleveland. In 1887 Cleveland appointed him associate justice of the United States Supreme Court, where he served until his death in 1893.

Sources

U.S. Congress. Senate. *Congressional Record.* 45th Cong., spec. sess. (See pp. 5–15.)

Blaine, James G. *Twenty Years of Congress.* Norwich, CT, 1886.

Burger, Nash K., and John K. Bettersworth. "Artificer of Reconciliation." In *Mississippi Heroes,* ed. Dean F. Wells and Hunter Cole. Jackson, MS, 1980.

Malone, Dumas, ed. *Dictionary of American Biography.* Vol. 9. New York, 1946; reprint of 1935 edition. (See pp. 551–54.)

Murphy, J. B. *L.Q.C. Lamar: Pragmatic Patriot.* Baton Rouge, LA, 1973.

Case 68

John T. Morgan

(1824–1907)

Alabama

Election Case
March 5, 1877 to March 8, 1877

Issues
Reconstruction: challenge to legislature's authority to elect

Result: Seated

Chronology:
Resolution submitted: Mar. 5, 1877
Senate vote: Mar. 8, 1877

Background

As the Reconstruction era drew to a close, Alabama Democrats effectively solidified their position in the state government. The party took advantage of the infighting among Republicans to gain control of political institutions throughout the state. Although the Senate had taken three years to resolve an earlier contested Alabama election during Reconstruction (See Case 62), there was far less difficulty in 1877 when the state sent to Washington John T. Morgan (D), a former general in the Confederate army.

Statement of the Case

On March 5, 1877, an objection was raised to seating John Morgan, and his credentials were ordered to lie on the table. The protest came from Alabama's other senator, Republican George E. Spencer, who charged that in 1876 state Democrats had succeeded in altering apportionment, setting registration requirements, and changing election laws in ways that effectively disenfranchised Republicans and black voters.

Response of the Senate

On March 8, Spencer again took the floor to deplore the government's indifference in failing to protect the rights of black people. He concluded forcefully, "Let the Senate of the United States, by its rejection of this applicant, give to the . . . good citizens of Alabama . . . the assurance that . . . the color line, the conflict of race, will rapidly disappear to be replaced by political issues which will tend only to the improvement and the happiness of the people."

While agreeing with Spencer that the 1876 election had been fraudulent, Oliver H.P.T. Morton (R-IN), chairman of the Privileges and Elections Committee, explained that he could not support Spencer because, in his judgment, Morgan had a sound prima facie case and therefore, according to

Senate precedents, should be seated. Any questionable matters could be investigated subsequently. Morton nevertheless quoted extensively from an investigative report the senators had received that morning that had uncovered widespread fraud in the Alabama election. He wryly noted that, if the current investigation received the same response the Senate had given to a similar report on 1873 voting frauds in Louisiana, Morgan would not be seated. Recognizing the changed mood of the Senate, however, he acknowledged Morgan's clear claim to the seat. The Senate agreed by voice vote, and Morgan was sworn in.

Conclusion

The seating of John T. Morgan marked the end of a particularly vitriolic era in Senate debate, the Reconstruction of the southern states. The composition of the Senate was changing, and a new generation of senators was turning its attention to other matters.

John Morgan belonged to the new era. A powerful advocate of American expansionism who fought to build a canal across Central America, he served in the Senate until his death in 1907.

Sources

U.S. Congress. Senate. *Congressional Record.* 45th Cong., spec. sess. (See pp. 24–31.)

Malone, Dumas, ed. *Dictionary of American Biography.* Vol. 13. New York, 1946; reprint of 1935 edition. (See pp. 180–81.)

V. Gilded Age: 1878–1900

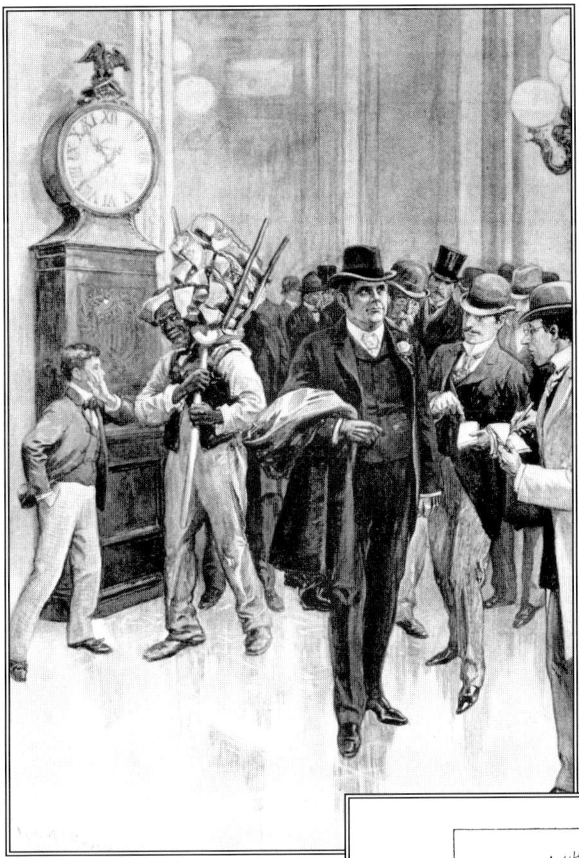

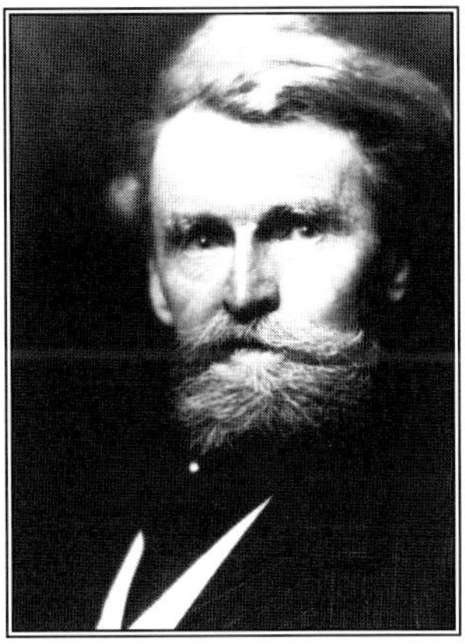

William A. Clark
(Cases 78, 89)
Library of Congress

Marcus A. Hanna *(Case 86)*
U.S. Senate Collection

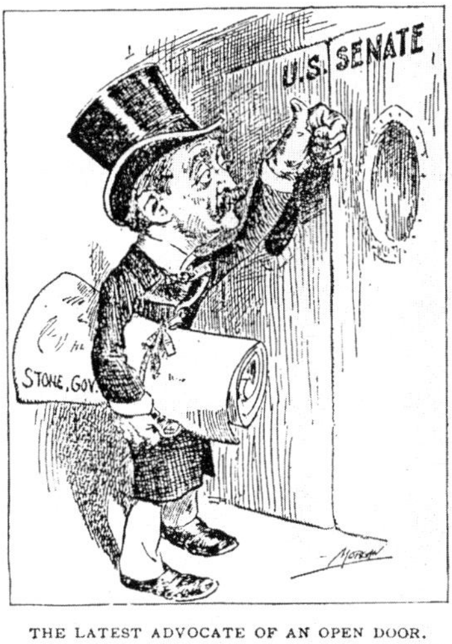

THE LATEST ADVOCATE OF AN OPEN DOOR.

MR. QUAY (to himself): "I wonder if the fellows will remember that I am on record against this sort of thing."—*The Times-Herald*, *Chicago.*

Matthew Quay *(Case 88)*
The Literary Digest, May 6, 1899

Case 69

La Fayette Grover

(1823–1911)

Oregon

Election Case
March 7, 1877 to June 15, 1878

Issues
Electoral misconduct: allegations of bribery and corruption

Result: Retained seat

Chronology:
Petition presented: Mar. 7, 1877
Referred to committee: Mar. 17, 1877
Committee report: June 15, 1878
No Senate action

Background

When the 1876 Samuel J. Tilden-Rutherford B. Hayes presidential contest failed to produce a victor, partisans of both sides feverishly attempted to manipulate electoral votes in several pivotal states, one of which was Oregon. There, Democratic Governor La Fayette Grover cooperated with plans to assist Tilden, his party's candidate. Using some technical pretext, Grover disqualified a Republican elector and substituted a Tilden man on the state's electoral commission. In a complex series of events, which included the illegal delivery of voting lists and certificates of election, the Democrats established a fraudulent electoral commission and cast their votes for Samuel Tilden. Ultimately, a national electoral commission voided the unlawful proceedings and gave the three Oregon votes to Hayes, but the role played by Governor Grover left bitter feelings among many Oregon citizens.

Statement of the Case

When La Fayette Grover was elected to a term in the Senate to begin March 4, 1877, his opponents in Oregon immediately prepared formal protests. Before Grover could be sworn in, his Oregon colleague, John H. Mitchell (R) presented a petition charging the senator-elect with bribery and corruption to secure his office. The petition also alleged that Grover had lied to the Senate's Committee on Privileges and Elections about granting the certificate of appointment to the substitute presidential elector.

Democratic and Republican senators alike, weary of the constant investigations of credentials, resisted denying Grover his seat. Even staunch Republican Roscoe Conkling (NY) called for Grover's admission. During the debate on March 8, 1877, he pointed out that there was a prima facie case for seating Grover and conducting any investigation afterwards. Oregon met all the conditions: the state was in the Union and had a single legislature that had carried out the election for U.S. senator; there was one undisputed governor who had issued unchallenged credentials to the senator-elect; and there was no question regarding the individual's qualifications. The Senate agreed that Grover should be seated, and he took the oaths of office that day.

On March 9, Grover asked the Senate to investigate the charges against him. A reluctant Senate, convinced the investigation would be both time-consuming and expensive, finally voted on March 17 to send the matter to the Committee on Privileges and Elections. It authorized the committee, if necessary, to send a subcommittee to Oregon to collect testimony and spend up to $10,000 for that purpose.

Response of the Senate

On June 15, 1878, the committee report reaffirmed the hesitancy members voiced fifteen months earlier when Grover requested the investigation. The committee stated that it found no evidence to sustain the charges against Grover. Concurring in this view, Eli Saulsbury (D-DE), a member of the subcommittee that had held hearings in Oregon, added a statement including some of the testimony to demonstrate that it vindicated Grover.

Apparently convinced that no evidence had been found to support the charges, the Senate took no further action on the matter.

Conclusion

La Fayette Grover completed his Senate term in 1883 and returned to the practice of law. He died in 1911.

Sources

U.S. Congress. Senate. *Congressional Record.* 45th Cong., spec. sess. (See pp. 22–23, 31–39, 42–46.)

———. Senate Report No. 540. 45th Cong., 2d sess., 1878.

Blaine, James G. *Twenty Years of Congress.* Norwich, CT, 1886.

Johnson, Allen, and Dumas Malone, eds. *Dictionary of American Biography.* New York, 1946; reprint of 1935 edition. (See p. 29.)

Case 70

Stanley Matthews

(1824–1889)

Ohio

Censure Case
June 5, 1878, to March 1, 1879

Issues
Allegations of corruption before Senate term

Result: Not censured

Chronology:
Request for investigation: June 5, 1878
Referred to committee: June 5, 1878
Committee report: Mar. 1, 1879
No Senate action

Background

The contested 1876 Rutherford B. Hayes-Samuel J. Tilden presidential election left in doubt the critical electoral votes from three states, among them Louisiana. Soon after the November election, with a political stalemate threatening the future of the country, both Republicans and Democrats sent influential citizens to observe the counting of disputed votes in the pivotal three states. Ohio Republican Stanley Matthews was selected, along with other political luminaries, to travel to New Orleans to supervise the vote counting for presidential electors, amid wheeling and dealing by both parties. When the election was still undecided by February 1877, Congress established a special bipartisan electoral commission, composed of five senators, five representatives, and five Supreme Court justices. Stanley Matthews served as counsel before the commission on behalf of Rutherford B. Hayes, who was ultimately declared to have been elected president.

Subsequently, in March 1877, the Ohio legislature elected Matthews to the United States Senate to fill a vacancy in the term ending March 3, 1879, and he took his seat without incident.

Statement of the Case

On June 5, 1878, Stanley Matthews asked the Senate to investigate allegations that, during his stay in New Orleans, he had acted in a fraudulent manner or had offered illegal rewards to any official in exchange for a Republican vote during the electoral count. The Senate agreed to Matthews' request and established a select committee of four Republicans and three Democrats to look into the matter. The allegations against Matthews stemmed from charges made by a Louisiana citizen, James E. Anderson, testifying in the House of Representatives. Anderson claimed that Matthews had offered him a government job in return for concealing his fraudulent actions in the presidential election.

Response of the Senate

The select committee was frustrated in its efforts to take direct testimony from Anderson. At his first appearance on June 13, 1878, he presented a note from the chairman of the House committee, asking that he be excused because he was needed at hearings in that body. When summoned on a second occasion, Anderson refused to give any evidence because the committee denied him the right to have counsel present. The obdurate Anderson turned aside every question and would not even give his age or occupation. Despite the rising agitation his stubborn demeanor caused among committee members, he then dared to bargain for his testimony. Anderson offered to cooperate if, in turn, Stanley Matthews would testify before the House committee. Indignant that Anderson should attempt to negotiate terms for his testimony, the committee members were doubly annoyed because the Senate had adjourned the previous day, leaving the committee without the power to cite Anderson for contempt.

When the committee again turned its attention to the inquiry in December 1878, it received a wire from Anderson in Nevada stating that he would testify if summoned. The committee instead decided to obtain a transcript of Anderson's House testimony and to examine Stanley Matthews in person. In contrast to Anderson's evasiveness, Matthews cooperated fully. He recalled every detail of his brief stay in New Orleans and recounted his conversations with clarity and precision. He said he hardly knew Anderson and had agreed to recommend him for a federal post, such as customs officer or consul, simply as a kind gesture to someone in need. Anderson told him he had been active as a loyal Republican over several years in Louisiana but had somehow incurred the enmity of party leaders in the state, forcing him to seek other employment. According to Matthews, Anderson did not say that he had committed illegal acts on behalf of the Republican cause in Louisiana or ask for any reward for such acts. He did, however, give to Matthews for safekeeping a document he had prepared that falsely described such illegal acts, having changed his mind about using it to threaten a local official. Matthews had provided the document to the House committee investigating Anderson's charges.

On March 1, 1879, the select committee reported to the Senate on the Matthews investigation. It unanimously found that Matthews had "no connection with any real or supposed frauds in the election in Louisiana" and had not engaged in any corrupt conduct. The committee did, however, call Matthews' efforts to obtain federal employment for Anderson in spite of his apparently questionable character "wrong and injurious to the public interest." The Senate, anxious to waste no further time on the 1876 election intrigues, took no action on the matter.

Conclusion

Stanley Matthews' Senate term ended two days after the committee reported. In 1881 President James A. Garfield appointed him to the Supreme Court, but the appointment encountered considerable Senate opposition because of Matthews' close ties to corporations and railroad interests. He was eventually confirmed by a vote of 24 to 23 and served on the Court until his death in 1889.

Sources

U.S. Congress. Senate. *Congressional Record.* 45th Cong., 2d sess. (See p. 4119.)

———. Senate Report No. 867. 45th Cong., 3d sess., 1879.

Malone, Dumas, ed. *Dictionary of American Biography.* Vol. 11. New York, 1946; reprint of 1935 edition. (See pp. 418–20.)

Urofsky, Melvin I. *The Supreme Court Justices: A Biographical Dictionary.* New York, 1994.

Case 71

Charles H. Bell

(1823–1893)

New Hampshire

Election Case (appointment)
March 18, 1879 to April 10, 1879

Issues
Right of governor to make appointment to a term not previously filled by a legislature

Result: Seated

Chronology:
Credentials presented: Mar. 18, 1879
Referred to committee: Mar. 19, 1879
Committee report: April 2, 1879
Senate vote: April 10, 1879

Background

In 1878, New Hampshire adopted a new state constitution that became effective in October of that year. As a result, the state conducted elections for two legislatures in one year: the first chosen in March 1878 to serve from June 1878 to May 1879; the second elected in November 1878 to serve from June 1879 to June 1881. During the Forty-fifth Congress, New Hampshire officials asked the United States Senate for an advance ruling on which of these legislatures would have the authority to select a senator. The Committee on Privileges and Elections declared and the Senate agreed that under the 1866 election law only the legislature chosen in November 1878 could elect a senator, since it would be the legislature elected "next preceding the expiration" of the senatorial term. This decision led to controversy in the Senate when one New Hampshire senator's term expired on March 3, 1879, three months before the legislature elected in November was due to meet in June. To fill the vacancy until the legislature could convene and hold an election, the state's governor appointed Charles H. Bell (R).

Statement of the Case

Charles Bell's credentials were presented to the Senate on March 18, 1879, on the first day of the new Forty-sixth Congress. In a Senate under Democratic control for the first time in nearly twenty years, William Wallace (D-PA) promptly challenged the legitimacy of the New Hampshire Republican's claim. Wallace argued that the governor had acted incorrectly when he appointed Bell to a vacancy caused by the expiration of a term of office.

Supporters and opponents of the claimant prepared to dissect all previous Senate cases where gubernatorial appointment had been made after a vacancy occurred. George F. Hoar (R-MA), a member of the Committee on Privileges and Elections, suggested that, since members appeared to know the details of each earlier challenge, the Senate might save time by keeping the matter out of committee and devoting one day to floor debate on the subject. The Senate ignored his efforts at efficiency and sent the credentials to committee on March 19.

Response of the Senate

On April 2, the Committee on Privileges and Elections reported that Charles Bell was not entitled to his seat. The new Democratic majority described the committee's advisory ruling in the previous Congress when the Republicans controlled the Senate as "not important in the settlement of the question now presented." The majority argued that the power of a governor to make a temporary appointment was limited to vacancies in a term that had already been filled by the legislature. This precedent, they asserted, was established in the 1825 case of James Lanman (See Case 12) and observed by the Senate in all subsequent cases. The Republican minority sharply disagreed, contending that the history of the Senate supported a governor's right to appoint when a legislature was unable to convene and that the intent of the U.S. Constitution was that vacancies should be filled. The only occasion that deviated from this interpretation, the minority continued, was the case of James Lanman cited by the majority. Although that case was so shrouded in confusion that members could not identify through available records the motivations behind the 1825 decision, one key point in the debate had been that the governor made the appointment before the vacancy actually occurred. That one case aside, the minority report argued, all precedents upheld the governor's appointment of Bell.

The reading of the reports launched a lengthy and heated floor debate, as members rehashed each earlier case of gubernatorial appointment. Former Supreme Court Justice David Davis (I-IL) argued for following the precedent in the Lanman case. He observed that, according to the memoirs of Thomas Hart Benton, who was in the Senate at the time, the Senate had ruled that governors could only fill unexpected vacancies. "It could not apply to a foreseen event bound to occur at a fixed period," Benton wrote. "Here the vacancy was foreseen; there was no contingency in it. It was regular and certain."

On April 10, after two long days of debate, Committee Chairman Eli Saulsbury (D-DE) once more restated the majority's view that a governor could not make an appointment to a term the legislature had not yet filled by election. He stressed that this was an important constitutional point that should be recognized as precedent for future Senate action. On the other hand, he declared that during the debates he had developed a high regard for the character, respectability, and intelligence of Charles Bell. He also observed that, because of the substantial Democratic majority in the Senate, seating the Republican Bell would be of little political consequence.

Saulsbury therefore, while retaining his opinion about the policy issue, encouraged his colleagues in this case to accept the governor's appointment. With an ambiance of magnanimity established, a few Democrats joined with Republicans to seat Bell by a vote of 35 to 28.

Conclusion

In the first Congress since the Civil War to have both houses controlled by Democrats, the majority party could afford to be generous. Democrats outnumbered Republicans by nine in the Senate, and Bell did not pose a serious threat, for he would serve only for three months until the legislature met and elected a successor. He returned to New Hampshire, becoming governor in 1881. He died in 1893.

Sources

U.S. Congress. Senate. *Congressional Record.* 46th Cong., 1st sess. (See pp. 2–3, 184–89, 273–98, 312–25, 341–55.)

———. Senate Report No. 1. 46th Cong., 1st sess., 1879.

Johnson, Allen, ed. *Dictionary of American Biography.* Vol. 1. New York, 1946; reprint of 1935 edition. (See pp. 153.)

Case 72

John J. Ingalls

(1833–1900)

Kansas

Election Case
March 19, 1879 to February 17, 1880

Issues
Electoral misconduct: charges of bribery and corruption

Result: Retained seat

Chronology:
Memorial received: Mar. 19, 1879
Referred to committee: Mar. 19, 1879
Committee report: Feb. 17, 1880
Senate vote: Feb. 17, 1880

Background

Although Kansas entered the Union in 1862, the internal organization of the state was not completed until 1888. Hotly disputed contests over the establishment of county seats and the marking of county borders kept political excitement high and affected all the business of the state legislature, including the selection of United States senators. After helping the Republicans win the 1878 legislative election, incumbent Senator John J. Ingalls (R) returned to Washington to await the outcome of the January 1879 senatorial election.

Statement of the Case

When Ingalls won a narrow victory, his opponents charged election fraud. On March 19, 1879, the day after Ingalls took his oath for a second term, the Senate received a memorial from one faction of the Kansas legislature protesting irregularities in the January election. The Senate referred the matter to the Committee on Privileges and Elections. Late in March, the committee received a report from the Kansas legislature on an investigation it conducted into the election. Armed with that material, the committee asked for and received authorization to carry out its own investigation. Ingalls then withdrew as a member of that committee, and the remaining members began the time-consuming task of summoning witnesses.

Response of the Senate

A brief Senate debate on the Ingalls case took place in January 1880, after several witnesses had been arrested and brought to the Senate chamber for failing to respond to the committee's summons. All three frontier residents were quickly relieved of charges of contempt when they explained their failure to appear earlier as due either to family emergencies or the fact that great distances and poor communications had delayed delivery of the summons.

Finally, on February 17, 1880, the committee reported on the testimony gathered, both in Washington and at a subcommittee hearing in Topeka. Witnesses had described bribes and blackmail arranged at the Topeka Tefft House, a favorite meeting spot for Kansas politicians. The tales of clandestine rendezvous among drunken legislators who schemed for Ingalls' election echoed the misconduct charges leveled in 1872 against then-Senator Samuel C. Pomeroy, which had led the legislature to choose Ingalls in that election (See Case 61). The committee majority stated that, while "bribery and other corrupt means were employed" in 1879 by those favoring Ingalls, no witness could conclusively tie Ingalls to the irregularities, and there was no proof that the questionable deals had altered the election results. A minority report agreed but added that Ingalls should be exonerated more forcefully, since the whole matter smacked of a plot to defeat the senator by falsely incriminating him. The Senate approved the majority report by voice vote that same day.

Conclusion

In 1882 the Senate adopted a resolution reimbursing Ingalls for the expenses of his defense.

Perhaps reflecting the prevailing view of Kansas elections, John Ingalls a decade later made the widely quoted statement in an 1890 newspaper interview: "The purification of politics is an iridescent dream. Government is force. Politics is a battle for supremacy.... The Decalogue and the Golden Rule have no place in a political campaign. The object is success." Renowned for his acid tongue, John Ingalls continued to serve in the Senate until 1891, the last four years as president pro tempore. He died in 1900.

Sources

U.S. Congress. Senate. *Congressional Record.* 46th Cong., 2d sess. (See pp. 234–41, 415.) 3d sess. (See pp. 814–15.)

———. Senate Report No. 277. 46th Cong., 2d sess., 1880.

Williams, Burton J. *Senator John James Ingalls: Kansas' Iridescent Republican.* Lawrence, KS, 1972.

Case 73

Elbridge G. Lapham and Warner Miller

(1814–1890) (1838–1918)

New York

Election Case
October 10, 1881 to December 13, 1881

Issues
Election irregularities

Result: Retained seats

Chronology:
Credentials presented: Oct. 10, 1881
Referred to committee: Dec. 8, 1881
Committee report: Dec. 12, 1881
Senate vote: Dec. 13, 1881

Background

Republican party infighting, halted temporarily for the 1880 presidential election, surfaced almost immediately when the victorious James A. Garfield in March 1881 seized control of patronage appointments from machine bosses. The president's actions particularly incensed Roscoe Conkling (R-NY) who, having supported Ulysses S. Grant against Garfield in the Republican convention, saw a bitter enemy appointed as collector of the port of New York. In fury, Conkling and his New York colleague Thomas C. Platt (R) decided to protest Garfield's disregard for the time-honored patronage system of "senatorial courtesy" by resigning from the Senate on May 16, 1881. Conkling convinced Platt that the New York legislature would support their gesture and rebuke Garfield by immediately returning them to the Senate. The once mighty Conkling, however, had misread the temper of his own state assembly, which deadlocked on the vote until the fifty-sixth ballot. Much to the embarrassment of Conkling and Platt, the legislature in July 1881 finally chose two members of the U.S. House of Representatives, Elbridge G. Lapham (R) to fill Conkling's seat and Warner Miller (R) for Platt's.

Statement of the Case

The fierce New York struggle moved to the Senate when the Conkling forces in the legislature submitted a memorial protesting the seating of Elbridge Lapham and Warner Miller during a special session on October 11, 1881. Despite a list of five specific charges against them, the Senate permitted the two to take their oaths of office without delay. Ten days later, the complainants submitted a second protest, charging procedural infractions in the election process and personal corruption by Lapham and Miller.

At the start of the regular session on December 8, 1881, the Senate referred the petitions to the Committee on Privileges and Elections.

Response of the Senate

Four days later, on December 12, Benjamin H. Hill (D-GA), who had been a bitter antagonist of Conkling's, presented a brief oral report in which the committee upheld the validity of the New York election. Hill explained that none of the three procedural charges, relating to the date of the election and questions regarding the quorum, had sufficient merit to invalidate the balloting. Since no evidence supported the charges of bribery and corruption, the committee also dismissed the request for an investigation of Lapham and Miller.

Without debate, the Senate on December 13, 1881, discharged the committee from further consideration of the matter.

Conclusion

In his anger, Roscoe Conkling had outsmarted himself. He retired from public life and practiced law in New York City until his death in 1888. Thomas Platt, who foolishly went along with Conkling's plan, returned to the Senate in 1897 and served until 1909. He died in 1910.

Elbridge Lapham served until the conclusion of his term in 1885. He died in 1890. Thomas Platt managed to prevent Warner Miller from being reelected to the Senate in 1886, but Miller remained active in state politics. He died in 1918.

Sources

U.S. Congress. Senate. *Congressional Record.* 47th Cong., spec. sess. (See pp. 70–71.)

Jordan, David M. *Roscoe Conkling of New York: Voice in the Senate.* Ithaca, NY, 1971.

Malone, Dumas, ed. *Dictionary of American Biography.* Vol. 11. New York, 1946; reprint of 1935 edition. (See p. 641.)

Case 74

Henry W. Blair

(1834–1920)

New Hampshire

Election Case
March 9, 1885 to March 10, 1885

Issues
Right of governor to make appointment to a term not previously filled by a legislature

Result: Seated

Chronology:
Credentials presented: Mar. 9, 1885
Senate vote: Mar. 10, 1885

Background

In 1878, New Hampshire changed its state constitution, creating some confusion in the procedure for selecting United States senators. In 1879, the Senate (then controlled by the Democrats) debated and resolved issues regarding the gubernatorial appointment of New Hampshire Senator Charles Bell (R) (See Case 71). When Henry W. Blair (R), who was elected in 1879 to replace Bell, was appointed by the governor in 1885 to fill a vacancy at the beginning of the new term, the Senate (now under Republican control) again debated essentially the same questions.

Statement of the Case

Henry Blair's first term expired on March 3, 1885, but the legislature was not due to meet until June. On March 9, he presented credentials for an appointment by the governor to serve for the three months until the legislature could convene and hold an election. George G. Vest (D-MO), who had opposed seating Bell, immediately protested that the earlier New Hampshire case had been decided incorrectly. He moved that the Committee on Privileges and Elections be charged to consider whether a governor had the right to fill a vacancy, not during a term but at the beginning of a senatorial term.

Response of the Senate

Republicans quickly responded that the identical issue had been resolved in the 1879 Bell case and that Blair had a prima facie claim and should be seated. Democrats, on the other hand—even some who had voted to seat Bell in 1879—now insisted that the issue was important enough to be reviewed.

George F. Hoar (R-MA) became the Republican champion in the debate, insisting that everyone understood that the governor's power of appointment did not encompass the full term but lasted only until the next session of the legislature. He suggested that the real strategy behind the attempts to postpone Blair's oath was to create an interruption in his senatorial service so that he would lose the position on committees that he had earned by his previous service.

Convinced by Hoar's arguments, the Senate then defeated the motion to refer to committee and, by a vote of 36 to 20, admitted Blair on March 10, 1885.

Conclusion

On June 17, the New Hampshire state legislature met and reelected Henry Blair to the full term ending in 1891. A supporter of education, woman suffrage, and disarmament, Blair after his Senate service practiced law in Washington, D.C. He died in 1920.

Sources

U.S. Congress. Senate. *Congressional Record.* 49th Cong., spec. sess. (See pp. 4–6, 16–26.)

Johnson, Allen, ed. *Dictionary of American Biography.* Vol. 1. New York, 1946; reprint of 1935 edition. (See pp. 334–35.)

Case 75

Henry B. Payne

(1810–1896)

Ohio

Election Case
April 27, 1886 to July 23, 1886

Issues
Electoral misconduct: charges of bribery and corruption

Result: Retained seat

Chronology:
Request for investigation: April 27, 1886
Referred to committee: May 11, 1886
Committee report: July 15, 1886

Background

In the 1880s, three strong-willed Ohio Republicans—Senator John Sherman, Governor Joseph B. Foraker, and party boss Marcus Alonzo Hanna—warily sparred with each other for state and national influence. The state's Democrats took advantage of the simmering rivalries to capture control of the state legislature in 1884. When deposed Republicans saw they had no chance to elect one of their own in the coming senatorial election, several threw their support to Democratic candidate Henry B. Payne, whose protectionist tariff policies meshed well with Republican fiscal goals.

Statement of the Case

On March 4, 1885, Henry Payne appeared and without challenge took his oath in the United States Senate. After the next Ohio election, majority control of the legislature swung back to the Republicans, who instigated an inquiry into charges that bribery and corruption were used in securing the Democratic nomination for Payne over the then-incumbent Democratic senator, George H. Pendleton. On April 27, 1886, one group of Ohio legislators submitted their committee's report to the U.S. Senate with a request for a full investigation into Henry Payne's 1884 election. The Senate referred the matter to the Committee on Privileges and Elections on May 11. Additional materials submitted by the legislature during the month of May were also referred to the committee.

Response of the Senate

On July 15, the committee returned three reports to the Senate. Two of these, although for different reasons, concluded that there was no basis for a Senate investigation. The majority report, signed by the four Democrats on the committee, noted that the original legislative committee report submitted in April simply transmitted to the Senate the testimony received, without including any specific charge. Then in May the legislature sent an additional resolution to the effect that, since "charges of bribery must be directly made" in order for the Senate to investigate, the legislature stated that the charges of corruption were true. The committee questioned the long delay between Payne's election and the submission of charges that had been common knowledge for more than two years. Since there was no question about either the Ohio legislature's authority to elect or the validity of Payne's credentials, the members feared that any credence the Senate gave to such "naked, unsupported charges" would only pave the way for future accusations and persecutions by any personal or political enemy of any senator. In the committee's view, "to deprive a sitting member of the Senate of his seat, the Senate must be satisfied by legal evidence that he was personally guilty of" or "had personal knowledge of" the bribery. After examining the testimony provided, the Senate committee found no evidence "personally inculpating" Henry B. Payne or justifying further investigation by the Senate.

The second report, signed by three committee Republicans, concurred with the first but observed that a senator could be deprived of his seat if evidence showed that the number of votes tainted by bribery was sufficient to have affected the outcome of the election, even if the member himself was not personally involved. The report added that, if bribery had occurred, it was up to the Ohio state government to seek indictments; yet, after interrogating fifty-five witnesses, the state had sought no further action against either Payne or other possible culprits. One author of this report, John A. Logan (R-IL), explained during floor debate that, in several previous cases where election bribery was charged, the Senate had refused to hold its own inquiry unless the legislature had already investigated the actions of its members, found evidence of wrongdoing, and prosecuted those responsible. As precedents, he cited the case of Humphrey Marshall in 1795 (See Case 3), that of Lewis Bogy (See Case 65), and the more recent cases of John J. Ingalls (See Case 72) and Elbridge Lapham and Warner Miller (See Case 73). Logan concluded by blaming an irresponsible press for making reckless, slanderous charges against many prominent politicians.

The minority report, signed by two other Republicans, conceded that the investigation by the Ohio legislature failed to find any evidence that the briberies had changed the election results but argued that the Senate should conduct its own investigation. During debate, Ohio's Republican senator John Sherman and committee members George F. Hoar (R-MA) and William P. Frye (R-ME) stressed the Senate's responsibility to ensure that justice was not denied either to Payne or to the people of Ohio. In fact, Sherman expressed surprise that Payne himself had not asked for an investigation. On the question of jurisdiction, Sherman contended that only the Senate could determine whether sufficient votes had been affected by bribery to invalidate the election. Of particular interest among the charges was one that Oliver H. Payne, a tycoon of Standard Oil Company and son of the embattled senator, had observed that his father's election had cost him $100,000. When Hoar brought the minority arguments to the floor debate, he urged a full investigation, declaring, "I will not say that the adoption of this majority report will be a disgraceful fact; that would not be parliamentary or courteous or proper; but I do say . . . it will be the most unfortunate fact in the history of the Senate."

On July 23, 1886, the Senate disagreed with Hoar's assessment, voting 44 to 17 to drop any further investigation of Payne. Fifteen Republicans joined with 29 Democrats in opposing a Senate inquiry.

Conclusion

Henry Payne continued to serve in a Senate that was increasingly dominated by businessmen and the friends of corporate interests. He completed his term in 1891 and died four years later.

Sources

U.S. Congress. Senate. *Congressional Record.* 49th Cong., 1st sess. (See pp. 3861, 4118, 7251–72, 7308–29, 7350–61.)

———. Senate Report No. 1490. 40th Cong., 1st sess., 1886.

———. Senate Miscellaneous Documents No. 106 and 141. 49th Cong., 1st sess., 1886.

Malone, Dumas, ed. *Dictionary of American Biography.* Vol. 8. New York, 1946; reprint of 1935 edition. (See pp. 325–26.)

Case 76

David Turpie

(1828–1909)

Indiana

Election Case
February 10, 1887 to May 15, 1888

Issues
Electoral misconduct

Result: Retained seat

Chronology:
Memorial submitted: Feb. 10, 1887
Referred to committee:
Feb. 16, 1887; Dec. 6, 1887
Committee report: May 14, 1888
Senate vote: May 15, 1888

Background

David Turpie's public career encompassed an era of national turbulence. In 1863, Indiana sent Turpie to the Senate as a replacement for Jesse Bright, expelled for his political indiscretion during the Civil War (See Case 40). After his brief Senate service, Turpie returned to Indiana, where he held a variety of state posts during the disorders of Reconstruction. In 1887, Indiana, a state that had seen its share of political party infighting and factionalism, sent Democrat David Turpie to the United States Senate for a second time.

Statement of the Case

On February 10, 1887, before the beginning of Turpie's term, members of the Indiana legislature submitted a memorial protesting his election. When Turpie's credentials for a term to begin March 4 were presented six days later, the Senate referred both sets of papers to the Committee on Privileges and Elections. The committee, however, asked to be discharged from consideration of the matter until it was reconstituted at the beginning of the new Congress, since the credentials and protest related to a Congress not yet in session. The Senate agreed.

On December 6, 1887, at the opening of the Fiftieth Congress, David Turpie appeared and was sworn in. That same day, his opponents filed a new protest, and all papers in the Turpie case were referred to the Committee on Privileges and Elections. The Indiana protest claimed that a lawfully elected Republican state senator had been ejected from the Democratic-controlled body and replaced by a Democrat for the express purpose of guaranteeing Turpie's election, and that a second ineligible Democratic legislator had voted in the election. According to Turpie's opponents in the legislature, the participation in the vote by illegally chosen members should invalidate Turpie's election.

Response of the Senate

On May 14, 1888, the committee issued a report in favor of Turpie, stating that even if the charges were true they were not sufficient to invalidate the election, since "the body in question was the constitutional senate of Indiana." In the floor debates, George F. Hoar (R-MA), the committee chairman, rejected the Indiana arguments. Hoar made a distinction between a case like the recent one of Henry Payne in 1886 (See Case 75), in which there were allegations of bribery and corruption in the election itself, and the present situation, where the question related to the makeup of the state legislature. Although in the Payne case Hoar had argued in vain that the Senate had a duty to investigate the charges of electoral corruption, in the current case he believed that the U.S. Senate had no right to determine who could cast a vote in the legislature. Henry Teller (R-CO) supported Hoar, adding, "It does not lie in the power of the Senate . . . [and] it never was intended by the framers of this Government that that question of the right of members of the Indiana State Legislature to sit in either body there would ever be a subject of discussion in this body."

On May 15, 1888, the Senate agreed. By voice vote, it discharged the committee from further consideration of the matter and dropped the inquiry.

Conclusion

In its report, the committee specifically did not preclude the Senate from refusing to admit a senator elected by "a legislative body which is itself the result of fraud or crime, which has overcome the true will of the people." If such a case were to arise, it would be "dealt with on its own merits." Such circumstances, of course, had occurred during the Reconstruction cases of the 1860s and 1870s, when the Senate did in fact scrutinize the composition of certain southern state legislatures to determine whether they met the criteria established in the Reconstruction acts. By the 1880s, however, Reconstruction was over, and the Senate would generally seat the senator chosen, as long as an election was carried out by a recognized state legislature according to the procedures set forth in the 1866 election act.

David Turpie retired from the Senate in 1899 and died in 1909.

Sources

U.S. Congress. Senate. *Congressional Record.* 49th Cong., 2d sess. (See pp. 1564, 2474.)

———. *Congressional Record.* 50th Cong., 1st sess. (See pp. 4145–47.)

———. Senate Report No. 1291. 50th Cong., 1st sess., 1888.

Case 77

Daniel B. Lucas v. Charles J. Faulkner

(1836–1909) (1847–1929)

West Virginia

Election Case
December 5, 1887 to December 14, 1887

Issues
Qualifications: whether the Senate should consider other than the constitutionally mandated qualifications to serve; challenge to legislature's authority to elect

Result: Faulkner seated

Chronology:
Credentials presented: Dec. 5, 1887
Referred to committee: Dec. 12, 1887
Committee report: Dec. 14, 1887
Senate vote: Dec. 14, 1887

Background

On March 5, 1887, West Virginia Governor E. W. Wilson called the state legislature into special session to consider a specific agenda. The governor's list of items to be covered did not include the selection of a United States senator, a task the assembly had failed to complete in its previous session. On the same day that he summoned the special meeting, Governor Wilson named Daniel B. Lucas, a poet, playwright, and staunch Democrat, to serve an interim term in the U. S. Senate until the next session of the West Virginia legislature.

Statement of the Case

When the Senate convened on December 5, 1887, two claimants appeared for the West Virginia seat. The first credentials presented were those of Daniel Lucas, followed by those of Charles J. Faulkner, also a Democrat, who was elected by the West Virginia legislature on May 5, 1887, during the special session. The governor signed Faulkner's credentials, indicating that he had only appointed Lucas for the interim before the legislature could elect. Lucas, however, protested Faulkner's claim, arguing that at the time of his May election Faulkner held a state judgeship. Under the West Virginia constitution, such a position would prevent his assuming any other political office, although he resigned from the position on the day he was elected to the Senate. Lucas also claimed that the legislature was not empowered to hold an election because the state's constitution precluded a legislature called by the governor from conducting any business not specifically listed in the agenda for the special session.

Because the conflicting credentials represented a challenge to the legality of the election and because one candidate might be disqualified, the Senate refused to seat either claimant until it resolved the matter. On December 12, 1887, the Senate referred the credentials and petitions to the Committee on Privileges and Elections, which promised to act promptly on the case.

Response of the Senate

Two days later, the committee returned a unanimous report favorable to Faulkner. The committee determined that West Virginia's constitutional limitation on the matters a legislature could deal with during a governor's special session restricted only state and not federal business. According to the committee, state law had no power to prohibit a legislature from carrying out a duty imposed by the U. S. Constitution, which specified that the legislature should fill a vacancy at its next meeting. Additionally, the committee interpreted West Virginia's restriction on the political offices that could be held by a justice to apply only at the state level. Any other interpretation, the committee argued, would allow a state to add to the U.S. Constitution's eligibility requirements for a United States senator, which the Senate had rigorously guarded since its formation. In support of this view, the committee cited the Senate's decision to the same effect in the 1855 case of Lyman Trumbull (See Case 28).

Without debate, the Senate agreed by voice vote that Charles Faulkner was entitled to his seat, and he came forward to take the oath of office.

Conclusion

On December 20, 1887, Charles Faulkner offered a resolution seeking compensation for Daniel Lucas, and on January 25, 1888, the Senate agreed to pay Lucas $1,000 for his expenses in contesting the seat.

In the Senate, Faulkner chaired the Committee on Territories. When he retired in 1899, he returned to the practice of law. He died in 1929.

Sources

U.S. Congress. Senate. *Congressional Record.* 50th Cong., 1st sess. (See pp. 1–5, 53, 54.)

———. Senate Report No. 1. 50th Cong., 1st sess., 1887.

Hinds, Asher C. *Hinds' Precedents of the House of Representatives of the United States.* Vol. 1. Washington, DC, 1907, sec. 632.

Johnson, Allen, and Dumas Malone, eds. *Dictionary of American Biography.* Vol. 5. New York, 1946; reprint of 1935 edition. (See p. 299.)

Malone, Dumas, ed. *Dictionary of American Biography.* Vol. 11. New York, 1946; reprint of 1935 edition. (See pp. 483–84.)

Case 78

William A. Clark v. Wilbur F. Sanders
(1839–1925) (1834–1905)

Martin Maginnis v. Thomas C. Power
(1841–1919) (1839–1923)

Montana

Election Case
January 16, 1890 to September 30, 1890

Issues
Challenge to legislature's authority to elect (rival legislatures)

Result: Power and Sanders seated

Chronology:
Credentials presented: Jan. 16, 1890
Referred to committee: Jan. 16, 1890
Committee report: Mar. 24, 1890
Senate vote: April 16, 1890

Background

The organization of the Montana state government and the selection of the first United States senators was marked by acute political strife, with charges of residency violations, fraudulent counting procedures, and drunken melees at polling places. Controversy over the makeup of the state legislature after the 1889 state election, in turn, cast doubt upon the legitimacy of senatorial credentials.

Statement of the Case

On January 16 and 23, 1890, the Republican-controlled Senate received credentials for two contesting pairs of newly elected Montana senators, Republicans Wilbur F. Sanders and Thomas C. Power and Democrats William A. Clark and Martin Maginnis, the latter of whom had served six terms as Montana's territorial delegate to Congress. At the core of the problem lay the existence of two legislative delegations from Silver Bow County—the copper-mining area around Butte—each claiming the right to sit in the Montana state assembly and participate in the selection of senators. Well acquainted with the intricacies of state legislative disputes, the Senate quickly referred all the Montana papers to the Committee on Privileges and Elections. At the same time, without discussion or objection, the Senate granted floor privileges to all four claimants.

Response of the Senate

The committee returned its report to the Senate on March 24, 1890. The committee's majority favored the seating of Republicans Wilbur F. Sanders and Thomas C. Power. The report explained that two bodies, each claiming to be Montana's lawful house of representatives, had held separate elections for the state's first U.S. senators. One house—consisting of Republicans—had met with half the senate and elected Sanders and Power. The other body—made up of Democrats—had met in a different location with the other half of the senate and elected Democrats William A. Clark and Martin Maginnis. Each body was made up of representatives whose credentials were unchallenged, plus five who claimed to represent Silver Bow County. The legitimacy of the bodies thus turned on whether the Republican or Democratic Silver Bow claimants had been properly elected, and specifically on the validity of the election in the county's precinct 34, a camp on a railroad line under construction. If the vote there was fair and proper, the five Democratic legislators were elected, but if the election was fraudulent and the votes from the precinct were thrown out, the winners were the Republican candidates. The county board of Silver Bow had excluded all the votes from that precinct as tainted, but a single judge later ruled that the votes should be counted. The dispute resulted in the two groups of five contesting legislators.

During its inquiry, the committee encountered a tangle of political misconduct that included voting by unnaturalized aliens and secret rather than public ballot counting. It therefore rebuked the new state for the "lawless and revolutionary methods" employed in organizing the first state assembly but nonetheless upheld the legitimacy of the Republican contingent from precinct 34. Although tempted to refuse to seat any of the claimants as a way of teaching the state a lesson and displaying its disapproval of the rowdy conduct, the majority decided that these would be inappropriate reasons for rejecting the claims of Sanders and Power.

The report of the minority and the ensuing floor remarks of its spokesman, David Turpie (D-IN), painted a different picture of the questionable events in Silver Bow County. The minority report stated that voters had been qualified, ballots cast, and votes counted in an entirely proper manner in precinct 34. The problem began, the minority believed, when the Republican-controlled board of county commissioners illegally ordered the returns from that precinct excluded from the count. If these votes had been included, the five Democratic legislators would have been elected. Since these legislative contestants had participated in the legislature that elected Clark and Maginnis, the minority contended that the Democratic senators should be seated.

The debate continued through March and into April. At one point, on April 9, Turpie launched a scathing attack on Republican contestant Thomas

Power, charging that the Montana politician had bartered with the canvassing judges to have the votes from Silver Bow County disqualified.[1] When angry Republicans urged a prompt vote, Democrats insisted on further delay to allow other members to speak. The debate thus dragged on for another week until April 16, when the members voted, 32 to 26, to seat Republicans Power and Sanders, who then came forward to take the oath of office.

Conclusion

In this case the Senate reaffirmed that when prospective senators appeared who claimed to have been elected by rival legislatures, neither should be sworn in on the basis that their credentials were prima facie evidence of election. Instead, all the contestants could be granted floor privileges until the resolution of the case.

Both William Clark and Martin Maginnis received compensation for their time and expenses. Power and Sanders each served only one term in the Senate. Sanders died in 1905 and Power in 1923. Clark subsequently served in the Senate in 1899 and from 1901 to 1907 (See Case 89).

Sources

U.S. Congress. Senate. *Congressional Record.* 51st Cong., 1st sess. (See pp. 2906–10, 2968–97, 3101–14, 3136–45, 3188–3200, 3228–49, 3279–92, 3378–94, 3419–35.)

———. Senate Report No. 538, 51st Cong., 1st sess. 1890.

Johnson, Allen, ed. *Dictionary of American Biography.* Vol. 4. New York, 1946; reprint of 1935 edition. (See pp. 144–46.)

Malone, Dumas, ed. *Dictionary of American Biography.* New York, 1946; reprint of 1935 edition. Vol. 12. (See p. 199.) Vol. 16 (See pp. 336–37.)

[1] Turpie's insulting remarks figured in a case three years later that appears in the 1972 Election book as Case 95 but is not included here because the matter was not referred to committee and the Senate took no action. In March 1893, Democrats angered by Republican attacks on one of their number hinted they planned to investigate Turpie's old charges against Power. Although the Montana senator demanded an investigation to clear his name, the Senate preferred to drop the matter.

Case 79

George L. Shoup and William J. McConnell
(1836–1904) (1839–1925)

William H. Clagett v. Fred T. Dubois
(1838–1901) (1851–1930)

Idaho

Election Case
December 29, 1890 to March 3, 1892

Issues
Election irregularities; form of credentials

Result: Dubois retained seat

Chronology:
Credentials presented: Dec. 29, 1890
Referred to committee: Dec. 29, 1890
Committee report: Jan. 5, 1891
Credentials presented: Dec. 7, 1891
Referred to committee: Dec. 8, 1891
Committee report: Feb. 2, 1892
Senate vote: Mar. 3, 1892

Background

In December 1890, the first legislature for the new state of Idaho convened to vote for two United States senators. When the legislature appeared deadlocked, one of the candidates, Fred T. Dubois (R), inquired of the Senate Judiciary Committee whether the state would be permitted to elect three senators, one to fill a very brief term ending March 3, 1891, one to succeed him in that seat for the full term, and one to serve either a two- or a four-year term. The committee chairman agreed to this approach, and negotiations began among the candidates to determine who would fill which seat. Ultimately, the legislature chose Republicans George L. Shoup and William J. McConnell to draw lots between the six-week and four-year terms. The legislature then elected Dubois to replace whoever drew the short term.

Statement of the Case

Although Shoup, who had been the state's first governor, signed the qualifying credentials for himself and the other two senators, the Senate raised no objections on that point and focused instead on whether the Idaho legislature had inappropriately tried to anticipate the Senate's action regarding the classes of the two new senators. When, on December 29, 1890, the credentials for Shoup and McConnell were presented, the Senate referred them to the Committee on Privileges and Elections but also permitted George Shoup, who was present, to be sworn in. A week later on January 5, 1891, the committee returned a brief, favorable report recommending that William McConnell also be sworn in. McConnell, having arrived in Washington, came forward and was seated as the second Idaho senator.

When the two drew lots to determine the length of term, Shoup won the four-year term, while McConnell was assigned to the brief term due to conclude on March 3, 1891.

On December 30, 1890, Fred T. Dubois had presented his credentials for the full term to begin on March 4, 1891, which were also referred to the Committee on Privileges and Elections. The committee quickly responded that the Senate did not consider matters for a future Congress and recommended that Dubois' papers be placed on file. On January 10, 1891, a memorial arrived from some Idaho legislators, contending that Dubois should not be seated and questioning whether a state legislature could elect a new senator before the Senate had determined when a term ended. The Senate referred this document to the Committee on Privileges and Elections.

In February 1891, the Idaho legislature held a second vote and selected Republican William H. Clagett to fill the term beginning March 4, 1891. The stated reason for the second election was that the Senate would ultimately challenge the validity of Dubois' election, but an equally crucial factor was the insistance on representation in the Senate by the mineral-rich northern portion of the state, which had little in common with the agricultural south.

Response of the Senate

The Senate did not turn its attention to the contest between Clagett and Dubois until the latter appeared to claim his seat on December 7, 1891, at the beginning of the regular congressional session. Members, agreeing that Dubois' credentials appeared in order, admitted him on December 8 but referred the credentials of both claimants to the Committee on Privileges and Elections.

On February 2, 1892, the committee returned a bipartisan majority report favorable to Fred Dubois, with a resolution denying Clagett's claim. The majority ruled that Dubois had been legally elected and that his election predated Clagett's. A minority report submitted by two Democratic committee members, on the other hand, agreed with Clagett's assertion that the Idaho legislature had not been organized until Tuesday, December 9, 1890, rather than Monday, December 8. Thus, under the 1866 election law requirement that a Senate election be held "on the second Tuesday after the meeting and organization" of a legislature, the election should not have been held on Tuesday, December 16, but a week later. The committee's majority rejected this claim, since at the time of the election no protest was lodged in the legislature that the body was not sufficiently organized to conduct business. The first indication of a question had appeared in the January 10 memorial received by the Senate, followed in February by adoption of a legislative resolution stating that a new election would be held, because the election of Dubois might not be valid.

During the debate that followed, the Senate granted Clagett a seat on the floor and two hours to defend his claim. Given his opportunity to speak,

Clagett asserted that he knew much about the admission process because, during his long life on the frontier, he had assisted with the entry of many new states. Despite his promise that this experience gave him a keen appreciation for the elements and purposes in the transformation from territorial to state government, Clagett only droned on about party pledges and trickery in Idaho. Dubois, from his advantageous position of sitting senator, reviewed the state legislature's 1890 decision to elect three senators at once, an action he insisted the assembly thought had several precedents.

On March 3, 1892, the Senate voted that Fred Dubois should retain his seat. The lengthy floor debate ultimately had required the Senate to rule on several related points.

- In the case of Shoup, the Senate, without objection, accepted credentials signed by a governor certifying his own election.
- The Senate did not delay the seating of McConnell and Shoup, even though the state assembly's joint convention proceedings were not included in the credentials but submitted separately.
- The Senate examined the credentials of McConnell and Shoup because of a question about which vacancy was to be filled in the assignment of classes to senators from the newly admitted state.
- In the case of Clagett and Dubois, the Senate ruled, in response to a point of order, that an amendment offered to a resolution to declare a member entitled to a seat is out of order if the amendment consists merely of a declaration of principles and does not state whether a contestant is or is not elected.
- This was one of the very few occasions on which the Senate granted a claimant who had not been seated the opportunity to present his case on the Senate floor.

The Senate also reiterated its traditional rulings on two other points: the Senate would not act upon credentials presented before the beginning of the Congress to which they apply but would simply place them on file; and the Committee on Privileges and Elections would examine federal and state constitutions and statutes to determine whether a state legislature was properly organized at the time of a senator's election.

Conclusion

One month later in April 1892, the Committee on Privileges and Elections recommended that William Clagett receive $4,000 and Fred Dubois $2,000 for expenses in prosecuting their claims to the Idaho seat.

In 1895 Clagett again unsuccessfully sought election to the United States Senate.

Fred Dubois lost his bid for reelection as a Silver Republican in 1896 but won in 1901 and then became a Democrat and served until 1907. From 1924 until his death in 1930, he served as a member of the commission that worked to prevent water boundary disputes between the United States and Canada.

McConnell remained in the Senate only until March 3, 1891, and then served four years as governor of Idaho. He subsequently held a post with the U.S. Immigration Service until his death in 1925.

George Shoup was reelected in 1894 and served in the Senate until 1901. He died in 1904.

Sources

U.S. Congress. Senate. *Congressional Record.* 51st Cong., 2d sess. (See pp. 843–48.)

———. *Congressional Record.* 52d Cong., 1st sess. (See pp. 1175–1202, 1229–44, 1384–1401, 1430–32, 1445–48, 1473–86, 1538–51, 1584–98, 1622–36, 1665–77.)

———. Senate Report No. 1904. 51st Cong., 2d sess., 1891.

———. Senate Report No. 1905. 51st Cong., 2d sess., 1891.

———. Senate Report No. 148. 52d Cong., 1st sess., 1892.

Lauterbach, Margaret. "A Plenitude of Senators." *Idaho Yesterdays* 21 (Fall 1977): 2–8.

Malone, Dumas, ed. *Dictionary of American Biography.* Vol. 9. New York, 1946; reprint of 1935 edition. (See p. 131.)

Case 80

Robert H. M. Davidson v. Wilkinson Call

(1832–1908) (1834–1910)

Florida

Election Case
December 7, 1891 to February 4, 1892

Issues
Conduct of election

Chronology:
Credentials presented: Dec. 7, 1891
Referred to committee: Dec. 8, 1891
Committee report: Jan. 25, 1892
Senate vote: Feb. 4, 1892

Result: Call retained seat

Background

In 1865 the Florida legislature elected Wilkinson Call (D) to the United States Senate; but the Senate, caught in the first confusion of early Reconstruction policies, denied him admission, and the state remained unrepresented in the Senate until 1868. When Florida again selected the former Confederate adjutant general in 1879, a more amenable Senate, willing to forget his Civil War service, seated Call.

Statement of the Case

Wilkinson Call's second term expired March 3, 1891, and on May 26 of that year the Florida legislature reelected him for the term that had begun on March 4.

On December 7, 1891, Call's credentials were presented, as were those of Robert H. M. Davidson (D), a former member of the U.S. House of Representatives, for the same seat. Davidson's supporters contended that, when the assembly voted for Call, fewer than a quorum of the members of one house had been present for the joint session. Considering that no valid election had taken place, the governor had appointed Davidson to fill the vacancy.

The Senate hesitated only a day before deciding upon its course of action. It permitted Wilkinson Call to take his seat and sent the credentials of both claimants to the Committee on Privileges and Elections.

Response of the Senate

On January 25, 1892, the committee returned a unanimous report stating that Call had been properly elected by the legislature and was entitled to his seat. Davidson had challenged the election on the ground that a quorum of the state senate was not present at the time of the election. The committee pointed out that, under the 1866 act governing Senate elections, the joint assembly of the two houses was a separate body to consist of "'a majority of all the members elected to both houses' without any reference to a quorum" of either house. Fifty-two of the 100 members of the Florida legislature were present and voted. Of these, 51 voted for Call, making a majority of the members of both houses. The committee therefore determined that, since the legislature had in fact elected Call, no vacancy existed for the governor to fill.

In the Senate debate on February 4, 1892, William E. Chandler (R-NH) presented a lengthy argument defending the constitutionality of the 1866 election statute. Following a discussion regarding various provisions of that law that did not relate to the present case, the Senate agreed with the committee that Wilkinson Call had been properly elected and should retain his seat.

Conclusion

In March 1892, the Senate agreed to pay Robert Davidson $1,250 for expenses he incurred while contesting the seat.

Wilkinson Call served in the Senate until 1897 and then returned to Florida to practice law. He died in 1910.

Sources

U.S. Congress. Senate. *Congressional Record.* 52d Cong., 1st sess. (See pp. 2–4, 512, 833–46.)

———. Senate Report No. 106. Parts 1 and 2. 52d Cong., 1st sess., 1892.

Case 81

Horace Chilton

(1853–1932)

Texas

Election Case (appointment)
December 7, 1891 to January 27, 1892

Issues
Challenge to governor's authority to appoint before vacancy occurred

Chronology:
Credentials presented: Dec. 7, 1891
Referred to committee: Dec. 7, 1891
Committee report: Jan. 25, 1892
Senate vote: Jan. 27, 1892

Result: Retained seat

Background

Early in 1891, Texas Senator John H. Reagan (D) resigned his seat, effective June 10, 1891. Upon receipt of that resignation, the state's governor, J.S. Hogg, appointed Tyler lawyer Horace Chilton (D) to fill the vacancy. Chilton, a Texas native and former newspaper publisher, presented himself to the Senate on December 7, 1891.

Statement of the Case

Although the Senate immediately seated Chilton, his credentials were challenged by George F. Hoar (R-MA). Hoar agreed that Chilton clearly had a prima facie right to the seat but questioned whether a governor could make an appointment before the effective date of a senator's resignation. Chilton's credentials bore the date April 25, 1891, but Reagan had not vacated his seat for another several weeks. At Hoar's request, the Senate referred the matter to the Committee on Privileges and Elections.

Response of the Senate

On January 25, 1892, the committee, composed of five Republicans and four Democrats, returned a unanimous report favorable to Horace Chilton. The committee had reviewed several similar cases that had occurred in earlier congresses and found six precedents related to the Chilton appointment. In three of these cases, the appointees were admitted without question. In the other three—Uriah Tracy of Connecticut in 1801 (See Case 6), James Lanman of Connecticut in 1825 (See Case 12), and Ambrose Sevier of Arkansas in 1836 (See Case 16)—a question was raised. Tracy and Sevier were seated, while Lanman was refused admission. The Lanman case was particularly perplexing because Senate records and contemporary documents did not fully clarify the basis for the Senate's decision. It was unclear whether Lanman was not seated because the governor had acted in advance of the actual vacancy or because a governor could not fill a vacancy at the beginning of a new senatorial term. This question had been extensively discussed during Senate consideration of the 1879 case of Charles H. Bell (See Case 71) and the Senate had decided the motivation in the Lanman case was too unclear to make it useful as a precedent. As a result, the committee concluded that these earlier unclear circumstances freed the 1892 Senate from any binding precedents.

Committee member George Hoar reversed his earlier objections, explaining that he had thought previous cases had indicated a governor could not make such an appointment but the committee had found this was not the case. He spoke sympathetically about the hardships inflicted on the distant western states if an executive was forced to wait until an actual vacancy before naming a replacement. In recent years, he noted, the Senate had generally resolved such doubtful questions in ways that would keep the body's seats full. For the good of the public interest, therefore, Hoar recommended that Chilton be permitted to retain his place. He cited the case of Bell and the 1885 case of Henry W. Blair (See Case 74), in both of which the Senate had decided that a governor could fill a vacancy at the beginning of a senatorial term if the legislature had failed to elect.

Eugene Hale (R-ME) asked whether a change in state executives between a resignation and its effective date would possibly place two claimants, each named by a different governor, before the Senate. Samuel Pasco (D-FL) added a yet more complicated hypothetical problem that might develop between the governor and the state legislature. Hoar swept aside their objections, asserting that they worried about dilemmas that might occur once in a thousand years. A rare contingency, Hoar concluded, should not dictate the usual.

On January 27, 1892, the Senate agreed that, if a senator resigned effective on some future date, a governor could anticipate the vacancy and name a replacement. Horace Chilton remained in the Senate.

Conclusion

Chilton served until a successor was elected in March 1892. Then, in 1894, the Texas legislature elected him to a full six-year term. After leaving the Senate in 1901, Chilton practiced law in Texas. He lived until 1932.

Sources

U.S. Congress. Senate. *Congressional Record.* 52d Cong., 1st sess. (See pp. 3, 510–11, 576–78, 635.)

———. Senate Report No. 105. 52d Cong., 1st sess., 1892.

Hinds, Asher C. *Hinds' Precedents of the House of Representatives of the United States.* Vol. 2. Washington, DC, 1907. (See sec. 1228.)

Case 82

John B. Allen	Asahel C. Beckwith	Lee Mantle
(1845–1903)	(1827–1896)	(1851–1934)
Washington	**Wyoming**	**Montana**

Election Case (appointment)
March 9, 1893, to August 28, 1893

Issues
Right of governor to make an appointment to a term not previously filled by a legislature

Result: Not seated

Chronology:
Credentials presented: Mar. 9, 1893
Referred to committee: Mar. 20, 1893
Committee report: Mar. 27, 1893
Senate vote: Aug. 28, 1893

Background

In the 1890s, economically strapped western and southern farmers turned to the Populist party in an effort to enhance their political influence. The party's power fragmented state politics in the West by cutting into both Democratic and Republican strongholds. As a result, three western states—Washington, Montana, and Wyoming—adjourned their regular legislative sessions without managing to elect a United States senator for the term beginning on March 4, 1893. In each of these states, the governor proceeded to name an individual to fill the vacant Senate seat until the next meeting of the legislature. In the meantime, the country was struggling with the economic chaos created by the Panic of 1893.

Statement of the Case

On March 9, 1893, Lee Mantle (R-MT) presented his credentials to the Senate. He was followed on March 15 by Asahel C. Beckwith (D-WY) and on March 20 by John B. Allen (R-WA), who had been serving as a senator since his state's admission to the Union in 1889 but failed to be reelected because of a deadlock in the legislature. The Senate seated none of the three westerners and referred the credentials to the Committee on Privileges and Elections. Once again, the Senate questioned the right of a state executive to appoint a senator when the legislature had failed to elect. Since the three claimants were appointed under essentially identical circumstances, the Committee on Privileges and Elections handled the cases as one action.

Response of the Senate

On March 27, 1893, a bipartisan majority of the committee returned favorable reports on the three claims. The reports upheld the power of a governor to appoint if the legislature had failed to elect a senator, on the constitutional principle that a state was entitled to be fully represented in the Senate. On the other hand, the committee's minority, also made up of both Republicans and Democrats, contended that a governor had no right to make an appointment at the beginning of a Senate term even if the legislature had not elected during its session.

The Senate debate on the contested appointments began on March 29 and continued throughout April. Then, during the extraordinary session of Congress called in August 1893 by President Grover Cleveland to consider repeal of the Sherman Silver Purchase Act, the subject was again discussed. The lengthy arguments employed by both sides reiterated many of the points covered in earlier discussions of a governor's right to appoint, including analysis of the constitutional intent of the founding fathers, discussion of parallel situations in the executive branch, and dissection of every previous Senate appointment by a governor.

On this issue, the divisions were closely tied to the demonetization of silver and thus were chiefly sectional, rather than running along party lines. In general, easterners supported the president's call for repeal of the Sherman Silver Purchase Act, believing that, if the government stopped buying silver, the drain on the nation's gold supply would be eased, helping to alleviate the panic. Those from southern and western states tried to block the change, so that the government would continue buying silver for coinage. It was generally expected that, if the three western senators were admitted, at least some of them would vote against repeal. The conflict severely split the Democratic party, but Republicans too were divided on the issue.

During August, temperatures and tempers mounted as both sides charged each other with "winding and turning and . . . splitting of hairs." George F. Hoar (R-MA), champion of the contestants, eloquently argued that the Senate would corrupt popular liberty and republican government if it disregarded its own precedents, which clearly favored the seating of the three. Opponents of admitting the claimants denied that the 1879 case of Charles Bell (See Case 71) had set a new precedent for accepting senators appointed by a governor at the beginning of a term, since in that case the legislature had not met and failed to elect, as in the western cases, but rather was not scheduled to convene until several months after the term began. In responding to a suggestion by Orville H. Platt (R-CT) that admitting the claimants could lead to some future hypothetical corrupt bargain with a governor, Hoar asked what corrupt influence could be greater than that which "will be brought to bear on the minds of the members of this body to seat or unseat men who have a rightful title to seats here according as they expect they will vote one way or the other on some exciting question pending." In spite of his impassioned conclusion, "I should feel myself degraded . . . if I voted to keep them out because I do not like the votes they are expected to give," Hoar did not prevail.

On August 28, 1893, the Senate voted, 32 to 29, to deny Lee Mantle and John Allen their seats. Asahel Beckwith had withdrawn his claim on July 11, 1893, but on September 19 was granted $2,000 for his expenses. That same day, the Senate agreed that both Mantle and Allen should receive $2,500 in compensation for their expenditures.

Conclusion

Some senators continued to suspect that Mantle, Beckwith, and Allen had been turned away for political rather than constitutional reasons. On September 27, 1893, Fred T. Dubois (R-ID) expressed concern that his western neighbors would not have full Senate representation during crucial silver and tariff discussions. He therefore submitted a resolution to postpone the votes on certain national financial issues until January 1894, in order to give the three states time to fill their vacant Senate seats. Despite his plea, the Senate took no action on his resolution, and each of the three states had only one senator from March 1893 to early 1895. In fact, the three additional silver votes would have made no difference to at least one issue, for at the conclusion of a western filibuster, the Senate on October 30 voted, by a comfortable margin of 43 to 32, to repeal the Sherman Silver Purchase Act.

Of the three contestants, only Lee Mantle returned to the Senate, elected by the legislature in January 1895 to fill the remainder of the disputed term. In 1896, during his Senate term, he organized and became chairman of the Silver Republican party but returned to the Republican party in 1900. An unsuccessful candidate for renomination in 1899, he entered the real estate and mining business in Butte, Montana. He died in 1934.

John Allen practiced law in Seattle until his death in 1903.

Asahel Beckwith continued his coal-mining and stock-raising businesses in Wyoming. He died in 1896.

Sources

U.S. Congress. Senate. *Congressional Record.* 53d Cong., spec. sess. (See pp. 15, 20, 33, 38–66, 68–74, 75–79, 80–89, 93–96.) 1st sess. (See pp. 198, 225, 289–90, 332–37, 393, 421–29, 676–89, 994–96, 1048, 1238, 1300–1301, 1569, 1776–77, 1828–38.)

———. Senate Reports No. 1, 2, and 3. 53d Cong., spec. sess., 1893.

———. *The Senate, 1789–1989: Addresses on the History of the United States Senate,* by Robert C. Byrd. S. Doc. 100–20. 100th Cong., 1st sess. Vol. 1, 1988. (See pp. 351–54.)

Case 83

Joseph W. Ady v. John Martin

(dates unknown) (1833–1913)

Kansas

Election Case
April 3, 1893 to February 28, 1895

Issues
Challenge to legislature's authority to elect (rival legislatures); Senate ruled on point of order

Result: Martin retained seat

Chronology:
Memorial received: April 3, 1893
Referred to committee: April 3, 1893
No Senate action
(floor debate Feb. 28, 1895)

Background

Kansas politics remained in turmoil long after the state's admission to the Union. Counties viciously competed with each other to attract settlers, and rival railroads openly connived for control of politicians, especially during unsettled political periods like Reconstruction or the Populist agitation of the 1890s. Thus, the predictable clashes erupted over the selection of a replacement for Republican Senator Preston B. Plumb, who died on December 20, 1891. Gubernatorial appointee Bishop W. Perkins (R) filled the seat for a year until the Kansas legislature, on January 25, 1893, finally managed to elect Democrat John Martin to the vacancy. Martin entered the Senate at the beginning of the Fifty-third Congress when the body was under Democratic control for the first time since 1881.

Statement of the Case

On March 4, 1893, John Martin presented credentials for the two years remaining in Plumb's term. Since his papers were in order, the Senate admitted him without objection, although George F. Hoar (R-MA) raised the possibility of a contest when he noted, "If there be any question as to his title upon the merits, the Senate can deal with it afterwards." On April 3, a memorial from Joseph W. Ady, claiming to be the duly elected senator, arrived and was referred to the Committee on Privileges and Elections. A few weeks later, seventy-seven members of the Kansas legislature filed a memorial that alleged the use of illegal procedures in John Martin's election and asserted that Joseph W. Ady was the correctly chosen candidate. The Senate directed the Committee on Privileges and Elections to investigate the charges.

Response of the Senate

The committee did not consider the Martin matter either during the brief special session of the Senate or during the extraordinary session of Congress that President Grover Cleveland called in the summer of 1893 to repeal the Sherman Silver Purchase Act. By March 1894, both Martin and Ady had provided the committee with records and other materials supporting their claims, but action was further delayed by the prolonged illness and death in April of Committee Chairman Zebulon B. Vance (D-NC), followed by a lengthy Senate adjournment from August to December. When the committee finally did consider the matter on January 29, 1895, the majority voted to postpone the case indefinitely. Infuriated by the extensive delay, and with only five weeks remaining in the disputed term, William E. Chandler (R-NH) on January 31 attempted to jar the matter loose. In the midst of Senate debate on an appropriation bill, he offered a privileged resolution that declared Kansas had no properly organized legislature at the time of Martin's election. When a point of order was raised, Vice President Adlai E. Stevenson ruled that the motion was not privileged and thus could not interrupt the business at hand; and the Senate sustained the decision.

On February 28, 1895, Chandler again raised the issue, chronicling the complicated events that surrounded the 1893 Kansas senatorial vote. When the Kansas legislature convened in January 1893, he explained, it consisted of a legal senate and two competing houses of representatives. Both the state senate and the governor recognized one of the houses, which joined with the senate in voting for Martin. In order to achieve a quorum, however, the presiding officer permitted two members of the rump house to vote but refused to accept the votes of the remaining members of that house. Out of this hodge-podge assemblage, John Martin received an undisputed majority of ballots. The rump house then held its own session and voted for Ady. Subsequently, the state supreme court ruled that the rump house was actually the legal one, and the other house disbanded. Chandler argued that these circumstances clearly indicated that Kansas had not had a properly organized legislature at the time of the election for U.S. senator.

In his intensely partisan speech, Chandler complained that the original Democratic Senate majority at the beginning of the Fifty-third Congress had been achieved by fraud and trickery. Again, objection was raised to Chandler's resolution as not being a privileged matter, but the Senate agreed to allow John Martin to respond and enter into the Congressional Record evidence in defense of his election. The angry Martin, however, used such bitterly intemperate language about the New Hampshire senator—saying that "he ought to be in the penitentiary" and calling him a "buzzard" who "vomited forth his filth on every occasion"—that the Senate had to cut short his remarks and formally call him to order.

There the matter rested. The Committee on Privileges and Elections produced no report on the question; the issue did not come to a floor vote; and John Martin retained his seat for the few days remaining in the term. The Senate did agree that Joseph Ady should receive $2,000 and John Martin $1,000 for their expenses in the contest.

Conclusion

Considerable partisanship was evident both here and in the simultaneous effort to unseat William N. Roach (D-ND) for actions before he entered the Senate,[1] because the narrow Democratic margin in the Senate appeared vulnerable. By the time of Chandler's February 1895 speech, deaths and other changes had brought enough Republicans into the chamber that unseating both Martin and Roach could have tipped the party balance. At that point, however, such machinations were hardly necessary, since the 1894 election had returned the Republicans to power in the new Senate that would convene on March 4, 1895.

John Martin, who chaired the Committee on Railroads during his brief Senate service, returned to Kansas and became clerk of the state supreme court. He died in 1913.

Sources

U.S. Congress. Senate. *Congressional Record.* 53d Cong., spec. sess. (See pp. 135, 139, 525.) 3d sess. (See pp. 1566–67, 2912–18, 2922–25.)

Lamar, Howard R., ed. *The Reader's Encyclopedia of the American* West. New York, 1977.

White, William Allen. *The Autobiography of William Allen* White. New York, 1946.

[1] The Roach incident appears in the 1972 Election book as Case 96 but is not included here because it never went to committee and the Senate took no action. A few weeks after William Roach entered the Senate in March 1893, Republicans urged the Senate to investigate newspaper reports that he had embezzled funds years earlier while working as a bank teller. The Senate declined to investigate.

Case 84

Henry A. du Pont

(1838–1926)

Delaware

Election Case
December 4, 1895 to March 1, 1897

Issues
Conduct of election; form of credentials; Senate refused to reverse previous action

Chronology #1:
Petition submitted: Dec. 4, 1895
Referred to committee: Dec. 4, 1895
Committee report: Feb. 18, 1896
Senate vote: May 15, 1896
Result: Not seated

Chronology #2:
Petition submitted: Jan. 12, 1897
Referred to committee: Jan. 12, 1897
Committee report: Mar. 1, 1897
No Senate action
Result: Not seated

Background

For months in early 1895, the Delaware legislature had been deadlocked among three Republican candidates in its effort to elect a United States senator. Then, on April 8, Delaware Governor Joshua Marvil died, throwing the state legislature into an election dispute involving Henry A. du Pont, railroad president and scion of that state's prominent entrepreneurial-political family. The central figure in the controversy proved not to be du Pont but William T. Watson, former speaker of the Delaware senate, who ascended to the governor's chair upon Marvil's demise. On May 9, 1895, Watson, claiming he had never given up his state senate seat when taking over the governorship, presided over and voted in the legislature's joint session, in an effort to defeat any Republican candidate for U.S. senator, of whom du Pont was the strongest. As a result, du Pont received 15 of the 30 votes cast in the joint assembly, one less than the majority needed for election. If Watson's vote against du Pont were disqualified, however, then du Pont had a majority of the 29 legitimate votes cast. Apparently believing this to be the case, one Republican senator declared du Pont elected.

Statement of the Case

On December 4, 1895, at the beginning of the Fifty-fourth Congress, supporters of Henry du Pont entered a petition on his behalf, claiming that he had been elected to the Senate for the term beginning March 4, 1895. Du Pont charged that Watson illegally performed dual functions, essentially destroying the traditional separation between the executive and legislative branches, when as governor he participated in the assembly's election.

Although du Pont possessed no credentials signed by the governor, he submitted a certificate of election signed by the speaker and the clerk of the Delaware house. Du Pont contended that he had won a majority vote if Watson's ballot was discounted. The Republican-controlled Senate referred du Pont's petition to the Committee on Privileges and Elections, together with several affidavits that arrived from Delaware during January 1896.

Response of the Senate

On February 18, 1896, a divided committee submitted its report. The Republican majority favored du Pont, holding that, since Watson's action violated both the Delaware constitution and U.S. laws, his vote should not count. Supporting du Pont's contention that he received a majority of the legally cast votes, the report declared that, of the two contradictory sets of evidence, the assembly's official journal entries of proceedings should take precedence over individual affidavits submitted by du Pont's opponents. The opponents contended that, before the senate entered the joint assembly for the U.S. Senate election, Watson had presided over legislative business and voted in the state senate on May 9 without any objection being raised. The journal, on the other hand, showed no such legislative action by Watson. Before the joint assembly adjourned, the legislators who had voted for du Pont had vigorously objected to Watson's participation in the vote, but Watson officially declared that the legislature had failed to elect a U.S. senator. While reaffirming a legislature's right to judge the qualifications of its own members, the committee majority ruled that the power was irrelevant in this case, because the Delaware constitution forbade an individual to serve simultaneously as governor and member of the legislature. The majority report also asserted that du Pont did not need a certificate of election signed by the governor since the speaker and clerk of the state house certified that he had received a majority of the legally cast votes.

The minority report, filed by the committee's Democratic members, specifically contended that the two offices of governor and state senator were not incompatible under the Delaware constitution, because Watson as senate speaker was only "exercising the office of governor" and did not become governor. As precedent the report cited the cases of three former senate speakers who had temporarily exercised the authority of governor and had then returned to the senate to complete their terms once a new permanent governor was chosen.

The report also stressed that it was the exclusive prerogative of the Delaware senate to determine the qualifications of its members and the U.S. Senate had no right to even consider the matter. Thus, since the Delaware constitution provided for 30 members in the combined houses of the legislature and 30 votes had been cast in the election, the United States Senate could not subtract the vote of one senator when nothing in the state record showed he had been judged unqualified by his own assembly.

In a Senate fiercely concerned with the delicate balance between parties and factions because of closely contested financial legislation, debates on the legitimacy of Republican Henry du Pont's claim proved lengthy and legalistic, as the floor orations continued for almost three months. The minute dissections of the Delaware constitution included repeated use of the terms "vacancy," "interim function," "devolving duty," and "exercise of office," yet when the matter came to a vote, the extensive constitutional analysis had done nothing to shift political loyalties. On May 15, 1896, by a party-line vote of 31 to 30, the Senate rejected du Pont's claim. Four Populists and one Silver party member joined with Senate Democrats to outvote the Republicans on the issue.

The case did not end there, however. On January 12, 1897, Henry du Pont brought his contest back to the Senate. In a new petition he charged that an error in the announced pairs in May 1896 had cost him a favorable decision and that the Senate had misunderstood the construction of the Delaware constitution. This petition went to the Committee on Privileges and Elections, which reported on March 1, 1897. Even though a majority of committee members still believed that the Senate should have seated du Pont, they did not find that there had been any mistake in counting the pairs. Since the claimant thus had no new evidence to present, the entire committee considered that the Senate's action in the case had been final. In a strong closing statement, the report cautioned the Senate to resist the temptation to reverse its own judgments or to vacate and award seats according to changing political majorities. The Senate took no action on the second report.

Conclusion

Du Pont's case, although unsuccessful for him, established several precedents. The Senate had agreed to investigate whether a claimant without credentials signed by the governor had a right to be seated. The committee determined that the journal of a state legislature showing that a candidate had been properly elected could serve as a substitute for such credentials. In addition, the committee ruled that, once the Senate had rendered a judgment in a case, the matter could only be reopened upon the submission of new evidence. During the debate, opponents of du Pont forcefully restated the principle that the Senate had no power to determine that a state legislator who was accepted by his own body could not vote in an election for U.S. senator.

In January 1898, the Senate awarded du Pont $1,855.45 for his expenses. At the conclusion of his case, he returned to his duties as as president and general manager of the Wilmington and Northern Railroad. In 1906 the legislature elected him to the United States Senate, where he served until 1917. Du Pont died in 1926.

Sources

U.S. Congress. Senate. *Congressional Record.* 54th Cong., 1st sess. (See pp. 29–30, 686, 956, 1065, 1096, 1675, 1781, 1827–61, 2419–38, 2477–85, 2595–2601, 2639–49, 2684–91, 2728–33, 2921–31, 3004–09, 3378–92, 3423–26, 3469–79, 3898–3912, 3943, 3954, 3981–96, 4031–39, 4768–72, 5169, 5226–36, 5286–96.) 2d sess. (See pp. 706, 1198–99, 1239–40, 2524–25.)

———. *Congressional Record*, 55th Cong., 2d sess. (See pp. 582–610, 720.)

———. Senate Report No. 289, 54th Cong., 1st sess., 1896.

———. Senate Report No. 1567, 54th Cong., 2d sess., 1897.

Hinds, Asher C. *Hinds' Precedents of the House of Representatives of the United States.* Vol. 1. Washington, DC, 1907. (See secs. 563, 564.)

Myers, Gustavus. *History of the Great American Fortunes.* New York, 1936.

Johnson, Allen, and Dumas Malone, eds. *Dictionary of American Biography.* Vol. 5. New York, 1946; reprint of 1935 edition. (See pp. 528–29.)

Case 85

Henry W. Corbett

(1827–1903)

Oregon

Election Case
March 15, 1897 to February 28, 1898

Issues
Right of governor to make an appointment to a term not previously filled by a legislature

Result: Not seated

Chronology:
Credentials presented: Mar. 15, 1897
Referred to committee: Mar. 15, 1897
Committee report: Jan. 26, 1898
Senate vote: Feb. 28, 1898

Background

In Oregon, the two major parties were closely matched from the state's admission in 1859 throughout the remainder of the nineteenth century, leading to frequent stalemates in the conduct of the state's business. This deadlock was particularly apparent during the 1897 meeting of the state legislature. When the contentious house finally achieved an organization on its second attempt, neither the senate nor the governor would recognize the body. The two legislative houses gathered in a futile and unproductive joint convention and were finally forced to disband without transacting any state business or electing a United States senator.

Statement of the Case

After the Oregon legislature dispersed, the governor appointed Henry W. Corbett (R), a successful entrepreneur who had served a term in the Senate from 1867 to 1873, to fill the vacant Senate seat. When Corbett presented his credentials on March 15, 1897, the Senate refused to seat him and referred his certificate, along with several related documents, to the Committee on Privileges and Elections. Once again, the Senate faced the issue of whether a governor could appoint a United States senator at the beginning of a term if the state legislature had failed to elect.

Response of the Senate

In the Fifty-fifth Congress, Republicans held a majority of ten in the Senate, but twelve members of three splinter parties, the Populists, Silver Republicans, and the Silver party, were sufficient to tip the balance against the mainstream Republicans on certain issues.

On January 26, 1898, a divided committee returned majority and minority reports. The committee's majority—made up of a Populist, a Republican, and several Democrats—opposed seating Henry Corbett, contending that the Oregon legislature "deliberately refused" to elect a U.S. senator. It also determined that the circumstances of Corbett's case were similar to those of several earlier claims, including that of Lee Mantle (See Case 82), in which the Senate had decided that the governor had no right to appoint when the legislature failed to complete an election at the beginning of a term. In support of this position, the report also cited the earlier cases of Kensey Johns (See Case 2) and James Lanman (See Case 12).

The minority report, signed by four Republicans including William E. Chandler (NH), the committee chairman, argued that the Constitution gave governors the right to fill vacancies even at the beginning of a Senate term. This report, however, failed to cite any Senate precedents for such a view.

The Senate debated the matter from late January until the end of February. On February 3, Donelson Caffery (D-LA), leader of the committee's majority, reiterated the Senate principle that "under no circumstances can the governor appoint to fill an original vacancy commencing at the beginning of a term." In this case, he noted, the legislature "had ample opportunity...to fill the vacancy." If the Senate were to seat a claimant appointed by a governor in such circumstances, it would be encouraging "legislatures to disregard their duty" and deliberately prevent an election to give a governor a chance to appoint a senator.

On February 7, Henry Corbett wrote to his supporter, committee chairman William Chandler, and defended his appointment on the basis that all states are entitled to equal representation in the Senate. He vehemently denounced the suggestion that some legislators might have conspired with the governor to block a senatorial election for the purpose of guaranteeing him an executive appointment. Such conduct, Corbett asserted, would be unthinkable for a governor who had served with distinction on the state supreme court and who lived "in a modest way in his little cottage, and all that he has...is his good name and reputation."

Corbett's letter failed to move his opponents. On February 9, Edmund Pettus (D-AL) again reviewed the precedents and reminded Republicans George F. Hoar (MA) and William Chandler that in the 1893 unsuccessful bid by Lee Mantle (D-MT) both of the New England senators had asked that the question of executive appointment be settled once and for all. Pettus concluded, "If we are forever to treat this question in a partisan sense, if we are forever to debate it, then the debate will only work injury to the country at large."

On February 26, toward the end of the debate, Joseph B. Foraker (R-OH) supported Corbett by contending that the Senate's decision in the Mantle case had been erroneous and should not be used as a precedent because it had been based more on the political circumstances of the effort to repeal the Sherman Silver Purchase Act than on legal principles. Foraker also charged that the Mantle case differed from Corbett's in that the Montana legislature had been organized and failed to elect, unlike the

Oregon legislature, which never succeeded in organizing itself at all and thus was in no position to hold an election.

On February 28, 1898, the Senate, by an overwhelming vote of 50 to 19, denied Corbett a seat.

Conclusion

Henry Corbett's claim brought to the Senate two problems that promised to recur as long as the selection of U. S. senators lay in the province of state legislatures: how could the U. S. Senate determine that a state had a legally organized legislature, and how could the Senate define the appointive authority of a state governor? A weary Senate recognized that, with each succeeding election, disputes at the state level were requiring increasing amounts of senators' time. In that way, the Corbett case helped to move the Senate toward much-needed reform in the area of election procedures.

Henry Corbett continued to pursue his business interests until his death in 1903.

Sources

U.S. Congress. Senate. *Congressional Record.* 55th Cong., 1st sess. (See pp. 11–12, 66, 460–461.) 2d sess. (See pp. 1017–18, 1243, 1382–89, 1535–43, 1585–88, 1611, 1763, 1828–32, 2119–33, 2160–84, 2219–23, 2225–30, 2262–75.)

———. *Congressional Record.* 56th Cong., 1st sess. (See pp. 2573–79.)

———. Senate Report No. 505, 55th Cong., 2d sess., 1898.

Johnson, Allen, ed. *Dictionary of American Biography.* Vol. 2. New York, 1946; reprint of 1935 edition. (See p. 435.)

Case 86

Marcus A. Hanna

(1837–1904)

Ohio

Election Case
May 28, 1898 to February 28, 1899

Issues
Electoral misconduct: charges of bribery

Result: Retained seat

Chronology:
Petition received: May 28, 1898
Referred to committee: May 28, 1898
Committee report: Feb. 28, 1899
No Senate action

Background

When John Sherman (R-OH) resigned from the Senate in 1897 to become secretary of state in the administration of President William McKinley, the Ohio governor appointed Marcus A. Hanna (R), the president's political patron and campaign manager, as his replacement. Hanna, a successful entrepreneur, took office on March 5, 1897, and in January 1898 the Ohio legislature elected him to the remaining year of Sherman's term, as well as to the full six-year term beginning on March 4, 1899.

Statement of the Case

Hanna took his oath of office for the new term without objection on January 17, 1898. Five months later, on May 28, a special committee of the Ohio legislature submitted to the Senate the results of an investigation into charges that several "agents" of Hanna had tried to secure the vote of one Ohio legislator through bribery. The Senate referred the matter to the Committee on Privileges and Elections.

Response of the Senate

On February 28, 1899, a majority of the committee reported in favor of Hanna and asked to be discharged from further investigation into the Ohio election. The committee members remained unconvinced by the meager evidence offered by Hanna's opponents and the failure to supply convincing witnesses. Although the state report made clear that an unsuccessful effort had been made to bribe the legislator, the attempt had been exposed before the election, and the legislator voted against Hanna. There was no evidence linking Hanna to the individual offering the bribe. The report mildly rebuked Hanna and some of his Ohio associates for failing to respond to subpoenas from the state investigation but declined to suggest the need for further inquiry within the Senate.

Three committee Democrats signed a minority report that urged additional Senate action. In an era before federal wiretapping regulations, the minority report included incriminating transcripts Hanna's foes secured when a stenographer eavesdropped on a hotel extension telephone to write down what purported to be conversations between the agent accused of bribery and Hanna's campaign headquarters.

Senators apparently agreed with the majority report, for the Senate ordered the reports to be printed and took no further action on the matter.

Conclusion

The issue reappeared briefly more than a year later, on June 5, 1900, in the midst of a debate on antitrust legislation. Richard F. Pettigrew, a Silver Republican from South Dakota, placed in the *Congressional Record* the majority and minority reports on the Hanna election case, as well as the records of the entire investigation by the Ohio legislative committee, running to forty-six double-columned pages of fine print. Hanna, who was on the Senate floor at the time, denied any connection with the controversy and pointed out that he had offered to testify before the Committee on Privileges and Elections but was assured it would not be necessary. He charged that, not only had he not instigated the conspiracy, but that it was really "a conspiracy on the part of the Democratic party and a few traitors in the Republican party...to prevent Ohio from having another Senator in the United States Senate."

Election practices in the late nineteenth century deteriorated to the point where senators knew the charge of bribery could easily be hurled at nearly any member. Painfully aware of the proliferation of abuses in the state caucuses and assemblies in all areas of the country, senators were reluctant to press the inquiry into Hanna's election.

Marcus Hanna continued to be a forceful presence in Republican politics and in the Senate until his death in 1904.

Sources

U.S. Congress. Senate. *Congressional Record.* 55th Cong., 2d sess. (See p. 2558.) 3d sess. (See pp. 6585–6635.)

———. Senate Report No. 1859. 55th Cong. 3d sess., 1899.

White, William A. *The Autobiography of William Allen White.* New York, 1946.

Johnson, Allen, and Dumas Malone, eds. *Dictionary of American Biography.* Vol. 7. New York, 1946; reprint of 1935 edition. (See pp. 225–27.)

Case 87

John T. McGraw et al. v. Nathan B. Scott

((dates unknown) (1842–1924)

West Virginia

Election Case
February 23, 1899 to April 27, 1900

Issues
Qualifications: residency; conduct of election: eligibility of state legislators

Result: Scott retained seat

Chronology:
Memorials presented:
Feb. 23, 1899, Dec. 6, 1899
Referred to committee: Dec. 6, 1899
Committee report: Mar. 20, 1900
Senate vote: April 27, 1900

Background

In 1898 West Virginia joined a growing list of states whose internal political strife hindered the effective selection of a United States senator. As the state assembly gathered to choose a senator for the term beginning March 4, 1899, the proceedings were overshadowed by rumors that the Republican minority in the house intended to withdraw, establish a separate body, and join with the Republican senate to unseat various Democrats. This conflict was but the most recent in a series of state controversies that included charges of fraudulent election practices in the counties, certificates granted to unlawful assembly members, and the use of threats and intimidation by high-ranking state officials. To quell the rising ill-will that threatened to halt all legislative business, five Democrats and five Republicans signed a joint agreement that limited controversies about membership in the legislature to four individuals who were contesting two seats, postponing a decision on those seats until after the election for U.S. senator, in which none of the four contestants would vote. An imperfect solution at best, the document temporarily quieted seating challenges, but it was in this still hostile legislative climate that a joint assembly of the two houses elected Republican Nathan B. Scott to the United States Senate.

Statement of the Case

Before Nathan Scott appeared to claim his seat, disgruntled Democratic West Virginia legislators, led by their defeated colleague, John T. McGraw, filed petitions on February 23 and March 2, 1899, challenging the seating of the new senator. When Nathan Scott arrived on March 4, 1899, with proper credentials signed by the governor, the Senate permitted him to take his seat.

As the Senate appeared to have ignored the original complaints against Scott, his challengers prepared a new list of allegations and submitted another petition on December 6, 1899, shortly after the regular first session of the Fifty-sixth Congress began. In their second attack, Scott's opponents listed several charges, apparently in the hope that the Senate would find at least one to be a disqualification. The petition stated that the joint agreement was illegal because it had been forced on the Democrats under threats of physical violence. According to the petitions, state Republicans had used this agreement to secure the election of Scott because under it the two Democratic state legislative contestants who were eventually seated had not been permitted to vote for U.S. senator. In addition, two Republican members of the state senate, who should have been unseated, voted for Scott. As a final complaint, the West Virginia Democrats insisted that Scott failed to meet the state's residency requirements because he was an inhabitant of the District of Columbia. The Senate referred this lengthy petition and all the earlier papers related to Nathan Scott to the Committee on Privileges and Elections.

Response of the Senate

On March 20, 1900, a majority of the committee returned a report favorable to Nathan Scott. Noting that Scott had been elected by a majority of the legislators who voted, and that a quorum of the joint assembly and a quorum of each house were present and voted, the report argued that the U.S. Senate could not review the decision of the West Virginia senate on seating its members. The Senate also could not reverse the signed agreement among the West Virginia legislators. Had the complaining parties proved force or intimidation by "revolutionary conspirators," the report asserted, the Senate could, as it had in the past, investigate charges of fraud and corruption. In the view of the committee majority, the West Virginia case simply did not represent such an extreme situation, particularly since the evidence showed that the five Democrats had signed and submitted the proposed agreement, which was then accepted by the Republicans, making it unlikely that the Democrats had acted under coercion by the Republicans. Regarding Scott's residence, the report noted that Scott lived in Washington, D.C., while discharging the duties of his office as U.S. commissioner of internal revenue but remained officially an inhabitant of Wheeling, West Virginia. All committee members agreed on this latter point. For all of these reasons, the committee's majority determined that Scott was entitled to his seat.

In a strongly worded minority report, Edmund W. Pettus (D-AL) vigorously dissented, complaining that the committee had refused to accept depositions from witnesses stating that a conspiracy interfered with the freedom of the West Virginia legislature's election of Scott.

The floor debate continued until late in April. Scott's opponents argued that the Senate had a responsibility to scrutinize elections that involved charges of bribery and corruption. They bemoaned the Senate's seemingly frivolous attitude toward the West Virginia constitution's eligibility qualifications. Scott's supporters countered that the journal entries for the legislative proceedings did not reveal threats or plots. They conceded that the records showed some members denied voting privileges; but this action, they contended, fell under the right of a state assembly to decide the eligibility of its own members. Despite repeated efforts by Pettus to delay action, the Senate on April 27, 1900, voted 52 to 3 to affirm Nathan Scott's right to retain his seat.

Conclusion

On May 25, 1900, the Senate agreed that John McGraw and Nathan Scott should each receive $2,850 in compensation for their expenses. Scott, whose earlier careers had included frontier miner and glass manufacturer, served in the Senate until 1911. He then engaged in banking in Washington, D. C., where he died in 1924.

Sources

U.S. Congress. Senate. *Congressional Record.* 55th Cong., 3d sess. (See pp. 2205–6, 2691–92.)

———. *Congressional Record.* 56th Cong., 1st sess. (See pp. 98, 132, 231, 3072, 4651–53, 4696–4710, 4742, 4750–60, 5734, 6015–16.)

———. Senate Report No. 679. 56th Cong., 1st sess., 1900.

Case 88

Matthew Quay

(1833–1904)

Pennsylvania

Election Case (appointment)
December 4, 1899 to April 24, 1900

Issues
Right of governor to make appointment to a term not previously filled by a legislature

Result: Not seated

Chronology:
Credentials presented: Dec. 4, 1899
Referred to committee: Dec. 4, 1899
Committee report: Jan. 23, 1900
Senate vote: April 24, 1900

Background

Matthew Quay, Pennsylvania Republican political boss, first came to the United States Senate in 1887. With the powerful machine he built in his home state, Quay had no problem securing reelection in 1893. By 1899, however, the anti-Quay faction, which included state Democrats, insurgent Republicans, and wealthy businessman John Wanamaker, had sufficient strength in the legislature to block a new term for Quay.

The struggle to select a senator overlapped with an unsavory trial that linked Quay to a mismanaged bank and the suicide of its cashier. Complaints from Quay supporters that the financial disclosures had been timed to coincide with the senatorial election in the state legislature appeared valid, for the embezzlement case was sent to the jury the very afternoon that the deadlocked assembly adjourned. The next day, April 21, 1899, Quay was acquitted of any complicity in the scandal. Quay returned to Washington, convinced that the state's governor, controlled by his machine, could be depended upon to give him an interim Senate appointment.

Statement of the Case

Matthew Quay, who enjoyed a bipartisan popularity among his Senate colleagues, received a warm welcome, although many expressed immediate doubts that the expected gubernatorial appointment would be legal. Predictably, when Quay's credentials were presented on December 4, 1899, Julius Burrows (R-MI) protested on the basis of numerous complaints he had received from Pennsylvania legislators. Quay was not seated, and the matter was referred to the Committee on Privileges and Elections.

Response of the Senate

On January 23, 1900, a divided committee presented a majority and minority report. The committee's majority—made up of three Democrats, one Populist, and one Republican—declared that Quay was not entitled to the seat. The report cited earlier Senate election decisions in reaffirming that the governor had no right to make an appointment if the legislature had an opportunity to elect a senator and failed to do so.

Four Republican senators signed a minority report contending that Quay was entitled to be seated until the next meeting of the legislature. They interpreted the language of the U.S. Constitution to mean that the governor could appoint whenever there was a vacancy in a Senate seat. They also believed that the previous Senate precedents cited by the majority did not apply in this case.

The committee's conflicting reports launched a three-month debate on the subject of Quay's claim. On March 2, 1900, George F. Hoar (R-MA), one of those signing the minority report, emerged as the Senate expert on the subject of contested gubernatorial appointments, a matter he had studied extensively during his years as chairman of the Committee on Privileges and Elections from 1881 to 1891 and again in 1897. In supporting Quay's claim and defending the gubernatorial action, Hoar contended that the Founding Fathers wanted to assure the continuity of representation for the states. Julius Burrows, however, challenged Hoar's views, insisting that the Constitution and precedents showed clearly that the governor could not appoint if the legislature had failed to elect. His argument on April 12, combined with considerable pressure from Pennsylvanians opposed to Quay, led the Senate to deny Quay his seat by a narrow vote of 33 to 32 on April 24, 1900.

Conclusion

The vote was not an easy one for many senators, who counted the Pennsylvanian as a close friend. Despite their feelings, however, constitutional issues, Senate precedents, and the national implications for the Republican party carried the day.

Quay continued to seek the Senate seat when the state legislature again addressed the issue in January 1901, and his state machine remained strong enough to ensure his election. Quay's reappearance in the Senate was subdued, for his health failed quickly. Unable to complete his term, he returned in 1904 to his Pennsylvania home, where he died on May 28.

Sources

U.S. Congress. Senate. *Congressional Record.* 56th Cong., 1st sess. (See pp. 1, 646, 1051, 2062–63, 2115, 2122, 2233, 2240, 2310–16, 2462, 2469, 2503, 2508, 2529–33, 2573, 2579, 2929–39, 2963–64, 3732–36, 3795–98, 3829–30, 3873–74, 3913–16, 3965–66, 4001, 4079–94, 4159, 4520–25, 4539–57, 4586–4613.)

———. Senate Report No. 153. 56th Cong., 1st sess., 1900.

Kehl, James A. *Boss Rule in the Gilded Age.* Pittsburgh, PA, 1981.

Malone, Dumas, ed. *Dictionary of American Biography.* Vol. 15. New York, 1946; reprint of 1935 edition. (See pp. 296–98.)

Case 89

William A. Clark

(1839–1925)

Montana

Election Case
December 4, 1899 to May 15, 1900

Issues
Electoral misconduct: bribery

Result: Clark resigned but later was again elected

Chronology:
Petition received: Dec. 4, 1899
Referred to committee: Dec. 4, 1899
Committee report: April 23, 1900
No Senate action

Background

In 1890 Montana copper mining czar William A. Clark failed in his first effort to become a United States senator (See Case 78). Undaunted, Clark continued to devote the full measure of his extensive economic and political power to achieving that goal. Enormous sums of money changed hands in Montana as Clark and his chief rival, Anaconda Company copper magnate Marcus Daly, sought to influence the economic structure of the state, the location of the capital, the direction of Democratic politics, and the selection of a United States senator. The blatant business and political competition between the Clark and Daly factions was but a continuation of the turmoil that had marred Montana politics since the organization of the state government in 1889.

Statement of the Case

Nine years after his initial disappointment in 1890, William Clark won the Senate seat he so avidly desired, presenting his credentials on December 4, 1899. The Senate admitted him immediately, although on the same day his opponents filed a petition charging that Clark had secured his election through bribery. The memorial asserted that Clark had spent far more on his election than the $2,000 permitted by an 1895 Montana law aimed at controlling political corruption. The Senate referred the matter to the Committee on Privileges and Elections, which quickly asked for and received authorization to conduct a full investigation into Clark's election.

Response of the Senate

On April 23, 1900, after hearing extensive testimony from ninety-six witnesses, the committee returned a report unanimously concluding that William Clark was not entitled to his seat. The testimony detailed a dazzling list of bribes ranging from $240 to $100,000. In a high-pressure, well-organized scheme coordinated by Clark's son, Clark's agents had paid mortgages, purchased ranches, paid debts, financed banks, and blatantly presented envelopes of cash to legislators. In addition, the winning margin in Clark's election had been secured by the votes of eleven Republican legislators under suspicious circumstances. Clark did not enhance his position when he admitted that he had destroyed all his personal checks that dealt with campaign transactions. The committee cited a number of previous bribery cases, especially that of Samuel C. Pomeroy and Alexander Caldwell in 1872–1873 (Case 61), as precedents for declaring an election void if bribery on behalf of the winner could be proved even if no proof was found that the candidate knew of the actions. The report also noted the precedent from the Pomeroy case that, if the winner "clearly participated in any one act of bribery or attempted bribery, he should be deprived of his office," even if "the result of the election was not thereby changed." While concurring in the committee's conclusion, two members tried to reduce the impact of the anti-Clark testimony by pointing to the unlimited sums that his rival, Marcus Daly, had invested in an effort to block Clark's election. Rather than exonerating Clark, however, that observation simply confirmed the way in which corruption totally pervaded Montana politics.

On May 15, 1900, as the Senate prepared to vote on Clark's right to retain his seat, the beleaguered senator rose to speak. Predictably, Clark complained about the procedures of the committee, the admissions and omissions of evidence, and the machinations of Marcus Daly. He contended that the Senate had lost sight of the principle of presumption of innocence and concluded lamely that the committee had not shown that bribery sufficient to alter the election results had occurred. At the conclusion of his remarks, Clark, clearly aware that he did not have the necessary votes to keep his seat, resigned.

This did not conclude the Montana case, for on May 19 the acting governor of Montana immediately appointed Clark to fill the Senate vacancy. When the governor learned of this action on his return to the state three days later, he telegraphed the Senate that Martin Maginnis would fill the Clark vacancy. Credentials for both Clark and Maginnis were presented to the Senate, which ordered them to lie on the table.

Conclusion

In January 1901 a newly elected Montana legislature—in which most of the winning candidates had received financial support from William Clark—elected him to the Senate for the same term he had filled earlier. Marcus Daly had died in November 1900, and this time no charges of corruption were raised. On March 4, 1901, Clark appeared and was seated without objection.

In this case, the Privileges and Elections Committee stressed that the Senate had a duty to itself and to the country to demonstrate by its action that senators cannot retain seats procured by corruption. It also saw an equal duty to Montana because the state had adopted the 1895 law in an effort to end corruption in its elections.

William Clark, having finally achieved his great ambition, served one term as United States senator. He retired from the Senate in 1907 and returned to his far-flung business ventures. While remaining notorious for the corruption of his 1899 election, Clark continued to add to his vast fortune. He died in 1925.

Sources

U.S. Congress. Senate. *Congressional Record.* 56th Cong., 1st sess. (See pp. 22, 85, 132, 231, 4537, 5536, 5732, 5850, 6698.) 56th Cong., 2d sess. (See pp. 29, 58, 93, 216, 219, 354–55, 419, 462–66, 2726, 2869, 3189, 3420–3435.)

———. Senate Report No. 1052. 56th Cong., 1st sess., 1900.

High, James. "William Andrews Clark: Westerner." *Arizona and the West* 2 (Autumn 1960): 245–64.

Hinds, Asher C. *Hinds' Precedents of the House of Representatives of the United States.* Vol. 1. Washington, DC, 1907. (See secs. 692–695.)

Lamar, Howard R. *The Reader's Encyclopedia of the American West.* New York, 1977.

Malone, Michael P. "Midas of the West: The Incredible Career of William Andrews Clark." *Montana: The Magazine of Western History* 33 (Autumn 1983): 2–17.

VI. PRE-DIRECT ELECTION: 1902–1913

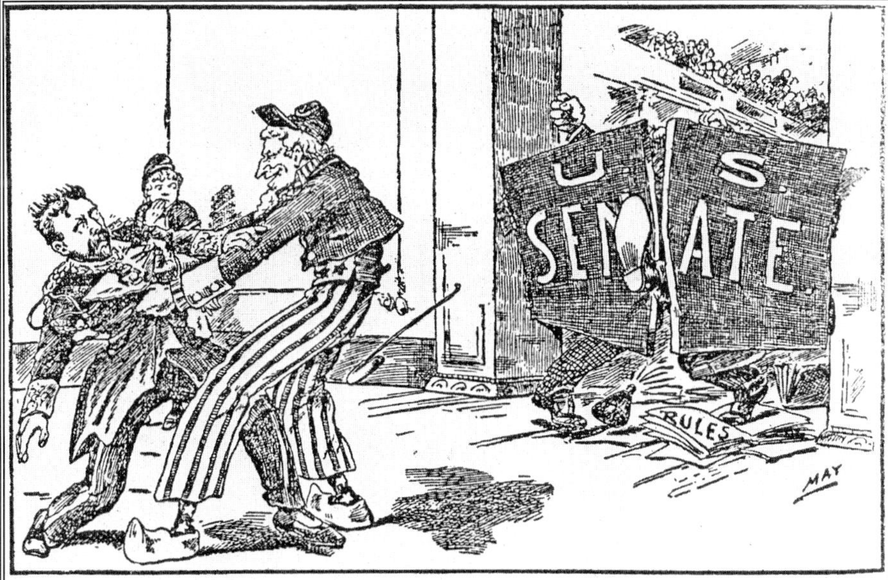

UNCLE SAM: "Come on in, Heinrich; they never touch visitors."
—*The Detroit Journal.*

A CARTOONIST'S VIEW OF THE TILLMAN-MCLAURIN FIGHT *(Case 90)*
The Literary Digest, March 9, 1902

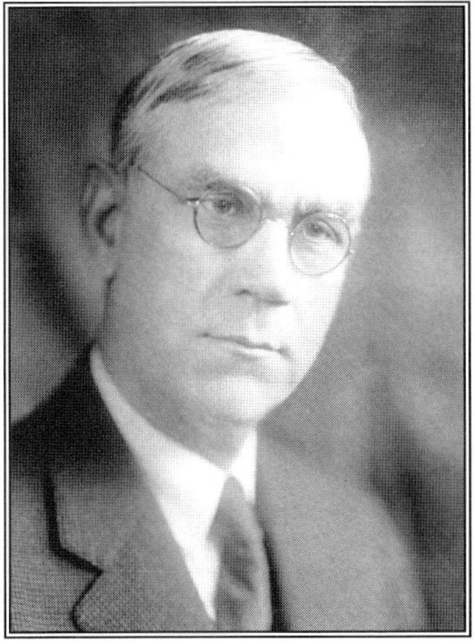

REED SMOOT *(Case 91)*
U.S. Senate Historical Office

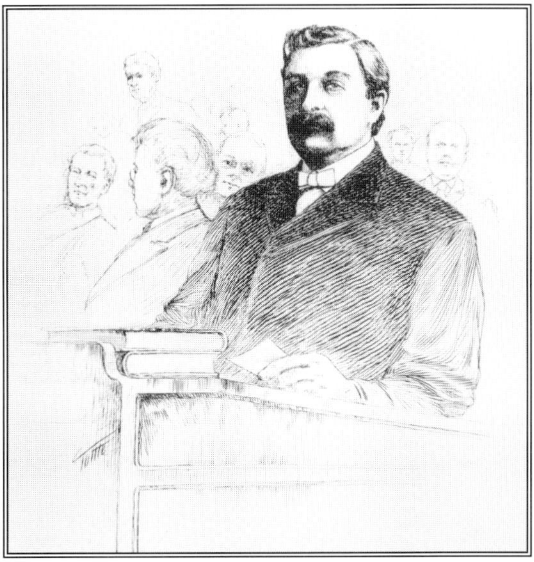

WILLIAM LORIMER *(Case 95)*
Library of Congress

Case 90

John L. McLaurin and Benjamin R. Tillman

(1860–1934) (1847–1918)

South Carolina

Censure Case
February 22, 1902 to February 28, 1902

Issues
Breach of comity; Senate's power to suspend a member

Result: Censured

Chronology:
Altercation on floor: Feb. 22, 1902
Referred to committee: Feb. 22, 1902
Committee report: Feb. 28, 1902
Senate vote: Feb. 28, 1902

Background

In 1896 South Carolina junior Senator John L. McLaurin (D) entered the Senate, joining his longtime close friend Benjamin R. Tillman (D-SC), who as governor and political boss of the state had helped to foster his career. Despite their political connection of many years, McLaurin, a man of somewhat erratic temperament, turned away from his old mentor and permitted himself to be courted by Senate Republicans. He may have been motivated by a desire to see South Carolina participate more fully in the nation's industrial progress, but his behavior infuriated the outspoken Tillman.

Statement of the Case

On February 22, 1902, the Senate debated a bill relating to the Philippine Islands. Benjamin Tillman, known to be less than courteous on the Senate floor, used the occasion to direct scathing remarks toward John McLaurin's empty chair, charging that his colleague had succumbed to "improper influences" in changing his position on the treaty to annex the Philippines. Tillman accused McLaurin of treachery for casting his vote with the Republicans to approve the treaty after publicly speaking against it. In return, Tillman charged, the majority Republicans had allowed McLaurin to control government patronage in South Carolina and granted him committee positions as a Republican. Word of Tillman's remarks quickly reached McLaurin in a committee meeting and, incensed, he dashed into the Senate chamber and denounced Tillman's statement as "a willful, malicious, and deliberate lie."

In response, the fifty-four-year-old Tillman jumped from his place and physically attacked McLaurin, who was forty-one, with a series of stinging blows. Efforts to separate the two combatants resulted in misdirected punches landing on other members. Such a blatant physical assault had not occurred during a Senate session since Henry S. Foote (D-MS) and Thomas Hart Benton (D-MO) had accosted one another in 1850 (See Case 22).

Response of the Senate

Immediately, the galleries were cleared, and the Senate went into closed session to discuss the altercation. After a two-hour debate in which both South Carolinians were unanimously "declared in contempt of the Senate," the matter was referred to the Committee on Privileges and Elections. When the Senate returned to open session, the president pro tempore, William P. Frye (R-ME), noted that, as long as the senators were in contempt, neither could be recognized to speak on the floor except at the request of another senator. At this point, a senator asked that they be permitted to speak, and Tillman and McLaurin apologized to their colleagues. They did so, however, in such unpleasant and bitter terms that the ruckus threatened to explode anew.

The clash occurred during a Saturday session. On the following Monday, as their behavior was considered in the committee and widely criticized in the press, the two senators found that, until the matter was resolved, their names were also to be omitted from roll-call votes. A piqued Tillman registered a written protest about this procedure in the *Congressional Record* on February 26, charging that it was unconstitutional to deprive South Carolina of its voice in the Senate. The following day both names were restored, because the president pro tempore believed that the full Senate, rather than the presiding officer, should make such a serious decision.

The culprits did not have long to wait for a resolution of the matter. On February 28 the committee reported that, although Benjamin Tillman was guilty of the graver offense in resorting to physical violence rather than simply using unparliamentary language as John McLaurin had, both senators should receive the same penalty. Declaring that the conduct of the two South Carolinians represented "an infringement of the privileges of the Senate, a violation of its rules and derogatory to its high character, tending to bring the body itself into public contempt," the committee explained that the legal effect of the Senate's contempt judgment had been "to suspend their functions as Senators," a punishment "clearly within the power of the Senate." The committee therefore recommended that both be censured and that the contempt order suspending them then be lifted. The Senate agreed and by a vote of 54 to 12 censured Tillman and McLaurin. Their punishment thus consisted of censure plus the brief suspension they had already endured. Twenty-two senators did not participate in the vote, perhaps indicating the strong sentiment among many members that McLaurin's outburst had been provoked by Tillman's intemperate language.

Conclusion

Although the Senate took no vote on the issue of suspension, all committee members had concurred that the Senate had the power to suspend as well as to expel a member found to be in contempt.

The breach of comity prompted members to change the rules of the Senate to provide stricter guidelines for the decorum of floor debate. On August 8, 1902, the Senate adopted this change (Rule XIX, secs. 2 and 3), stating, "No Senator in debate shall, directly or indirectly, by any form of words impute to another Senator or to other Senators any conduct or motive unworthy or unbecoming a Senator" and "No Senator in debate shall refer offensively to any State of the Union."

Under continuing political attack by Benjamin Tillman in South Carolina, John McLaurin served only until the end of his term in 1903 and did not seek reelection to the Senate. Instead, he practiced law in New York City for a time, later returning to South Carolina. There he served in the state senate and as state warehouse commissioner before retiring to private life. He lived until 1934.

Although Tillman continued to serve in the Senate until his death in 1918, he fell ill in 1908. As repeated strokes and a progressive paralysis marked his declining years, political control of South Carolina gradually slipped from his hands.

Sources

U.S. Congress. Senate. *Congressional Record.* 57th Cong., 1st sess. (See pp. 1063, 2015–43, 2087–90, 2203–7, 3329, 3819.)

———. Senate Report No. 574 and Senate Document No. 228. 57th Cong., 1st sess., 1902.

Haynes, George H. *The Senate of the United States.* Vol. 1. Boston, 1938. (See pp. 187–88.)

Hinds, Asher C. *Hinds' Precedents of the House of Representatives of the United States.* Vol. 2. Washington, DC, 1907. (See sec. 1665.)

Simkins, Francis Butler. *Pitchfork Ben Tillman: South Carolinian.* Baton Rouge, LA, 1967; reprint of 1944 edition.

Case 91

Reed Smoot

(1862–1941)

Utah

Election Case / Expulsion Case
February 23, 1903 to February 20, 1907

Issues
Qualifications: whether there could be a religious disqualification for Senate membership

Result: Retained seat / Not expelled

Chronology:
Memorial received: Feb. 23, 1903
Referred to committee: Jan. 27, 1904
Committee report: June 2, 1906
Senate vote: Feb. 20, 1907

Background

Members of the Church of Jesus Christ of Latter-day Saints, commonly known as Mormons, had fled to the desert isolation of Utah following the 1844 murder of the church's founder, Joseph Smith. Mormons and non-Mormons faced the 1896 admission of Utah to the Union with some dread as both groups had grown comfortable with the physical distances separating their communities. Non-Mormons, largely uninformed about the cultural and economic institutions of the Mormon church, disliked the way in which it tended to blur business and political distinctions. Outsiders often demonstrated their distrust of the church by expressing repugnance for plural marriage, even though the Mormon church had officially terminated the practice in 1890, after Congress enacted laws making polygamy illegal. Utah's election of Reed Smoot, a prominent Mormon, to the United States Senate sparked a marathon investigation that became the focus for Americans' fear, ignorance, and suspicion of Mormonism.

Statement of the Case

On February 23, 1903, the credentials for Reed Smoot (R-UT) were presented and placed on file. On the same day, a memorial from several Salt Lake City residents asked that Smoot, a well-known and influential Mormon manufacturer and banker, not be permitted to take his seat. The protesters were a small group of businessmen and Protestant ministers who opposed Mormon economic policies in Utah.

On March 5, 1903, Reed Smoot appeared and took his oath of office, under the Senate's policy that a senator whose credentials were in order would be seated and any challenges dealt with afterward. The arrival of the Mormon senator, a member of the church's powerful Quorum of Twelve

Apostles, attracted national attention and unleashed a torrent of complaints against him. Petitions with thousands of signatures flooded the Senate from Protestant churches, women's organizations outraged by polygamy, and others influenced by newpaper attacks on Smoot. The protesters charged that the Mormon leadership, including the Quorum of Twelve, held supreme authority over both spiritual and temporal matters for its members and frequently interfered in Utah politics. They also complained that the leaders continued to believe in, encourage, and practice polygamy, even though it was illegal.

The deluge of petitions and resolutions moved the Senate on January 27, 1904, to order an investigation into the hierarchy of the Mormon church. A central issue was whether Smoot, as one of the Quorum of Twelve, had taken a church fealty oath that made him ineligible to sit in the United State Senate. The Senate referred the matter to the Committee on Privileges and Elections.

Response of the Senate

The committee plunged into an investigation that lasted more than two years, gathering testimony that filled five volumes. The scope of the investigation expanded far beyond Smoot and became a full dissection of the structure and machinery of the Mormon church, as well as the temporal and religious concerns of Mormons. Arguments against Smoot centered on three points: he was a member of a church that encouraged polygamy; he had taken a religious oath that disqualified him from the Senate; and he was a member of a religion that united church and state.

The Smoot forces argued that since 1890 the Mormon church had not "controlled or attempted to control elections in Utah," and Smoot had never taken any oath including "an obligation of hostility to the United States," as had been alleged. They also correctly observed that other Mormons—although none holding such high positions in the church—had already been elected to and served in the U.S. Congress. More directly relevant to the matter at hand was the argument that none of the practices of the Mormon church had any bearing on Smoot's constitutional qualifications to be a United States senator.

Despite this significant point, the committee on June 1, 1906, voted 7 to 5 that Smoot was not entitled to his seat. On June 11 a divided committee filed majority and minority reports. The majority recommended that Smoot be removed from office, having concluded that he perceived his first loyalty to be the maintenance of the corporate and spiritual interests of Utah's Mormons. For its part, the minority report contended that testimony before the committee failed to substantiate any of the charges against Smoot. The lengthy proceedings never included personal attacks on the senator, whose character was above reproach.

When the Senate reconvened in December 1906 after its summer recess, the Smoot case took center stage. Privileges and Elections Committee Chairman Julius C. Burrows (R-MI) led the attack against Smoot, tying him and the Mormon church to support for polygamy. Smoot, however, gained some eloquent defenders, among them noted orator Albert J. Beveridge (R-IN), one of those signing the committee's minority report. Not only was Smoot not himself a polygamist, Beveridge asserted, but "the evidence shows that, from the first, Reed Smoot has been the leader of the younger, wiser, and more modern element of his Church that oppose that insult to marriage." He then closed with a stirring call for religious tolerance.

On February 20, 1907, the ordeal of Reed Smoot—during which he conducted himself with grace and dignity—finally reached a conclusion. After deciding to require a two-thirds vote to declare Smoot not entitled to his seat, the Senate first voted down a move to expel him, 27 yeas to 43 nays, and then refused by a vote of 28 yeas to 42 nays to deny the Utah senator his right to remain in the Senate.

Conclusion

The investigation into Reed Smoot's right to a Senate seat had in many ways been an American trial of the Mormon church. In permitting Smoot to retain his seat, the U.S. Senate took a stand in support of religious freedom for all Americans. In practical terms, the staunch support of Republican President Theodore Roosevelt had helped to ensure the margin of victory by encouraging wavering Republican senators to stand firm.

Reed Smoot served in the Senate for thirty years. At his death in 1941, he was third in line for the presidency of the Church of Jesus Christ of Latter-day Saints.

Sources

U.S. Congress. Senate. *Congressional Record.* 57th Cong., 2d sess. (See pp. 2496, 2689.)

———. *Congressional Record.* 58th Cong., 1st sess. (See p. 1.) 2d sess.(See pp. 1100, 1239, 5628.)

———. *Congressional Record.* 59th Cong., 1st sess. (See pp. 3238, 7715, 8318–38.) 2d sess. (See pp. 241–348, 933–45, 1486–1501, 1933–34, 2681–89, 2934–39, 3268–81, 3404–30, 4222, 4448–52.)

———. Senate Report No. 4253. 59th Cong., 1st sess., 1906.

Arrington, Leonard. *Great Basin Kingdom: Economic History of the Latter-Day Saints, 1830–1900.* Lincoln, NE, 1958.

Garner, James W. "The Case of Senator Smoot and the Mormon Church." *North American Review* 184 (1907): 46.

Holsinger, M. Paul. "For God and the American Home: The Attempt to Unseat Senator Reed Smoot, 1903–1907." *Pacific Northwest Quarterly* 60 (July 1969): 154–60.

Merrill, Milton R. *Reed Smoot: Apostle in Politics.* Logan, UT, 1990.

Case 92

Joseph R. Burton

(1852–1923)

Kansas

Expulsion Case
January 24, 1904 to June 4, 1906

Issues
Corruption: convicted of illegally accepting compensation for services before a federal agency

Result: Resigned before Senate could act

Chronology:
Indictment: Jan. 24, 1904
Conviction: Mar. 28, 1904
Conviction overturned: Jan. 16, 1905
2d conviction: Nov. 26, 1905
Conviction upheld: May 21, 1906
Referred to committee: May 22, 1906

Background

On January 24, 1904, a federal grand jury in Missouri indicted Senator Joseph R. Burton (R-KS) on charges that he had received five checks for $500 each from the Rialto Grain and Securities Company of St. Louis in return for interceding with the United States postmaster general and the chief post office inspector on a mail fraud investigation. Such activity violated an 1864 law prohibiting members of Congress from receiving compensation for services performed before a federal agency. The law also provided that anyone found guilty would be "rendered forever thereafter incapable of holding any office . . . under the Government of the United States." Burton's indictment came about during a general investigation of corruption in the Post Office.

Burton denied any wrongdoing and explained that he had accepted the fees to become general counsel to Rialto because he had lost heavily in the recent financial panic and needed the $500 monthly salary. Burton had accompanied the president of Rialto, Hugh Dennison, to a meeting with the chief post office inspector to determine whether or not the Post Office had issued a mail fraud order against the company. Burton claimed to have told the inspector that "other Senators and Representatives had built up large private practices during their terms of office, and that I in a small way desired to emulate them. I told him that I was general counsel for the Rialto Company of St. Louis and asked him as a general matter of friendship to tell me if at any time I did wrong." Burton added that both he and the chief post office inspector were from Kansas.

Statement of the Case

When Joseph Burton was convicted on March 28, 1904, he appealed to the Supreme Court, which ruled in January 1905 that Missouri did not have jurisdiction to try Burton for checks that he had received in Washington and cashed at the Riggs Bank there. In July of that year, Burton was again indicted by a federal grand jury in St. Louis on more limited charges. He was convicted once more, in November 1905, and sentenced to six months in prison and a $2,500 fine. Again, he appealed to the Supreme Court.

After each of his convictions while his appeals were pending, Burton remained a member of the Senate and continued to draw his salary. He did not, however, enter the Senate chamber to participate in Senate business. According to press accounts, other senators let it be known they would not act to expel him until after he had exhausted his appeals in the courts but that if he appeared on the Senate floor he would forfeit his claim to their sympathy. On May 21, 1906, the Supreme Court upheld Burton's second conviction. In its opinion the Court indicated that conviction in the case "did not operate, ipso facto, to vacate the seat of the convicted Senator nor compel the Senate to expel him or to regard him as expelled by force alone of the judgment." (*Burton* v. *United States*, 202 U.S. 344) The Court also declared that the law's prohibition of anyone convicted under it from serving again in the U.S. government did not apply to U.S. senators, who were selected by the states. It was therefore up to the Senate to take its own action against Burton.

In response to this ruling, the Senate the next day directed the Committee on Privileges and Elections to examine the legal effect of the Supreme Court's decision and make a recommendation, but on June 4, before the committee could issue a report, Burton resigned from the Senate.

Conclusion

Joseph Burton served five months of his six-month sentence in the Iron County Jail, Ironton, Missouri. He claimed to have rejected a presidential pardon, although the United States attorney insisted that no pardon was ever offered. When Burton left prison in March 1907, he was met by a delegation of prominent lawyers and political leaders who escorted him back to Abilene where he was given a triumphant reception. Burton charged that President Theodore Roosevelt had instigated the government's prosecution of him because he had broken with the president on the issue of Cuban trade reciprocity. "Roosevelt never forgave me," said Burton, and for that reason he was "hounded for years for a crime I never committed." Burton died in 1923.

Sources

U.S. Congress. Senate. *Congressional Record*. 59th Cong., 1st sess. (See pp. 7211, 7821.)

Hinds, Asher C. *Hinds' Precedents of the House of Representatives of the United States*. Vol. 2. Washington, DC, 1907. (See sec. 1282.)

Case 93

Charles H. Dietrich

(1853–1924)

South Dakota

Censure Case
February 1, 1904 to April 14, 1904

Issues
Authority to investigate conduct prior to a member's term

Result: Not censured

Chronology:
Request for investigation: Feb. 1, 1904
Referred to committee: Feb. 1, 1904
Committee report: April 14, 1904
No Senate action

Background

In 1878 South Dakota miner and merchant Charles H. Dietrich moved to Hastings, Nebraska, where he found lucrative business opportunities in meeting the needs of the burgeoning agriculture and livestock industries there. Establishing close financial ties with many German immigrants in the state, he became president of the German National Bank in 1887. In 1900 Dietrich was elected governor of Nebraska.

Statement of the Case

In May 1901, after his selection by the state legislature for the position of United States senator in March of that year, Charles Dietrich (R) resigned his gubernatorial office and came to Washington. On December 2, 1901, he presented himself in the Senate and took his oath without objection. No charges were ever made against the regularity of Dietrich's election.

On February 1, 1904, Dietrich submitted a resolution asking that the Senate investigate allegations of improprieties in certain postal appointments in Nebraska while he was governor. These alleged episodes, all of which predated Dietrich's election as senator, included charges that he accepted bribes in return for naming a postmaster and that he profited from the leasing of post office facilities in Hastings, Nebraska. Dietrich had been formally indicted on December 28, 1903, but the charges were dismissed on January 4, 1904. The Senate approved Dietrich's resolution, and the president pro tempore appointed a special five-member committee to conduct an inquiry.

Response of the Senate

The authority of the Senate to investigate allegations of criminal conduct that occurred prior to a member's election had been hotly debated in 1893 when charges were raised against William D. Roach (D-ND) (See footnote to Case 83). It was a topic about which the Senate clearly felt uncomfortable, and the issue was no more palatable because the investigative request came from the individual himself. After looking into the matter, the special committee on April 14, 1904, issued a unanimous report that exonerated Dietrich from any wrongdoing and discredited any charges published against him. No accusations against Dietrich were made on the Senate floor. No debate occurred after the report, and the Senate took no further action in the matter.

Conclusion

Charles Dietrich served only a single term in the United States Senate. He retired in 1905 and died in 1924.

Sources

U.S. Congress. Senate. *Congressional Record.* 57th Cong., 1st sess. (See p. 41.) 2d sess. (See pp. 1447, 1468, 1499, 1652, 1821, 4800–4801.)

———. Senate Report No. 2152. 58th Cong., 2d sess., 1904.

Case 94

John W. Smith

(1845–1925)

Maryland

Election Case
March 26, 1908

Issues
Conduct of election; immediate seating if credentials in order

Result: Seated

Chronology:
Credentials presented: Mar. 26, 1908
Senate vote: Mar. 26, 1908

Background

John W. Smith, a native of Maryland's eastern shore and a businessman of comfortable means, rose through the ranks of the state's Democratic machine politics to capture a succession of offices. In a career that spanned more than forty years, Smith served as a member of the state assembly, president of the state senate, and governor of Maryland. In 1908 Smith—who had become the unofficial Democratic leader of the state after the death in 1906 of his patron Senator Arthur P. Gorman (D-MD)—was elected to the United States Senate for the term beginning March 4, 1909. When the incumbent senator, William P. Whyte, died in March 1908, the Maryland assembly selected Smith to fill the remaining year of that term as well.

Statement of the Case

On March 26, 1908, John Smith's credentials were presented to the United States Senate, stating that the legislature had elected him the previous day. Julius C. Burrows (R-MI), chairman of the Committee on Privileges and Elections, raised an objection on the grounds that the Maryland election violated provisions of the 1866 federal election law regulating elections to fill vacancies. The statute in question, he declared, stipulated that a state legislature could not fill a vacancy until the second Tuesday after notice that one existed. Since William Whyte had died Tuesday, March 17, 1908, his replacement could not be selected until March 31, but John Smith's credentials showed the election was completed six days earlier, on March 25. Burrows asserted that every election to fill a vacancy since passage of the 1866 law had conformed to the requirement to wait until the second Tuesday and that Smith therefore should not be seated.

Smith's Maryland Democratic colleague Isador Rayner, however, pointed out that no one was contesting the election and that the Maryland legislature was required by the state's constitution to adjourn before the next Tuesday. Thus, delaying the election would leave the state without its full representation in the Senate. Rayner interpreted the statute simply to mean that a legislature must not elect a senator until the second Tuesday after it was organized. After that day, it could fill a vacancy whenever one occurred. At any rate, he concluded, the Senate precedent was to seat a senator who arrived with proper credentials and to conduct an inquiry afterward.

Response of the Senate

A resolution to delay the seating of John Smith failed by a vote of 28 to 34. Smith then came forward and took his oath of office.

The Senate thus agreed with Rayner that it would seat a senator-elect with regular credentials and no challengers. The early date of the election did not alter the essential validity of the procedure, and the Senate took no further action on the matter.

Conclusion

Smith held his Senate seat until 1921. In his final campaign, Smith's advancing age, his advocacy of prohibition, and factionalism among Democrats helped sweep Republican Ovington E. Weller to victory. Smith died in 1925.

Sources

U.S. Congress. Senate. *Congressional Record.* 60th Cong., 1st sess. (See pp. 3349, 3938–55.)

Walsh, Richard, and William L. Fox, eds. *Maryland: A History, 1632–1974.* Baltimore, 1974.

Case 95

William Lorimer

(1861–1934)

Illinois

Election Case
May 28, 1910 to July 13, 1912

Issues
Electoral misconduct: bribery and corruption

Result: Unseated

Chronology:
First investigation
Request for investigation: May 28, 1910
Referred to committee: June 1, 1910
Committee report: Dec. 21, 1910
Senate vote: Mar. 1, 1910

Second investigation
Referred to committee: June 4, 1911
Committee report: May 20, 1912
Senate vote: July 13, 1912

Background

William Lorimer, a self-educated immigrant from England who arrived in the United States as a youngster, climbed from extreme poverty to affluence and prestige. He acquired wealth through his brick manufacturing and real estate businesses and power through his political organizing skills and machine connections in Illinois. The vibrant and forceful Lorimer, affectionately known as the "blond boss," was first elected to the U.S. House of Representatives at thirty-three. He entertained his constituency with bands, circuses, and moving pictures, and they rewarded him by repeatedly reelecting him to the House, where he served from 1895–1901 and 1903–1909. In 1909 Lorimer, a Republican, sought a seat in the United States Senate and was elected after months of deadlock in the legislature with the help of many Democratic votes.

Statement of the Case

On June 18, 1909, William Lorimer presented his credentials and was seated in the Senate. Nearly a year later on May 28, 1910, Lorimer asked the Senate to investigate allegations by the *Chicago Tribune* that he had obtained his seat by bribery and corruption, charges that he vehemently denied. The Senate referred the matter to the Committee on Privileges and Elections on June 1, 1910, and on June 20 the Senate agreed with a committee request to conduct a full-scale investigation into Lorimer's campaign activities.

Response of the Senate

First Investigation

When the committee reported on December 21, 1910, a majority report exonerated Lorimer. In previous bribery cases, the report noted, the Senate had held that an election would only be invalidated if the senator involved had participated in or sanctioned an act of bribery or if bribery committed without his knowledge or sanction affected enough votes to change the outcome of the election. In this case, a subcommittee had held hearings in Chicago and received no testimony that implicated Lorimer himself in any acts of bribery, although four legislators claimed to have received bribes to vote for him. Several of these, however, had later changed their stories and denied receiving any bribes, and the three legislators accused of giving the bribes also denied any involvement. The committee therefore found no reason to believe that the Democrats who voted for Lorimer had been bribed to do so.

One committee member, Albert J. Beveridge (R-IN), even though belonging to Lorimer's party, refused to sign the majority report and submitted his own minority report. In it he contended that the four legislators had repeatedly testified under oath that they had been bribed and that they were found to have "unusual sums of money in bills of large denominations" right after the bribes were said to have occurred. The fact that the three legislators accused of giving the bribes denied the charge he considered unconvincing, since they would naturally not want to admit to a crime. Thus, he considered that seven of the votes for Lorimer were tainted by bribery, enough to invalidate the election, since Lorimer had won by only six more than a majority of those voting. Beveridge also differed with the majority report regarding the precedents from previous cases, asserting that it was time to establish a new precedent that "if only one case of bribery be clearly established in the election of a Senator," even without the knowledge of that senator, "this invalidates the entire election." Such a policy, he declared, would send a clear message to legislators to clean up elections. "Our business," he continued, "is to guard the purity of election." Adding that he found it unlikely that Lorimer, who carefully oversaw all aspects of his campaign, was truly ignorant of the efforts at bribery, Beveridge concluded that Lorimer's election was invalid. In separate reports, three other committee members joined Beveridge in this conclusion. When news that Beveridge was preparing a dissent leaked to the press, a deluge of supporting mail descended on the Indiana senator, since progressives viewed his denunciation of Lorimer as a holy crusade.

The Senate debate began on January 18, 1911, and continued for six weeks. When Beveridge rose to deliver his oration against the majority report, packed galleries awaited him. At the completion of his attack, divided into two segments titled "The Issue" and "The Evidence," Beveridge had demolished Lorimer's case and denied his colleagues an easy dismissal vote.

Despite the power of Beveridge's logic, the Senate on March 1, 1911, refused, by a vote of 40 yeas to 46 nays, to declare Lorimer's election void.

The committee's recommendation had unleashed a torrent of protest across the nation. During the long Senate investigation, public sentiment against Lorimer mounted as the Illinois press relentlessly chronicled the flagrant campaign abuses of his supporters. The American public, riding the crest of progressive reform, heightened its condemnation of William Lorimer when, at the investigation's midpoint, former President Theodore Roosevelt refused to be seated with the senator at a Chicago banquet table.

Second Investigation

Beveridge's Senate term ended on March 3, 1911, but the public uproar over Lorimer's campaign tactics lingered. On April 6, 1911, at the beginning of the Sixty-second Congress, Robert M. La Follette (R-WI) urged the Senate to reopen the case on the basis of reports in the Chicago newspapers indicating that $100,000 had been spent on bribes to secure Lorimer's election. Six weeks later, the Illinois state senate buttressed La Follette's position with a report tying Lorimer and high-ranking Illinois executives to the campaign corruption. After considerable debate, the Senate on June 7, 1911, authorized a special committee of eight members of the Privileges and Elections Committee to conduct a second investigation into the 1909 Lorimer election.

Almost a year later, on May 20, 1912, the committee returned a majority and a minority report of its findings. After hearing 180 witnesses and amassing eight volumes of testimony, the majority stated that it had "failed to find any evidence that a fund" was raised to be spent in connection with Lorimer's election, nor did they find evidence of "any corrupt practices" in that election. Once again, the majority argued that, despite the extensive testimony about illegal money transactions, no evidence directly linked Lorimer to the wheeling and dealing. The three minority members dismissed arguments from Lorimer's counsel that the matter had already been adjudicated by the 1911 Senate vote. They contended that the second investigation added substantive new information about the scope of Lorimer's involvement and established "conclusively that at least ten of the votes cast" for Lorimer were corruptly obtained. Led by Albert Beveridge's replacement, Indiana Democrat John Worth Kern, the minority therefore demanded that Lorimer's election be ruled invalid.

The Senate debated the two reports extensively before finally voting on July 13, 1912. By a vote of 55 to 28, a progressive-minded Senate agreed with the minority and declared William Lorimer's election invalid.

Conclusion

William Lorimer was the last senator to be deprived of office for corrupting a state legislature, since in May 1912 the Seventeenth Amendment providing for direct election of U.S. senators was finally passed by Congress and sent to the states for ratification. In May 1913 the amendment became part of the U.S. Constitution, and in November of that year the first senator was elected under its provisions, permanently ending the role of state legislatures in the election of U.S. senators.

The special investigating committee attempted to provide $35,000 for the ousted senator's expenses incurred from two investigations, but Congress adjourned without acting on the resolution, and the matter was not taken up at any future session.

William Lorimer, unrepentant and undaunted, returned to Chicago, where a loyal population greeted him with festive celebrations. Soon after, however, his financial affairs faltered. Although unsuccessful in his efforts to be elected to the Senate in 1916 and in 1918 to the House of Representatives, Lorimer continued to circulate among powerful business and political associates. He died in 1934 at the age of 74.

Sources

U.S. Congress. Senate. *Congressional Record.* 61st Cong., 1st sess. (See p. 3437.) 2d sess. (See pp. 7019–70, 7190, 7528–37, 8452, 8501.) 3d sess. (See pp. 547–52, 654–57, 665–68, 716–28, 767, 1041–58, 1279–90, 1413–25, 1487–88, 1524–35, 1886–96, 1980–90, 2050–66, 2187–89, 2246–51, 2474–90, 3258–3306, 3521–88, 3650–58, 3753–60, 4113–14, 1632–33.)

———. *Congressional Record.* 62d Cong., 1st sess. (see pp. 101, 793, 924, 1430–31, 1482, 1490–95, 1547–57, 1600–1605, 1609–10, 1628–46, 1654–82, 1693, 1698, 1732–34.) 2d sess. (See pp. 6790, 7594–97, 7700–7706, 7775–87, 7845–48, 8671–82, 8685–96, 8723–74, 8812–48, 8882–8901, 8936–49, 8968–87.)

———. Senate Report No. 942. 61st Cong., 3d sess., 1910.

———. Senate Report No. 769. 62d Cong., 2d sess., 1912.

Bowers, Claude. *Beveridge and the Progressive Era.* New York, 1932. (See pp. 406–9.)

Haynes, George H. *The Senate of the United States.* Vol. 1. Boston, 1938. (See pp. 132–35.)

Starr, Harris E., ed. *Dictionary of American Biography.* Supp. 1. New York, 1946. (See pp. 511–12.)

Case 96

Isaac Stephenson

(1829–1918)

Wisconsin

Election Case
June 30, 1911 to March 27, 1912

Issues
Electoral misconduct: bribery and corruption

Result: Retained seat

Chronology:
Request for investigation: June 30, 1911
Referred to committee: June 30, 1911
Committee report: Feb. 12, 1912
Senate vote: Mar. 27, 1912

Background

Isaac Stephenson, a successful Wisconsin businessman, plunged into Republican politics soon after the party's 1854 formation in the Dairy State. He served in a variety of local offices, and in 1883 Wisconsin voters sent him to the United States House of Representatives, where he remained for three terms. In May 1907 Stephenson was elected to fill a vacancy in the U. S. Senate, and in 1909 he was reelected to the full term beginning on March 4, 1909.

Statement of the Case

On March 15, 1909, Isaac Stephenson presented his credentials for the new term and was seated without objection. More than two years later, on June 30, 1911, the Wisconsin legislature notified the U. S. Senate that it considered Stephenson's claim to the seat invalid, because a state investigation into the 1909 election had found evidence of bribery and corruption by Stephenson both in the state's direct primary in 1908 and in his 1909 election by the legislature. State investigators reported, for example, that Stephenson's primary campaign expenditures exceeded $107,000. In the years before passage of the Seventeenth Amendment providing for direct election of senators, a number of states adopted the system of holding a popular primary to enable voters to express their preference for U.S. senator. Although the results of such primaries were not legally binding, in practice state legislators were inclined to follow the popular mandate when they formally elected a senator.

The Senate referred the Wisconsin communication to the Committee on Privileges and Elections that same day, and on August 15 the Senate authorized the committee to investigate Stephenson's campaign.

Response of the Senate

On October 2, 1911, a subcommittee began hearings in Milwaukee, Wisconsin, that lasted for twenty-five days and amassed over two thousand pages of printed testimony. One hundred twenty-four witnesses, often with flippancy and boldness, described receiving and spending campaign funds, destroying financial records, and removing campaign correspondence to a secret location outside the state.

On February 12, 1912, a divided committee reported to the Senate. The majority report sustained Stephenson's right to his seat. It dismissed as insignificant several technicalities in the election procedures of the Wisconsin legislature, none of which had substantive bearing on the outcome of the election. It also preferred not to review activities during the direct primary, because under the U.S. Constitution such state primaries were "no part of an election of a United States senator." Regarding the conduct of Stephenson himself, the report defended his campaign expenditures, such as the purchase of newspaper advertising, payment of poll workers and other campaign aides, and the maintenance of a headquarters in a local hotel, as acceptable campaign tactics rather than as evidence of corrupt practices. The committee mildly rebuked the senator for failing to require his associates to keep adequate records and for the lavish expenditure of money, but the report concluded that other candidates who spent less did so because of a lack of funds rather than a higher degree of morality. The committee noted that in 1911 the Federal Corrupt Practices Act had limited to $10,000 the amount a Senate candidate could spend on his campaign and Wisconsin had adopted a $7,500 limit, but neither law had been in effect at the time of Stephenson's election.

A minority report vehemently disagreed with these points. Although the direct primary had no legal force in the election of senators, the report noted that many legislators felt morally bound to vote for the individual who won the primary. Thus, if success in the primary was achieved by corrupt means, the actual election by the legislature would also have been affected. Mindful of a rising public outcry against expensive campaigns, the report's authors emphasized the undisputed testimony that seventy agents, charged to distribute funds on Stephenson's behalf, openly toured the state for that purpose, and Stephenson himself had ordered $2,500 given to a local game warden. Based on such uncontroverted evidence, the minority report told the Senate that corruption was used in the primary, which "directly contributed to destroy the purity and freedom of the election," and concluded that Stephenson's election was invalid.

Long and emotional floor debates followed the distribution of the reports, as supporters and opponents of Stephenson read into the *Congressional Record* extensive excerpts from the testimony gathered by the committee. Stephenson's champion, George Sutherland (R-UT) made the distinction that it was possible to spend a great deal of money for legitimate purposes in a primary election, such as the $11,000 Stephenson had expended for postage. While senators might disapprove of such exorbitant expenditures, they were not in themselves evidence of corruption. Sutherland concluded by pleading that, at the age of eighty-three, Stephenson probably had only a short time left to live and should be permitted to finish his life with his honor intact. "Yet a few more days and he must pass on, leaving nothing of permanent value behind him, unless it be the record of an honored and honorable name." Unmoved by these entreaties, opponents like Miles Poindexter (R-WA) denounced the majority report. Poindexter told his colleagues that, since Stephenson supplied the money that was spent, common sense made it obvious that he must have known about the flagrant transactions. At the close of the debate, Francis Newlands (D-NV) offered a line of reasoning that may have assisted many in their voting decision when he condemned Stephenson's campaign practices but pointed out that, since the Wisconsin election, public opinion had grown much stronger against activities prohibited by recent laws that had not been illegal in 1908. He therefore added, "I am unwilling to judge the acts of four years ago either by the political or the moral standards of today." When on March 27, 1912, the Senate voted 40 to 34 that Stephenson should retain his seat, spectators in the gallery burst into enthusiastic applause, for which they were promptly chided by the presiding officer.

Conclusion

This case, like that of William Lorimer (See Case 95), was being considered by the Senate at a time when public sentiment was running high against the use of money and questionable practices during state legislatures' election of senators and while Congress was debating the Seventeenth Amendment, which became law in 1913.

Although Stephenson's advanced age helped to save him from losing his seat, he did not expire quite as promptly as George Sutherland had predicted. Stephenson served in the Senate until 1915 and lived in retirement for another three years before his death in 1918.

Sources

U.S. Congress. Senate. *Congressional Record.* 62d Cong., 1st sess. (See pp. 2599, 3860, 3938.) 2d sess. (See pp. 1946–53, 2182–87, 2189–95, 2233–39, 2281–92, 2608–09, 2656–69, 2703–18, 2762–74, 3777, 3803–11, 3817–27, 3829–31, 3865–96.)

———. Senate Report No. 349. 62d Cong., 2d sess., 1912.

Malone, Dumas, ed. *Dictionary of American Biography.* Vol. 17. New York, 1946; reprint of 1935 edition. (See pp. 582–83.)

Case 97

Clarence W. Watson and William E. Chilton

(1864–1940) (1858–1939)

West Virginia

Election Case
August 26, 1912 to February 11, 1913

Issues
Electoral misconduct: charges of bribery

Result: Retained seats

Chronology:
Petition submitted: Aug. 26, 1912
Referred to committee: Aug. 26, 1912
Committee report: Feb. 11, 1913
Senate vote: Feb. 11, 1913

Background

Politics and industry blended in West Virginia in a union that often crossed party lines and blurred the distinctions between Democrats and Republicans. Senator Stephen B. Elkins dominated the Republicans while his father-in-law and business associate, Henry Gassaway Davis, controlled the Democrats. In 1911 this interconnection of political and industrial interests contributed to the election of two Democratic West Virginia senators, Clarence W. Watson and William E. Chilton.

Statement of the Case

On February 2, 1911, Clarence Watson took his seat for a term that ended March 3, 1913. Four days later, the credentials of William E. Chilton were presented for the other West Virginia seat for a term that began on March 4, 1911. On April 4, 1911, the first day of the Sixty-second Congress, Chilton took his seat.

Stephen B. Elkins had died in January 1911, ending the iron grip he had maintained on West Virginia political and industrial life. Since he had dominated the state's governors, it was not surprising that after his death the state's executive sought to flex his own political muscle. Accordingly, more than a year after the seating of Watson and Chilton, the West Virginia governor filed a petition charging that the two—both well connected to state industrialists—had secured their nominations through bribes paid by rail and oil corporations. The charge was based on the claim by one member of the West Virginia legislature that prior to the 1911 Democratic caucus he had accepted $1,000 as inducement to vote for the two senators. The Senate referred the matter to the Committee on Privileges and Elections.

Response of the Senate

On February 11, 1913, the committee returned a unanimous report favorable to Watson and Chilton. The report concluded that the only evidence of improper conduct stemmed from the account of the legislator, L. J. Shock, who had subsequently recanted the charges in a letter he sent to Clarence Watson on January 8, 1913. In it he stated: "I have let the talking go on because I hated to be put in a wrong light. The truth is that I set up the whole business. Nobody tried to buy my vote.... So far as I know, your election and Chilton's was honest and fair." The committee deemed the written retraction sufficient to recommend dismissing the charges. Any other allegations in the West Virginia petitions the committee considered to be nothing more than political rumors calculated to arouse suspicion and create prejudice during a campaign and thus unworthy of Senate consideration. The Senate accepted the recommendation for dismissal and took no further action.

Conclusion

Clarence Watson left the Senate at the completion of his term in 1913. He then ran a coal company and owned a training stables. He died in 1940. William Chilton served in the Senate until 1917. When narrowly defeated in 1916, he contested the election, but the Senate determined that his opponent should retain the seat (See Case 100). A forceful attorney and a dynamic public speaker, Chilton failed in his subsequent attempts at reelection to the Senate. He died in 1939.

Sources

U.S. Congress. Senate. *Congressional Record.* 61st Cong., 3d sess. (See pp. 1797, 1969.)

———. *Congressional Record,* 62d Cong., 1st sess. (See p. 2.) 2d sess. (See pp. 11862–65. 3d sess. (See pp. 2635–37, 3001.)

———. Senate Report No. 1206. 62d Cong., 2d sess., 1913.

Case 98

Henry D. Clayton and Franklin P. Glass

(1857–1929) (1858–1934)

Alabama

Election Case (appointment)
August 20, 1913 to February 4, 1914

Issues
Interpretation of 17th Amendment

Result: Not seated

Chronology:
Clayton
Credentials presented: Aug. 20, 1913
Referred to committee: Aug. 20, 1913
Credentials withdrawn: Oct. 21, 1913

Glass
Credentials presented: Nov. 22, 1913
Referred to committee: Nov. 22, 1913
Committee report: Jan. 21, 1914
Senate vote: Feb. 4, 1914

Background

On May 31, 1913, the Seventeenth Amendment officially became part of the United States Constitution. This long-awaited, badly needed change removed the selection of United States senators from the state legislatures and placed the elective power directly in the hands of the voting citizens. Less than three months after its effective date, the new amendment came under close scrutiny when the death of Alabama Senator Joseph F. Johnston required the Senate to analyze the meaning of the amendment regarding vacancies that occurred during the transition period.

Statement of the Case

On August 12, 1913, Alabama Governor Emmet O'Neal appointed U.S. Representative Henry D. Clayton (D) to fill the vacancy in Johnston's seat until the Alabama assembly gathered for its next regular session in 1915. Eight days later, on August 20, Clayton's credentials were presented to the United States Senate.

Senators found themselves in disagreement over the governor's right to appoint Clayton under the provisions of the new amendment. Some senators questioned the governor's right to appoint anyone to a seat that should have been filled through a special election by Alabama voters. Alabama state officials and their supporters in the Senate, however, contended that the third clause of the Seventeenth Amendment provided that a vacancy in the term of a member selected before the 1913 direct election change would be filled according to the regulations in the original Constitution. The Senate referred the matter to the Committee on Privileges and Elections.

On October 21, 1913, the other Alabama senator, J.S. Bankhead (D) announced that Henry Clayton had decided to decline his appointment, having been asked by President Woodrow Wilson to remain in the House of Representatives. Clayton therefore asked that his credentials be withdrawn.

On November 7, 1913, Governor O'Neal named a replacement, newspaper publisher and Wilson supporter Franklin P. Glass (D), to fill the vacancy caused by the death of Johnston. The presentation of these credentials on November 22 raised the same issue that had blocked Henry Clayton's seating. Glass was not seated, and the Senate sent his credentials to the Committee on Privileges and Elections.

Response of the Senate

On January 21, 1914, the majority of the committee returned a report unfavorable to Glass' claim, which rested entirely upon the construction given to the Seventeenth Amendment. In a minority report, the supporters of Glass argued, as they had for Henry Clayton, that Johnston had been elected to the Senate before adoption of the amendment, and that a vacancy in his seat demanded a replacement under the rules by which he was elected. They further asserted that the Seventeenth Amendment was not self-executing and that, until Congress or the individual states enacted legislation to establish election procedures, senators had to be chosen in the original manner.

The majority report dismissed these arguments unequivocally, holding that, with the passage of the Seventeenth Amendment, a governor needed the express permission of the state legislature to make a temporary appointment. The report also dismissed the notion that the amendment was not self-executing, noting that, if it were not, states could continue indefinitely to select senators under the old system. Finally, it concluded that the Alabama governor already possessed the authority to call a special election and did not need additional enabling legislation. Proponents of immediate enforcement rejected Alabama's contention that it was denied equal representation in the Senate because of the length of time required to organize a special election, observing that, in any event, there would always be some hiatus in a state's Senate representation after the death of a senator.

After two days of intense debate that centered on minute interpretations of constitutional language, the Senate on February 4, 1914, concurred with the majority report and voted 34 to 30 to deny Franklin Glass a seat.

Conclusion

After the refusal of the United States Senate to accept either of his appointees, Governor O'Neal issued a writ of election, and the people of Alabama elected Frank S. White (D) to fill the unexpired portion of Johnston's term. Sworn in on May 22, 1914, White served until the end of the term in 1915. He then returned to his law practice in Birmingham, where he died in 1922.

Henry Clayton remained in the House of Representatives until 1914, when he was appointed U.S. district judge in Alabama. He died in 1929. Glass continued his newspaper and civic activities in Alabama and served on the U.S. Board of Mediation from 1933 until his death in 1934.

Sources

U.S. Congress. Senate. *Congressional Record.* 63d Cong., 1st sess. (See pp. 3492, 3553, 3736, 5708, 5965–66.) 2d sess. (See pp. 2010–13, 2254–55, 2793–2817, 2864–86, 9000.)

———. Senate Report No. 164. 63d Cong., 2d sess., parts 1 and 2, 1914.

Link, Arthur S., ed. *The Papers of Woodrow Wilson.* Vol. 28. Princeton, NJ, 1978. (See p. 160.)

Starr, Harris E., ed. *Dictionary of American Biography.* Supp. 1. New York, 1946. (See pp. 179, 346–47.)

VII. Direct Election and the 1920s: 1914–1929

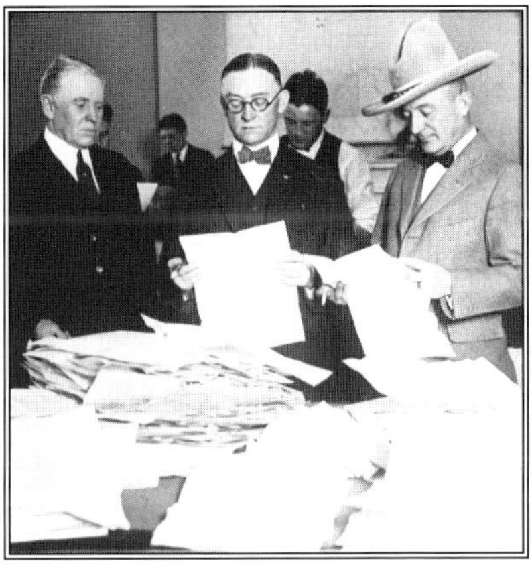

Members of the subcommittee investigating the Peddy-Mayfield contested election *(Case 103)*
U.S. Senate Historical Office

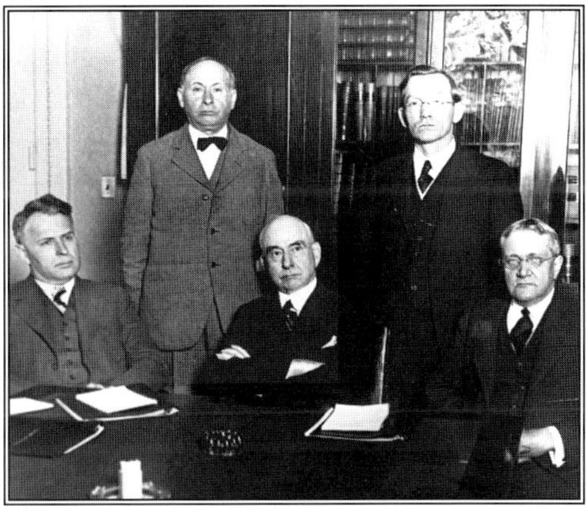

The subcommittee of the Committee on Privileges and Elections who recounted the ballots in the Wilson-Vare election *(Case 109) (Left to right, seated, Frederick Steiwer, Charles W. Waterman, George Moses; standing, T.H. Caraway, Sam G. Bratton.) January 30, 1928. U.S. Senate Historical Office*

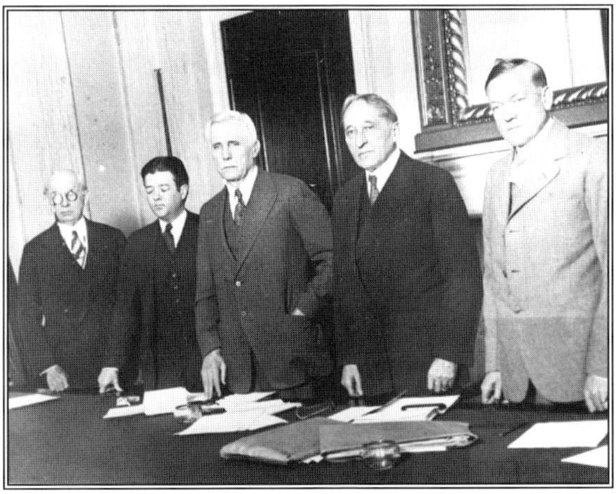

Special Committee to Investigate Senatorial Elections *(Case 109) (Left to right, Guy G. Goff, Robert M. La Follette, Jr., James A. Reed, chairman, William H. King, Charles McNary.) January 4, 1929. U.S. Senate Historical Office*

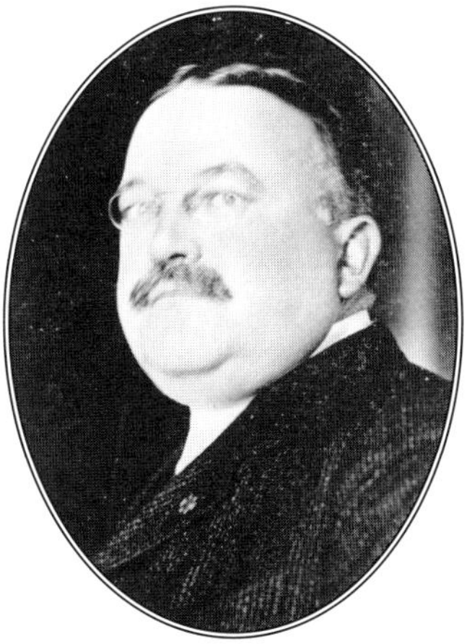

Truman H. Newberry
(Case 102)
U.S. Senate Historical Office

Case 99

William Purnell Jackson v. Blair Lee

(1868–1939) (1857–1944)

Maryland

Election Case
December 5, 1913 to January 28, 1914

Issues
Interpretation of the 17th Amendment

Result: Lee Seated

Chronology:
Credentials presented: Dec. 5, 1913
Referred to committee: Dec. 5, 1913
Committee report: Jan. 19, 1914
Senate vote: Jan. 28, 1914

Background

In January 1910 the Maryland state assembly elected Isidor Rayner to a United States Senate term that would end March 3, 1917. On November 25, 1912, Rayner died, and Republican reform governor Phillips Lee Goldsborough promptly named a party colleague, William Purnell Jackson, to fill the vacancy on a temporary appointment.

Statement of the Case

On May 31, 1913, the Seventeenth Amendment, providing for direct popular election of senators, became part of the Constitution. In accord with the new amendment's provisions, Governor Goldsborough issued a writ of election for the vacancy that Jackson filled under the temporary appointment. When Maryland held the special election on November 4, 1913, the winner, Democrat Blair Lee, became the first popularly elected United States senator.

Lee's election was quickly challenged by supporters of William P. Jackson on the grounds that, since he had been appointed under the original constitutional provision, he was entitled to hold his seat until the regularly scheduled adjournment date of the Maryland state assembly. Jackson argued that, under the terms of his appointment, he held his place until the assembly elected a replacement, or if it failed to do so, until it adjourned. Jackson thus claimed that he had the right to remain in the Senate until April 7, 1914, the latest date he could have remained a senator if the Seventeenth Amendment had never been passed.

In response to the challenge, the Senate deferred seating Blair Lee when his credentials were presented on December 5, 1912, and referred the matter to the Committee on Privileges and Elections.

Response of the Senate

On January 19, 1914, the committee returned a majority report favorable to Blair Lee. This report argued that Jackson's tenure had always been uncertain because his appointment was temporary. Since the passage of the Seventeenth Amendment ended the state legislature's authority in the matter of senatorial selection, there was no longer any basis for his contention that he should hold office until the legislature adjourned. The majority thus concluded that Jackson's right to a seat terminated on the election of a qualified successor, "without regard to the manner of such election." The bipartisan majority also emphasized the legality and propriety with which the Maryland special election had been conducted and praised the correctness of this first popular election. The report congratulated the Maryland governor for his willingness to comply with every aspect of the new regulation, including the endorsement of credentials when the election was won by a member of the opposing political party.

In two minority reports, three Republican committee members tried to bolster Jackson's case by arguing that the governor could not call an election without action by the legislature to set the time and manner of the election, and the Maryland legislature had adopted no regulation since ratification of the Seventeenth Amendment. The minority also contended that the amendment itself stated that it should not affect the term of any senator chosen before it took effect.

The Senate debated the intention and the meaning of the Seventeenth Amendment for two days. Then, on January 28, 1914, it voted 53 to 13 to accept the reasoning of the majority report that Jackson's claim was always a temporary one and that Blair Lee had been elected in accord with the requirements of the new constitutional amendment. Lee then came forward and took the oath of office.

Conclusion

This case and that of Franklin P. Glass that was resolved a week later (See Case 98) were the last in which the Senate wrestled with the role of the state legislatures in electing U.S. senators. All future election disputes were governed by the provisions of the Seventeenth Amendment.

William Purnell Jackson continued his political career in Maryland and served as the state treasurer for two years. He died in 1939. Blair Lee served in the Senate until 1917. He then returned to a distinguished career in the practice of law until his death in 1944.

Sources

U.S. Congress. Senate. *Congressional Record.* 63d Cong., 2d sess. (See pp. 233, 1917–18, 2014–15, 2252–53, 2319–29, 2414–26.)

———. Senate Report No. 160. 63d Cong., 2d sess., 1914.

William E. Chilton v. Howard Sutherland

(1858–1939) (1865–1950)

West Virginia

Election Case
March 14, 1917 to June 29, 1918

Issues
Campaign financing

Chronology:
Request for investigation: Mar. 14, 1917
Referred to committee: Mar. 14, 1917
Committee report: June 26, 1918
Senate vote: June 29, 1918

Result: Sutherland retained seat

Background

In 1916 U.S. Senator William E. Chilton (D) and U.S. Representative Howard Sutherland (R) squared off for a closely contested Senate race in West Virginia. Each possessed impressive business and political contacts throughout the state as well as a solid record of public service. Chilton, as the incumbent seeking his second Senate term, appeared to have the advantage, but the final count gave the victory to the Republican challenger Sutherland by slightly more than five thousand votes.

Statement of the Case

On March 5, 1917, Howard Sutherland was seated in the Senate without objection. A week later, however, on March 14, Furnifold Simmons (D-NC) presented a petition from his defeated party colleague, Chilton, requesting an investigation into the West Virginia election. Chilton charged that Sutherland's campaign expenditures in the primary election exceeded the limit set by West Virginia law and that the registration rolls included the names of thousands of nonresidents and deceased persons, whose names were used in repeat voting for Republican candidates. The Senate referred the petition to the Committee on Privileges and Elections.

Response of the Senate

In December 1917, while the committee was still reviewing the case, Chilton wrote to equivocate his charge, announcing that he lacked the evidence to substantiate the accusations of voting irregularities. Since he had neither the time nor the money to gather the necessary proof, Chilton withdrew that portion of his complaint. In doing so, he claimed patriotic motives, insisting that, with the onset of the First World War, he did not wish to tie up the Senate in a domestic political skirmish. Given the lack of evidence and the fact that Sutherland denied the charges of corruption, the committee ended its consideration of possible voting irregularities and focused instead on the matter of Sutherland's campaign expenditures.

On June 26, 1918, the committee reported that all parties agreed that Sutherland had complied fully with requirements for filing and publishing campaign expense accounts. After a review of all the financial statements, both Chilton and Sutherland concurred that the Republican had spent in the primary campaign $51.63 more than state law permitted. Chilton did not claim that this cash had been dispensed for bribes or corruption but only that it exceeded West Virginia campaign limitations. In view of that charge, the committee examined the corrupt practices law of West Virginia, which required that an individual be convicted before he could be ejected from office. Since Sutherland had not been arrested, tried, or convicted, this section of the West Virginia law had no application in his case. The committee therefore held that there was no reason to deprive Sutherland of his seat and added that, even though he had duly filed reports before the election showing the excess expenditure, no one had challenged his right to run in the general election.

Without debate, the Senate, on June 29, 1918, unanimously accepted the committee's recommendation that Howard Sutherland should retain his seat.

Conclusion

Despite the small sum involved in these charges, the committee thoroughly examined state and federal statutes governing election finances. The final report emphasized that all state and federal laws related to election procedures "should be strictly complied with." The committee also made clear that it had exonerated Sutherland because the amount in this particular case was trivial, but this action should not "be regarded as a precedent for disregard of state laws limiting expenditures."

William Chilton made two additional unsuccessful efforts to return to the Senate—once in 1924 and again in 1939, the year he died. Howard Sutherland unsuccessfully sought the Republican nomination for president as a favorite-son candidate in 1920, then returned to his Senate duties until the conclusion of his term. Defeated for reelection in 1922, he resumed his West Virginia business activities. From 1925 to 1933, he served in Washington, D.C., as alien property custodian, overseeing German property seized by the United States in World War I. He died in 1950.

Sources

U.S. Congress. Senate. *Congressional Record.* 64th Cong., 2d sess. (See p. 4369.)

———. *Congressional Record.* 65th Cong., spec. sess. (See pp. 2, 71.) 2d sess. (See pp. 8308, 8499.)

———. Senate Report No. 525. 65th Cong., 2d sess., 1918.

Casdorph, Paul D. "Howard Sutherland's 1920 Bid for the Presidency." *West Virginia History* 35 (October 1973): 1–25.

Case 101

Robert M. La Follette

(1855–1925)

Wisconsin

Expulsion Case
September 29, 1917 to January 16, 1919

Issues
Freedom of speech in wartime

Chronology:
Petition received: Sept. 29, 1917
Referred to committee: Sept. 29, 1917
Committee report: Jan. 16, 1919
Senate vote: Jan. 16, 1919

Result: Not expelled

Background

Shortly after America's entry into World War I, members of the Nonpartisan League, an organization of farmers that promoted cooperatives and an alliance with labor against the power of large corporations, gathered in St. Paul, Minnesota. On September 20, 1917, Wisconsin Senator Robert M. La Follette (R) delivered a keynote address to the convention that included a call for increased taxation of the wealthy, a fervent attack on corporations, and a stinging denunciation of America's participation in World War I. Delegates' cheers repeatedly interrupted the emotion-charged oration, and upon La Follette's return to Wisconsin, enthusiastic supporters continued to praise him for his outspoken remarks.

Statement of the Case

Not all Americans considered the senator's performance appropriate during a national crisis of world war, and the prowar press raised a public furor over the speech. On September 29, 1917, the Senate received a petition from the Minnesota Commission of Public Safety, formally taking exception to La Follette's St. Paul address and asking the Senate to expel the popular Wisconsin progressive. The commission charged that La Follette was "a teacher of disloyalty and sedition, giving aid and comfort to our enemies."

The Senate was keenly aware that La Follette's critics included not only some of the nation's most powerful entrepreneurs but also President Woodrow Wilson, who made no secret of his hatred for the popular senator. It therefore decided to refer the matter to the Committee on Privileges and Elections.

Response of the Senate

In early October committee chairman Atlee Pomerene (D-OH) sent La Follette a copy of the speech, asking whether it was a correct copy. In a forceful reply, La Follette asserted that the transcript Pomerene had sent him was grossly inaccurate, and he demanded to know whether the committee considered any of the statements he had made to be false. Noting that he had delivered the address extemporaneously, La Follette enclosed a transcript prepared by the official reporter of the Nonpartisan League, which he declared to be correct, although it did not include all of the questions from the audience.

Also in early October, La Follette delivered a dramatic speech on the Senate floor on the subject of "Free Speech in Wartime." In it he cited many authorities in his own defense and in support of "the right of the people to discuss the war in all its phases and the right and the duty of the people's representatives in Congress to declare the purposes and objects of the war." His remarks were well received by those opposed to the wartime suppression of free speech, although bitterly denounced by the press and prowar senators. Following the same theme in a brief prepared for the committee, La Follette's legal counsel reviewed several previous wars that had been opposed by members of Congress whose patriotism was unquestioned, including Abraham Lincoln, Henry Clay, and Daniel Webster. The brief also noted that, eight months after the speech to the Nonpartisan League, no one had yet questioned the accuracy of any statement made in it. The brief asserted firmly: "Whether . . . right or wrong in opposing the declaration of war . . . is immaterial. He had a right to his views, and he had a right to express them."

The committee's investigation dragged on for fourteen months. It became evident that a hostile press had in fact distorted the content of the speech. Although La Follette had delivered a blistering attack on corporate economic interests, for example, a press report that the senator had defended the sinking of the *Lusitania* was not substantiated, and the Associated Press submitted a statement to the committee apologizing for inaccuracies in the story it distributed.

Time worked in La Follette's favor, for the conclusion of the war helped to defuse the issue, and in the 1918 election the Republicans narrowly gained control of the Senate. On January 16, 1919, in the final session of the outgoing Democratic-controlled Congress, the committee majority, unable to find witnesses who would testify against La Follette and anxious to end the matter, recommended dismissing all charges, because the speech "does not justify any action by the Senate." Committee chairman Pomerene, however, who continued to represent the bitter interests of President Wilson, offered a brief minority report acknowledging that so far only scant evidence had been found against La Follette. Nonetheless, Pomerene urged the Senate to pursue the investigation on the basis that the senator had made an inflammatory speech opposing the war while the nation struggled under a military emergency.

The Senate, however, was ready to be rid of the issue. La Follette's friends objected to the investigation on principle, while his opponents feared that further prosecution would only add to his astounding popularity. All took a dim view of a policy that might lead a Senate majority to censure expressions of opinion made by the minority outside the Senate and not in the exercise of legislative duty. These considerations combined to make the Senate unwilling to pursue a subject whose importance had dwindled to little more than a personal vendetta by President Woodrow Wilson. On January 16, after only a brief debate, the Senate voted 50 to 21 to dismiss all charges against Robert La Follette.

Conclusion

Three years later, the Senate awarded La Follette $5,000 for his legal expenses in the case. La Follette, a champion of the rights of the people—who received 16 percent of the popular vote when he ran for president on the Progressive party ticket in 1924—died in Washington in 1925. As a funeral train carried the senator to his home in Wisconsin, thousands of Americans lined the rails to pay homage to a public servant who had worked tirelessly on their behalf.

Sources

U.S. Congress. Senate. *Congressional Record.* 65th Cong., 1st sess. (See p. 7491.) 3d sess. (See pp. 1506–27.)

———. *Hearings before a Subcommittee of the Committee on Privileges and Elections.* Part 1. 65th Cong., 1st sess. Part 2. 65th Cong., 2d sess., Vol. 188.

———. Senate Report No. 614. 65th Cong., 3d sess., 1919.

———. *The Senate, 1789–1989,* by Robert C. Byrd. Vol. 3. *Classic Speeches, 1830–1993.* S. Doc. 100–20, 100th Cong., 1st sess., 1994. (See pp. 519–40.)

Thelen, David P. *Robert M. La Follette and the Insurgent Spirit.* Boston, 1976.

Weisberger, Bernard A. *The La Follettes of Wisconsin.* Madison, 1994. (See pp. 208–10.)

Henry Ford v. Truman H. Newberry

(1863–1947) (1864–1945)

Michigan

Election Case/Expulsion Case
September 17, 1918 to January 12, 1922

Issues
Campaign financing; recount of ballots

Result: Newberry retained seat but later resigned/Not expelled

Chronology:
Petition filed: Sept. 17, 1918
Referred to committee: Sept. 17, 1918
Committee report: Sept. 29, 1921
Senate vote: Jan. 12, 1922

Background

A growing national concern about the need to regulate the use of money in political campaigns mushroomed as a result of the 1918 senatorial contest in Michigan. Each of the candidates—Truman H. Newberry, the Republican industrialist, and Henry Ford, the Democratic automobile magnate—was a person of enormous wealth. Henry Ford, asked to run by President Woodrow Wilson, entered both the Republican and Democratic primaries. Wanting to ensure that Ford, with his wider name recognition, did not win both primaries, the Newberry organization plunged into the Republican primary contest with vigorous rhetoric and an unrestrained budget that was used especially to buy advertising and other publicity. Newberry's campaign charged Ford with pacifism, anti-Semitism, and extreme efforts to keep his son, Edsel, from military service. As a result, in the August 1918 primary Newberry gained the Republican nomination, while Ford won the Democratic contest. In the general election campaign, Henry Ford's prestige failed to offset the impact of the Newberry attack, and on November 5, 1918, Truman Newberry won the Michigan seat.

A groundswell of protest erupted from the many citizens offended by the Newberry campaign's blatant spending practices, both in the August primary and the November general election. Newspapers called for Newberry's removal, and Republican associates advised him to resign. Choosing to brush aside these warnings, Newberry took the oath of office on May 19, 1919, at the beginning of the Sixty-sixth Congress, in which Republicans had a narrow two-vote majority.

Statement of the Case

Truman Newberry's Senate problems had begun even before the Michigan general election, when, on September 17, 1918, a resolution was introduced in the Senate calling for an investigation into the Michigan primary. The complaint was based on a report filed by Newberry's campaign committee stating that it had received and spent more than $175,000[1] on the election, far in excess of the $3,750 limit imposed by Michigan law and the Federal Corrupt Practices Act on the amount of his own money a Senate candidate could spend on his campaign. Then, on January 6, 1919, Henry Ford filed a petition with the Senate, formally contesting the election and asking for a recount. The Senate referred the September resolution and Ford's petition to the Committee on Privileges and Elections at the time each was received.

On the day after Newberry assumed his seat, Henry Ford filed a second petition. He again contested the election and charged Newberry with making unlawful expenditures and intimidating voters. The Senate referred the complaint to the Committee on Privileges and Elections and then, on December 3, 1919, adopted a resolution officially calling for an investigation into the election.

In the meantime, Newberry's problems acquired a new dimension when he and 134 campaign associates were indicted on November 29, 1919, and charged with violations of federal and state campaign laws. Despite Newberry's assertions that he knew nothing of illegal contributions and disbursements, a massive array of evidence, gathered by the U.S. Department of Justice with the help of agents financed by Henry Ford, indicated otherwise. Found guilty on March 20, 1920, Newberry appealed to the Supreme Court, which overturned the conviction by a 5-to-4 ruling on May 2, 1921. The justices narrowly struck down as unconstitutional the power of a federal statute to control state primaries, but they unanimously agreed that the judge in the case had given erroneous instructions to the jury. The favorable ruling concluded Newberry's difficulties in criminal court but not in the Senate.

Response of the Senate

On September 29, 1921, the Committee on Privileges and Elections reported that it had carried out a recount of the general election ballots and determined that Truman H. Newberry had been legally elected senator. A majority of the committee also concluded that the charges of fraud and voter intimidation were unfounded. After reviewing the testimony in the court case regarding Newberry's campaign expenditures, the majority found that no evidence sustained "the charge of improper use of money at the primary or the general election." During the primary campaign, Newberry had been away from Michigan, serving as a naval officer in New York City. According to the committee majority, the large amounts spent on Newberry's behalf were not his own funds but were contributed by his relatives and friends without his solicitation or knowledge. Although condemning the expenditure of

[1] This amount becomes more impressive to a modern reader if it is converted to 1991 dollars, in which it amounts to more than $1.5 million.

so much money—totalling at least $195,000—the majority noted that "there was no concealment whatever...and it was spent entirely for legal and proper purposes." The report therefore exonerated Newberry and recommended that the Senate declare him a duly elected senator.

A minority report signed by three Democrats contended, however, that Newberry had in fact known about the excessive expenditures and that much of the money had been transferred from his bank accounts. As a result, the minority concluded that, because of the illegal actions of the campaign, the Senate should declare Newberry not elected.

The Senate conducted an extensive debate on the matter in November and December 1921 and January 1922. Newberry and his defenders told the Senate that he regretted the large expenditures but had known nothing about them and therefore had not testified either at the trial or before the Senate committee. His opponents, however, strongly believed that the vast expenditures could not have occurred without his knowledge. Progressive Senator George W. Norris (R-NE), for example, took a satirical approach, announcing that "they had a public sale up in Michigan [for] a seat in the United States Senate." A vote to clear Newberry, he claimed, would lead to a Senate made up primarily of wealthy men, which, he added sarcastically, would "insure a high-class membership."

On January 12, 1922, the Senate adopted the majority view. It "severely condemned" Newberry's excessive expenditures as "harmful to the honor and dignity of the Senate" but voted, 46 to 41, that he was a duly elected senator from Michigan. The vote divided generally along party lines, with independent and radical Republicans joining Democrats against Newberry while regular Republicans supported him. This vote concluded the formal Senate action in the Newberry-Ford contest.

Conclusion

Even after the January 1922 Senate vote, Henry Ford, single-minded when angered, appeared unwilling to accept the decision as final. Faced with this threat of a possible renewed challenge from Ford, and also with the results of the November election, which sharply reduced the number of regular Republicans likely to support him if the question came to another Senate vote, Newberry resigned his Senate seat on November 18, 1922. He returned to his business in Michigan, where he lived until his death in 1945.

The case of Truman Newberry focused national attention on the peculiar power of the monied candidate. Although Henry Ford did not win the election, he, too, had enjoyed the special political benefits of his wealth. When he felt personally insulted by the Newberry campaign, Ford was able to marshal his vast resources to pursue his grievance in the courts. In some ways the contest was an intensely personal one between two bitter antagonists. In a larger sense, however, Ford could not have succeeded in his vendetta without the lingering spirit of progressivism that made the public anxious to rid political campaigns of financial corruption. When the Supreme Court's ruling in the case of *Newberry* v. *United States* severely weakened progressive-inspired attempts to control federal campaign expenditures, Congress in 1925 passed a new Federal Corrupt Practices Act designed to correct some of the defects of earlier legislation. Despite these endeavors, financial irregularities in congressional campaigns continued to occur throughout the next several decades.

Sources

U.S. Congress. Senate. *Congressional Record.* 65th Cong, 2d sess. (see pp. 10386–95.) 3d sess. (See pp. 437–40, 1061–67, 1607, 2118–22, 2260, 2805–18, 2875, 3449, 4209–16.)

———. *Congressional Record.* 66th Cong., 1st sess. (See pp. 3, 33–40, 62–68, 1262.) 2d sess. (See pp. 65–66.)

———. *Congressional Record.* 67th Cong., 1st sess. (See pp. 1008–18, 5866, 7633–35, 7746–7814, 7834–49, 7894–7913, 7952–74, 8040–59, 8089–8104, 8122–23, 8165–66.) 2d sess. (See pp. 101–4, 142, 218–29, 614–27, 771–77, 820–22, 830–32, 867–68, 874–94, 934–50, 955–79, 988–1006, 1037–62, 1089–1116, 1810–12, 1946, 2054–57, 2062, 2100, 4065–66, 5160, 6883–85, 11734–40, 11949.)

———. Senate Report No. 277. 67th Cong., 1st sess., 1921.

Newberry v. *United States* (1921), 256 U.S. 232.

Ervin, Spencer. *Henry Ford vs. Truman H. Newberry.* New York, 1935.

Garraty, John A., and Edward T. James, eds. *Dictionary of American Biography.* Supp. 4. New York, 1974. (See pp. 291–304.)

James, Edward T., ed. *Dictionary of American Biography.* Supp. 3. New York, 1973. (See pp. 549–51.)

McCusker, John J. *How Much Is That in Real Money? A Historical Price Index for Use as a Deflator of Money Values in the Economy of the United States.* Worcester, MA, 1992. (See pp. 330, 332.)

Norris, George. *Fighting Liberal: The Autobiography of George Norris.* New York, 1945.

George E.B. Peddy v. Earle B. Mayfield

(dates unknown) (1881–1964)

Texas

Election Case
February 22, 1923 to February 3, 1925

Issues
Recount of disputed ballots; Senate review of state primary election regulations

Result: Mayfield retained seat

Chronology:
Petition filed: Feb. 22, 1923
Referred to committee: Jan. 3, 1924
Committee report: Feb. 2, 1925
Senate vote: Feb. 3, 1925

Background

After the end of Reconstruction, the Republican party in Texas remained a shadow organization well into the twentieth century. Democrats enjoyed years of almost total state control as on several occasions Republicans failed to field a slate of candidates. However, in the 1922 Senate election George E. B. Peddy, running as both a Republican and an Independent, rallied sufficient support to challenge Democrat Earle Mayfield. Mayfield, a lawyer with strong support from business and railroad interests throughout Texas, claimed victory on November 7, 1922.

Statement of the Case

On February 22, 1923, George Peddy filed a petition protesting Mayfield's seating for the term to begin March 4. Peddy, in a complex list of complaints, charged irregularities in both the Texas Democratic primary and runoff and in the general election. His allegations included the use of fraudulent ballot counting procedures, excessive expenditure of money, and the flagrant participation of the Ku Klux Klan on behalf of Mayfield. Peddy specifically requested a recount of the general election.

When the Sixty-eighth Congress convened on December 3, 1923, Earle Mayfield appeared and took his oath of office. One month later, on January 3, 1924, the Senate authorized the Committee on Privileges and Elections to conduct an investigation into unlawful practices in the Democratic primary and the general election.

Response of the Senate

On February 2, 1925, the committee announced the result of its year-long investigation, which had included not only taking testimony but also recounting the general election ballots. Reviewing the ballots that had been transported to Washington, D.C., from Texas, the committee recorded thousands of irregularities for both candidates, in which ballots lacked numbers, the signatures of election judges, or the official stamp. Despite the clear and widespread violations by both parties, the committee decided the irregularities could not have altered the outcome of the election, since Mayfield received 221,596 votes to 117,599 for Peddy.

Although the committee discussed a number of the other irregularities cited by Peddy that dealt with state election laws and regulations, it chose not to challenge the authority of the state. For example, the report noted that the Texas attorney general had for the first time enforced a state election statute stating that a candidate's name could only appear on the ballot if he were nominated in a primary election. Since Peddy, like all previous Republican senatorial candidates, was selected through a convention process, his name was kept off the ballot. This action the committee believed to be within the authority of the state, even though the statute had not previously been enforced. The committee also refused to challenge a complicated Texas law that denied a primary vote to any party member who had not voted for the regular party ticket at the last preceding general election.

The committee also discussed but failed to confront the role played by the Ku Klux Klan in the 1922 election. The report noted that the committee found no evidence that the Klan spent illegal amounts of money on behalf of Mayfield. Although acts of voter intimidation had occurred during the primary election, the committee believed they had affected only local races and had had no impact on the general election for senator. The committee also noted that no evidence connected Mayfield with these actions by the Klan.

The report concluded with a recommendation that the contest against Mayfield be dismissed. The Senate agreed unanimously without debate.

Conclusion

In this unusual case, the Senate encountered the difficult problem of investigating a state's primary election procedures, a province long regarded as sacred to local control. It is hardly surprising that in this first inquiry, conducted during the era when the Ku Klux Klan was at the peak of its national power, the Senate chose to avoid some of the issues. However, because these matters were central to the constitutional right of U.S. citizens to vote without intimidation, the Senate would be called upon to consider similar topics again in the future.

Earle Mayfield served only one term. In 1928 he was defeated for renomination by Tom Connally, who attacked him for his connection to the Klan. Mayfield returned to Texas, where he practiced law and remained active in Democratic politics. He died in 1964.

Sources

U.S. Congress. Senate. *Congressional Record.* 67th Cong., 4th sess. (See pp. 1868, 4251.)

———. *Congressional Record.* 68th Cong., 1st sess. (See pp. 3, 422, 488–91.) 2d sess. (See p. 2929.)

———. Senate Report No. 973. 68th Cong., 2d sess., 1925.

Welch, June Rayfield. "Earle Mayfield Was the Klan Candidate." In *The Texas Senator.* Dallas, 1978.

Case 104

Burton K. Wheeler

(1882–1975)

Montana

Censure Case
April 9, 1924 to May 23, 1924

Issues
Senate review of charges against a member under indictment

Result: Not censured

Chronology:
Request for investigation: April 9, 1924
Referred to committee: April 9, 1924
Committee report: May 14, 1924
Senate vote: May 23, 1924

Background

Burton K. Wheeler built a successful reputation in Montana law and politics, distinguishing himself as an avid supporter of progressive principles. A spirited public speaker, Wheeler spent four years as U. S. attorney for Montana before seeking the governorship in 1920. Although badly defeated in that race, Wheeler was elected as a Democrat to the United States Senate in 1922.

Statement of the Case

Wheeler was seated without incident in December 1923. In January 1924 he spearheaded an investigation into the reasons Attorney General Harry M. Daugherty had failed to prosecute government officials implicated in the Teapot Dome scandal. As a result, Daugherty resigned in March. Soon after, on April 9, 1924, Wheeler learned that he had been indicted by a grand jury in Montana on charges of violating a statute that prohibited members of Congress from being paid to represent clients in cases in which the United States government was an interested party. Rising on a question of personal privilege, Wheeler asserted that he had been framed in order to block his continuing investigation of the Justice Department and asked the Senate to look into these charges against him. Granting his request, the Senate that same day authorized creation of a special committee to investigate the matter.

Response of the Senate

On May 14, 1924, a report by a bipartisan majority of the committee exonerated Wheeler. The investigation, led by William E. Borah (R-ID), showed that, during January and February 1923, Burton Wheeler, then a senator-elect, handled several cases of litigation for a Montana client. None of the lawsuits in question remotely involved the United States government, and all were adjudicated in the Montana state courts. Before he accepted the client, Wheeler had carefully explained that he could deal only with state litigation. It was the sense of the committee that Wheeler observed both the letter and the spirit of the law and that the charges should be dismissed.

A minority report filed by South Dakota Republican Thomas Sterling disagreed. He contended that the evidence submitted to the grand jury had been sufficient to warrant an indictment against Wheeler. Sterling pointed out that the senator's client was involved in drilling for oil and gas on federal public lands in Montana and had several proceedings under consideration by the Department of the Interior and other federal agencies. According to the indictment, witnesses indicated that Wheeler was hired to assist with these matters and that, once he took office as senator, he met with officials of the Interior Department. Sterling charged that, in declaring that Wheeler had broken no law, the committee majority was in essence prejudicing the court case. He urged the Senate to take no action until the court had completed its work.

During the three days of debate that followed, Borah defended Wheeler, who had met with the Interior Department solicitor, a friend from Montana, but had not discussed the client's request for a drilling permit. In Washington Wheeler had done nothing that went beyond his capacity as a senator assisting a constituent, and in fact the solicitor had recommended to the client a regular Washington attorney to handle the permit question. According to Borah, much of the evidence presented to the grand jury was based on hearsay, while the committee heard testimony from individuals familiar with the terms of Wheeler's actual contract but who were never called by the grand jury.

At the close of the debate, the Senate, by a vote of 56 to 5, agreed with the committee's recommendation exonerating Wheeler.

Conclusion

Nearly a year later, in April 1925, the jury acquitted Wheeler in the Montana court case. Meanwhile, Wheeler's role in the Daugherty investigation and his vindication by the Senate increased his public visibility as a reformer. During the 1924 presidential campaign, Wheeler ran as the vice presidential candidate of the Progressive party on the ticket headed by Robert M. La Follette. In a year when many voters, especially in the West, were disenchanted with the two major parties, the third party candidates, while falling far short of success, did win more than 16 percent of the popular vote in the presidential election. Wheeler spent the next twenty-five years in the Senate, where his isolationist principles led to frequent clashes with the Roosevelt administration. After leaving the Senate in 1947, Wheeler practiced law in Washington, D.C. He died in 1975.

Sources

U.S. Congress. Senate. *Congressional Record.* 68th Cong., 1st sess. (See pp. 5948–57, 5995, 8975–84, 9080–98, 9144–57, 9253–60, 9269–79.)

———. Senate Report No. 537. 68th Cong., 1st sess., 1924.

Ruetten, Richard T. "Senator Burton K. Wheeler and Insurgency in the 1920's." In *The American West: A Reorientation,* edited by Gene M. Gressley. University of Wyoming Publications 32. Laramie, WY, 1966.

Ruetten, Richard T. "Burton K. Wheeler and the Montana Connection." *Montana: The Magazine of Western History* 27 (July 1977): 2–19.

Wheeler, Burton K., with Paul F. Healy. *Yankee from the West.* Garden City, NY, 1962.

Daniel F. Steck v. Smith W. Brookhart

(1881–1950) (1869–1944)

Iowa

Election Case
January 8, 1925 to April 12, 1926

Issues
Recount of disputed ballots; incumbent unseated

Result: Brookhart unseated and Steck seated

Chronology:
Petition received: Jan. 8, 1925
Referred to committee: Mar. 10, 1925
Committee report: Mar. 29, 1926
Senate vote: April 12, 1926

Background

Smith W. Brookhart, an Iowa progressive Republican, first entered the Senate in 1922 to fill an unexpired term. Running for the full term in 1924, incumbent Brookhart narrowly triumphed over the Democratic challenger, Daniel F. Steck. During the confusing campaign, the Republican State Central Committee withdrew its support for Brookhart after he refused to back the Coolidge presidential ticket, although he did not actually endorse the Progressive party's presidential candidate, Senator Robert M. La Follette. One Republican organization went so far as to distribute sample ballots showing an "x" in the Republican column with another "x" beside Daniel Steck's name in the Democratic column to encourage regular Republicans to vote for Steck. When it became clear that the winning margin would be very small, both Republican and Democratic state chairmen requested a recount. Completed in late November, the recount showed Brookhart the winner by a plurality of less than 800 votes, and he was declared elected.

After the 1924 election, Senate Republicans retaliated against their insurgent colleagues, excluding from their party conference Brookhart, La Follette, and two other progressive Republicans who had failed to support the Coolidge campaign. The party also stripped these senators of their committee appointments.

Then, in January 1925 before the beginning of the new Congress, Daniel Steck served notice that he would challenge Brookhart's seating in March. The Iowa Republican State Central Committee also contested the election, declaring that Brookhart was not a member of the Republican party.

Statement of the Case

When the Sixty-ninth Congress convened on March 4, 1925, Brookhart was seated without incident. Six days later, on March 10, the Senate referred the election challenge to the Committee on Privileges and Elections.

Steck charged illegalities at the polls. According to his complaint, thousands of ballots were unlawfully counted for Brookhart, while many of his own were thrown out or fraudulently altered.

The Iowa Republicans took a different approach in their challenge, insisting that Brookhart had pretended to be a party member until after the deadline for removal of names from the ballot. Then, for the remainder of the campaign, he toured the state supporting the principles and the candidates of the La Follette Progressive party. The Iowa committee argued that state Republicans had in good faith voted for a person they assumed was a regular party member. On this basis Iowa Republicans asked for Brookhart's removal from office and the seating of Democrat Daniel Steck.

Response of the Senate

On May 16, 1925, before the committee could begin its work, the committee chairman, Selden P. Spencer (R-MO), died, and Richard P. Ernst (R-KY) assumed the chair. A subcommittee made up of two Republicans and two Democrats finally met to commence the investigation on July 20, 1925.

According to an agreement reached with the attorneys for Brookhart and Steck, the committee had all of the more than 900,000 ballots transported from Iowa to Washington for a recount, which was carried out during the summer and fall of 1925. Among the disputed ballots were a number on which the voters had apparently attempted to copy exactly a sample ballot that had been prominently featured in local newspapers, showing an arrow pointing to the box marked for Daniel Steck. Since the arrows constituted an extraneous mark that was illegal under Iowa law, these ballots had been excluded from the original count. Each was examined during the recount in an effort to ascertain what the true intent of the voter had been. Where it seemed clear the voter had meant to vote for Steck, the vote was counted for him.

Upon completion of the recount, the majority of the committee on March 29 issued a report finding that, in a four-person race, Daniel Steck had received a plurality of 1,420 votes. Stating that its only objective had been to decide which candidate had won a plurality, the committee's report declared that Smith Brookhart had not been elected and that Steck should be seated. Although the committee acknowledged that some ballots arrived in Washington with broken seals and that there were some discrepancies between the number of names on the polling lists and the number of ballots received, it stood by its determination that Steck had won.

In a minority report, one committee member, Hubert D. Stephens (D-MS), vigorously protested that the ballots had not been properly examined and secured in Iowa before being sent to Washington; that some 3,500 fewer ballots were received than the number of people on record as voting; that the majority refused to count for Brookhart some 1,300 straight Republican ballots, even though they were properly marked according to Iowa law. The committee refused to count these ballots for Brookhart because voters had also marked individual candidates in the Republican column but had failed to place a mark beside Brookhart's name. Stephens therefore concluded: without a recount Brookhart had carried the election; in those counties where ballots corresponded with names on the polling lists, Brookhart had a majority; and in a count of the legal ballots before the Senate, Brookhart had a majority.

The Senate debate on the subject consumed seven days. The many speeches focused on Iowa state election laws and the manner in which ballots were marked in the state. Walter George (D-GA) supported Steck's claim with the pronouncement that when there is "a naked conflict arising between the ballots and numbers of names on the poll lists, the ballots are always the higher and better evidence." When the committee majority contended that they were not constrained by Iowa election law, Brookhart's supporters maintained that there was no precedent for the Senate overruling state election laws in reviewing contested elections.

Meanwhile, Iowa supporters of Steck had been lobbying senators, including Brookhart's state Republican colleague, long-time incumbent Albert B. Cummins, to vote against the senator. On April 12, 1926, in a 45 to 41 vote that crossed party lines, the Senate unseated Smith Brookhart and replaced him with Democrat Daniel Steck. Neither Brookhart nor Cummins voted on the resolution.

Conclusion

On April 28, the Senate awarded $15,000 to Steck and $10,000 to Brookhart in compensation for their expenses in the case.

The forces behind the unusual decision to unseat an incumbent in favor of a contestant are somewhat clarified by a speech that George Norris (R-NE), Brookhart's fellow insurgent Republican, delivered just three months after Brookhart's removal. In reference to another contest, Norris discussed the Brookhart case and said that no one had questioned the legitimacy of Brookhart's nomination but that his independent spirit had offended party regulars. Iowa Republicans who supported Steck brought their complaint to Washington and enlisted high-level Republicans in the executive branch, the Republican national chairman, and Republican senators to cajole and threaten members to vote against Brookhart. Norris concluded: "The result was that this powerful partisan political combination brought about by Republican leaders nullified the voice of the voters of Iowa, threw out a Republican, and put in a Democrat."

Daniel Steck remained in the Senate until 1931. In 1933 he became an assistant to the United States attorney general, a post he held until three years before his death in 1950.

Smith Brookhart, turned out of the Senate by the manipulations of his own party, was soon vindicated. Returning to Iowa, he immediately ran in the June 1926 Republican primary for the state's other Senate seat and defeated his former colleague Albert Cummins. When Cummins died in late July,

Brookhart did not run in the special election to fill the remaining few months of the term but concentrated on winning the general election for the full term. He returned to the Senate in March 1927 and served until 1933. He then became a foreign trade advisor in the Agricultural Adjustment Administration before returning to the practice of law. Smith Brookhart died in 1944.

Sources

U.S. Congress. Senate. *Congressional Record.* 68th Cong., 2d sess. (See pp. 1430, 5259.)

———. *Congressional Record.* 69th Cong., spec. sess. (See pp. 4, 68–69, 73.) 1st sess. (See pp. 6501, 6859–76, 6939–44, 6947–62, 7097–7116, 7166–83, 7243–52, 7281–7302, 8342, 10563–64, 12900–901.)

———. Senate Report No. 498. 69th Cong., 1st sess., 1926.

Briley, Ronald F. "Smith W. Brookhart and the Limitations of Senatorial Dissent." *The Annals of Iowa* 48 (Summer/Fall 1985): 56–79.

James, Edward T., ed. *Dictionary of American Biography.* Supp. 3. New York, 1973. (See pp. 107–8.)

Lowitt, Richard. *George Norris: The Persistence of a Progressive, 1913–1933.* Urbana, IL, 1971. (See pp. 384–85.)

McDaniel, George William. "The Republican Party in Iowa and the Defeat of Smith Wildman Brookhart, 1924–1926." *The Annals of Iowa* 48 (Spring 1987): 413–434.

Case 106

Magnus Johnson v. Thomas D. Schall

(1871–1936) (1878–1935)

Minnesota

Election Case
February 2, 1925 to June 16, 1926

Issues
Charges of campaign misconduct; Senate refused recount

Result: Schall retained seat

Chronology:
Petition filed: Feb. 2, 1925
Referred to committee: Mar. 10, 1925
Committee report: June 6, 1926
Senate vote: June 16, 1926

Background

In Minnesota conflicts between agrarian and industrial interests helped spark several third-party movements that repeatedly threatened the political security of entrenched Republicans. The Farmer-Labor party succeeded in electing a member, Magnus Johnson, to fill a United States Senate vacancy in 1923. When the articulate Swede—whose earlier professions included glassblower, lumberjack, and farmer—ran for reelection in 1924, however, Republican challenger Thomas Schall defeated him by fewer than eight thousand votes.

Statement of the Case

On February 2, 1925, with only a month remaining in his term, Johnson notified his colleagues that he intended to contest Schall's seating at the beginning of the new Congress in March. Six days after Schall appeared and took his oath, the Senate ordered the Committee on Privileges and Elections to investigate Johnson's charges. Johnson had submitted a long list of allegations, including excessive campaign expenditures, false and defamatory statements made about Johnson, illicit promises of political appointments, violation of franking privileges, unlawful distribution of a scurrilous campaign newspaper, and coercion of campaign contributions from bootleggers and other miscreants.

Response of the Senate

On June 8, 1926, after holding twelve days of hearings in Washington, D. C., the Committee on Privileges and Elections recommended that Johnson's request for a recount be denied, the contest dismissed, and charges against Schall dropped. The testimony of eight pro-Johnson witnesses had failed to provide evidence connecting Schall with any wrongdoing.

In reviewing the accusations that Schall violated the Minnesota corrupt practices law, the committee noted that Johnson had not filed a formal contest in Minnesota district court, as provided for under that law. The Senate investigation, the committee noted, could not be expected to "act as a substitute for a district court." While the committee would have regarded a court judgment seriously, the report stressed that such a state action would not be binding upon the Senate, which is the sole judge of its members' qualifications.

On June 16, 1926, the Senate accepted the unanimous opinion of the committee that Schall retain his seat.

This action, however, did not fully mollify Thomas Schall. When objection was raised to the expense of printing the full set of hearings, Schall, who was blind, had the clerk read a lengthy prepared statement in order to place on the official record his rebuttal in strong language of "these unfounded, baseless slanders" against him. The intensity of the Minnesotan's concern convinced his colleagues, and the Senate ordered the hearings to be printed.

Conclusion

On July 2, 1926, the Senate authorized a $15,500 payment to Thomas Schall for his expenses in defending his seat. In 1932 his reelection was unsuccessfully challenged by another defeated candidate (See Case 116). Schall remained in the Senate until his death in 1935.

Magnus Johnson later served in the U.S. House of Representatives from 1932 to 1935. He died in 1936.

Sources

U.S. Congress. Senate. *Congressional Record.* 68th Cong., 2d sess. (See pp. 248, 2844.)

———. *Congressional Record.* 69th Cong., spec. sess. (See pp. 68, 73–74.) 1st sess. (See pp. 10912, 11351–53, 11799, 12633.)

———. Senate Report No. 1021. 69th Cong., 1st sess., 1926.

Schuyler, Robert L., ed. *Dictionary of American Biography.* Supp. 2. New York, 1958. (See pp. 347–48.)

Starr, Harris E., ed. *Dictionary of American Biography.* Supp. 1. New York, 1946. (See pp. 649–50.)

Case 107

Holm O. Bursum v. Sam G. Bratton

(1867–1953) (1888–1963)

New Mexico

Election Case
January 8, 1925 to April 30, 1926

Issues
Charges of voting fraud;
Senate refused recount

Result: Bratton retained seat

Chronology:
Resolution introduced: Mar. 9, 1925
Referred to committee: Mar. 10, 1925
Committee report: April 30, 1926
Senate vote: April 30, 1926

Background

The November 4, 1924, elections in New Mexico included closely contested races for the governorship and the United States Senate. Narrow Democratic victories for these positions prompted the two defeated Republicans to join forces in a challenge that began in the state courts and extended to the U. S. Senate. The defeated incumbent senator, Holm O. Bursum, hoped that evidence of general voting irregularities and tallying procedures throughout the state would convince the local courts to invalidate the election. Not content to depend entirely upon a ruling of the New Mexico state courts, Bursum informed the Senate in January 1925 that he planned to contest the March seating of his opponent, Sam Bratton, a former state judge.

Statement of the Case

When Bratton appeared in the Senate on March 4, 1925, the oath of office was administered without delay. Five days later the machinery for an investigation into Bratton's election began to grind slowly into action. On March 10 the Senate referred the matter to the Committee on Privileges and Elections, but Bursum waited until October 1925 to submit a formal statement of protest. In his petition Bursum charged that Bratton's plurality of 2,797 votes had been secured by altering returns, illegal voting by students at their colleges instead of in their home precincts, denying the vote to Indians, and illegally extending the vote to aliens, minors, and ex-convicts.

Response of the Senate

On April 30, 1926, the committee returned a report favorable to Bratton. The report noted that, after initiating the charges, Holm Bursum repeatedly delayed presenting his evidence to the committee despite its attempts to contact him. In somewhat testy tones, the committee explained that finally in late

November 1925 Bursum's attorney appeared and withdrew the various charges of ballot mutilations, voting fraud, and residential violations. Instead, Bursum sought to rest his case entirely upon a ballot recount, stating that he would drop his challenge if the recount did not substantiate his claim.

The committee agreed to this procedure and granted Bursum three weeks to produce his evidence and affidavits. When they arrived, the long-awaited documents and photographs convinced the committee that, although some discrepancies in the tallies ultimately reduced Bratton's margin of victory, they did not alter the election outcome. In fact, the only significant irregularity was created by election officers totalling the tally sheets, and their mathematical errors had been corrected later by the state canvassing boards. These mistakes did not constitute misconduct, and the committee did not consider them sufficient to warrant a recount that would have no bearing on the election results.

The committee saw no need to recommend spending substantial public funds and weeks of time to conduct a recount, since Bursum had failed to provide evidence to substantiate his original charges of wholesale and deliberate illegalities on the part of election officials. Bursum lost on every front. On April 30, 1926, the Senate concurred with the unanimous findings of the committee and declared Sam Bratton entitled to retain his seat.

Conclusion

Holm Bursum pursued a newspaper career in Washington and in New Mexico until his death in 1953. Sam Bratton served in the Senate until 1933, when he resigned to become a judge on the United States Circuit Court of Appeals. He died in 1963.

Sources

U.S. Congress. Senate. *Congressional Record.* 68th Cong., 2d sess. (See pp. 1121, 1429.)

———. *Congressional Record.* 69th Cong., spec. sess. (See pp. 4, 68, 72.) 1st sess. (see p. 8482.)

———. Senate Report No. 724. 69th Cong., 1st sess., 1926.

Case 108

Gerald P. Nye

(1829–1971)

North Dakota

Election Case (appointment)
December 7, 1925 to January 12, 1926

Issues
Interpretation of 17th Amendment

Result: Seated

Chronology:
Credentials presented: Dec. 7, 1925
Referred to committee: Dec. 7, 1925
Committee report: Dec. 16, 1925
Senate vote: Jan. 12, 1926

Background

The governor of North Dakota appointed progressive newspaper publisher Gerald P. Nye to fill temporarily the Senate vacancy caused by the death of Edwin F. Ladd in 1925. Nye had run unsuccessfully for the United States House of Representatives in 1924 as an Independent on the same ticket with Progressive party presidential candidate Senator Robert M. La Follette but would enter the Senate as a Republican. Questions immediately arose regarding the power of the state's governor to make temporary appointments since the 1913 adoption of the Seventeenth Amendment to the United States Constitution.

Statement of the Case

North Dakota Governor A. G. Sorlie appointed Nye on November 14, 1925, to fill the Senate seat until a special election could be held on June 30, 1926. The earlier constitutional arrangement permitting gubernatorial appointments during a legislative recess had been slightly altered by the second clause of the direct election amendment to empower a governor to make temporary appointments only if the state legislature had specifically extended that authority to the executive.

On December 7, 1925, Lynn Frazier (R-ND) presented Gerald Nye's credentials. Aware that the wording of the North Dakota state constitution would prompt a challenge to Nye's seating, Frazier immediately asked that the matter be referred to the Committee on Privileges and Elections. The Senate agreed with this request, and Nye was not seated while the committee studied the constitutional issues involved.

Response of the Senate

The committee acted promptly and, on December 16, 1925, returned a report unfavorable to Nye. The majority of the committee reasoned that, under the Seventeenth Amendment, a state legislature must adopt legislation granting the appointment power to the governor.

A review of the North Dakota constitution showed that, although it authorized the governor to fill a vacancy in "any office," the state document did not fulfill the United States constitutional requirement of specifically assigning appointive powers in the case of a United States senator. The committee further noted that forty-six states had passed laws expressly recognizing the language and the limitations of the Seventeenth Amendment. Since North Dakota was one of only two states that had failed to adopt such legislation, the committee maintained that the state assembly had not complied with the requirements of the Seventeenth Amendment for conferring the appointive power upon the North Dakota governor.

Hubert D. Stephens (D-MS) submitted a minority report that supported Nye's claim. Stephens argued that a North Dakota statute amended in 1917, since ratification of the Seventeenth Amendment, permitted the governor to fill "all vacancies" and meant exactly that. He dismissed as ridiculous the contention that the North Dakota assembly had not been aware of the amendment's provisions when it established the state law. Stephens, a Democrat, explained his support for the North Dakota Republican by asserting that he considered the right of a state to Senate representation as sacred and inviolable.

The Senate debated the case for five days. Opponents and proponents raised a variety of issues, including whether a senator is a state or federal officer, the authority of state constitutions, precedents in other disputed cases of gubernatorial appointments, the legislative intent of the North Dakota assembly, the right of a state to full representation in the Senate, court decisions in other cases, and interpretations of the Constitution. What was really at stake, however, was the objection of the regular Republicans to seeing an addition to the ranks of the progressive Senate Republicans.

The case was finally decided by an alliance of Democrats and progressive Republicans in favor of seating Nye. On January 12, 1926, by a vote of 41 to 39 with fifteen abstentions, the Senate agreed with the minority report of H. D. Stephens. Gerald Nye came forward, took his oath of office, and began a long Senate career.

Conclusion

The publicity surrounding his case proved beneficial to Nye, who had been relatively obscure at the time of his appointment. Having gained wide name recognition in North Dakota, he went on to win the special election in June and in November 1926 was elected to a full term. He served in the Senate until 1945. An ardent isolationist, he attained a national reputation in 1934 when he headed a special committee investigating the munitions industry. After his retirement from the Senate, he remained in Washington, D.C., where he practiced law and held a variety of federal posts until his death in 1971.

Sources

U.S. Congress. Senate. *Congressional Record.* 69th Cong., 1st sess. (See pp. 376, 904, 1408, 1615–34, 1681–1700, 1749–54, 1814–40, 1884–93.)

———. Senate Report No. 3. 69th Cong., 1st sess., 1925.

Cole, Wayne S. *Senator Gerald P. Nye and American Foreign Relations*. Minneapolis, 1962.

Leonard, Robert James. "From County Politics to the Senate: The Learning Years for Senator Nye." *North Dakota History* 39 (Summer 1972): 14–23.

Rylance, Daniel. "A Controversial Career: Gerald P. Nye, 1925–1946." *North Dakota Quarterly* 36 (Winter 1968): 5–19.

William B. Wilson v. William S. Vare

(1862–1934) (1867–1934)

Pennsylvania

Election Case
May 19, 1926, to December 6, 1929

Issues
Campaign financing; voting fraud; recount of disputed ballots; right of Senate to investigate matters related to its membership

Result: Neither Vare nor Wilson seated

Chronology:
Special committee created: May 19, 1926
Referred to special committee: May 19, 1926
Committee reports: Dec. 22, 1926; Feb. 22, 1929
Petition received: Jan. 8, 1927
Referred to Privs. & Elects. Committee: Mar. 3, 1927
Committee report: Dec. 5, 1929
Senate vote: Dec. 6, 1929

Background

When Pennsylvania voters went to the polls for a primary election on May 18, 1926, they did so under the full glare of a critical national press. For weeks reports emanated from Philadelphia that money and machine politics were playing a substantial role in the campaign, as wealthy families supported various competing candidates for governor and senator. When the primary votes were counted, the senatorial nominees were Republican William S. Vare, a former U.S. representative and the wealthy boss of the Philadelphia political machine, and the unopposed Democrat William B. Wilson, who had been the first U.S. secretary of labor and was also a former U.S. representative.

Statement of the Case

In the Senate on May 19, 1926, Byron P. Harrison (D-MS) spoke for those appalled by the newspaper stories about the conduct of the Pennsylvania primary. Harrison pointed to reports that a staggering $2 to $5 million had been poured into the campaign and reminded his colleagues that in an earlier election a far smaller amount expended by Michigan's Truman Newberry (See Case 102) had been labeled excessive. Senators agreed with Harrison and appointed a special committee chaired by James A. Reed (D-MO) to investigate campaign expenditures and evidence of corruption in the recent primary and in the forthcoming November general election. Under the terms of the resolution adopted, the committee investigated both the Pennsylvania election and the primary election campaign of Frank L. Smith in Illinois (See Case 110).

Response of the Senate

Special Committee

The five-member special committee of the Sixty-ninth Congress conducted its hearings and investigations throughout the summer of 1926. Witnesses led the three Republican and two Democratic senators through a maze of local politics and factions. Before the committee could finish sifting through the morass of evidence grudgingly provided by a series of hostile witnesses, William S. Vare easily won the November general election for the Senate term beginning on March 4, 1927.

On December 22, 1926, the special committee filed an interim report that, although incomplete, outlined the enormous expenditures in the campaign, in some cases made by coalitions formed between a candidate for governor and one for senator. The committee found that in the primary campaign, $187,000 had been spent on behalf of Governor Gifford Pinchot, most of the money being contributed by the candidate, his wife, and relatives. On behalf of the team of winning Republican gubernatorial candidate John S. Fisher and George Wharton Pepper, the defeated incumbent senator, $1.8 million was spent, $75,000 of it contributed by Secretary of the Treasury Andrew Mellon and members of his politically influential Pittsburgh family. The combination of William Vare and losing gubernatorial candidate Edward E. Beidleman spent some $785,000, $71,000 of it in Vare's personal funds.[1] In contrast, William Wilson, the Democratic nominee for senator, spent only $10,000 on his campaign. At the time, Pennsylvania campaign laws placed no limit on the amount a candidate could spend, although they did specify the purposes for which money could legitimately be spent. In addition, the Supreme Court had ruled in the 1918 Newberry case that the Senate had no power to judge primary elections, and the amended Corrupt Practices Act specifically did not apply to primary elections. The report noted that the committee had not yet had time to review the expenditures in the general election, partly because of its work on the Illinois election of Frank Smith. It therefore offered no conclusions or recommendations.

Thus far, the committee had focused on the primary election. Then, on January 8, 1927, William B. Wilson, the unsuccessful Democratic candidate in the general election, formally filed a petition charging corruption and voting irregularities by Vare supporters in that election. If only the legitimate ballots of qualified voters were counted, Wilson contended, he, rather than Vare, would have been elected. In a petition filled with emotion, Wilson asserted that in Philadelphia, where Vare controlled the Republican machine, the

[1] The outrage these expenditures aroused may become clearer to the modern reader when they are converted to current dollars. In 1991 dollars, the Vare-Beidleman expenditures would amount to roughly $6 million and Vare's personal contribution to about $548,000.

November senatorial election had been a "grotesque and fantastic travesty." Wilson's allegations included padded registration lists, "phantom" voters who were actually dead or imaginary, criminal misuse of campaign funds, and voter intimidation. He urged the Senate to take immediate steps to preserve the ballots and other evidence in order to conduct an investigation.

Already disturbed by the special committee's information about excessive expenditures in the primaries, the Senate on January 11 authorized the committee to take possession of the ballot boxes, tally sheets, and other records from the November Pennsylvania election, and the committee moved promptly to request the materials from the state. The special committee, however, soon found its efforts hampered by Senate procedural regulations. In the waning days of the Sixty-ninth Congress, which ended on March 4, 1927, Pennsylvania Republican David A. Reed filibustered to block passage of a resolution that would continue the special committee into the Seventieth Congress. The Senate's failure to act left the committee without authority for nine months, since the new Congress would not convene until December. After the Committee to Audit and Control the Contingent Expenses of the Senate rejected the special committee's funding requests and the sergeant at arms refused to execute directives from the investigators, the committee dispatched a representative to confiscate election returns in certain Pennsylvania districts. When state officials balked at releasing the election records, the Senate committee turned to the federal courts for a mandatory injunction to free the desired ballot boxes. The case of *Reed* v. *County Commissioners* eventually reached the Supreme Court, which in 1928 ruled that the Senate, vested with the constitutional authority to enforce its own process, had the right "to secure information upon which to decide concerning elections." In the meantime, committee members arranged with representatives of Vare and Wilson for the federal courts in Pennsylvania to impound and retain the ballots and election records until Congress convened in December 1927. It was not until February 1928 that the committee finally received the election records.

Privileges and Elections Committee

While these developments significantly delayed the conduct of the special committee's investigation for most of 1927, the Committee on Privileges and Elections was pursuing the matter of Vare's credentials. On January 8, 1927, Governor Gifford Pinchot, in a statement that deviated from the traditional language of qualifying credentials, declared that William Vare "appears to have been chosen." The reform-minded Pennsylvania governor, however, declined to certify that the senator-elect had been honestly nominated or honestly elected. Rather, Governor Pinchot spoke of a nomination "partly bought and partly stolen" and of frauds that "tainted both the primary and the general election." A few days later, Pinchot's term expired. His successor, John S. Fisher, promptly forwarded a second, conventional set of credentials for

William S. Vare. On March 3, 1927, the Senate referred both sets of credentials to the Committee on Privileges and Elections. In reporting to the Senate the next day, the last before adjournment of the Sixty-ninth Congress, the committee chose to ignore the Pinchot statement and ruled the Fisher credentials valid. This report specifically made no assessment of Vare's final right to claim his seat, for the Senate agreed that such a judgment would be the prerogative of the Seventieth Congress at the beginning of Vare's term.

Both committees

When Vare's credentials were presented at the convening of the Seventieth Congress on December 5, 1927, his opponents moved quickly to block his seating, and he was not permitted to take the oath of office. This procedure was unusual, since generally senators-elect with valid credentials were permitted to take their seats while an investigation proceeded.

After several days of discussion, the Senate on December 9 extended the existence and powers of the special committee and directed it to conduct additional hearings. The Senate also granted Vare floor time to speak in his own behalf. Concurrently, the Committee on Privileges and Elections was authorized to review the matter of William Wilson's petition against William Vare, and each of the committees was empowered to consider evidence gathered by the other.

Special Committee (continued)

The additional investigation by the special committee focused on the general election. Committee staff reviewed the election records, including a tedious examination of voter lists, ballots, and tally sheets. It also heard testimony from the Philadelphia district attorney regarding his prosecution of election fraud in the 1926 election for senator. He testified that Vare's ward leaders provided financial and moral support to those charged with fraud and endeavored to obstruct his investigations. He described a pervasive pattern of election corruption over a period of years. In the process of its hearings, the committee offered Vare an opportunity to present evidence that would refute the earlier unfavorable partial report, but Vare failed to do so.

As it delved deeper into the general election in Philadelphia and Pittsburgh, the committee found ample evidence of corruption, including thousands of cases of fraudulent registrations. "The fraud pervading the actual count by the division election officers is appalling," the committee charged, adding that a Philadelphia voter had only a 1-in-8 chance of having his or her ballot counted correctly. More than two thousand people voted who were not registered, and hundreds of repeat voters were found, as well as evidence of stuffed ballot boxes.

Even after Vare responded that he had no counter-evidence to present when the testimony concluded on May 8, 1928, the committee offered him one more opportunity to produce additional information at a hearing on May

19. On that day, the committee received a letter from Vare in which he claimed an "attack of acute indigestion" forced his absence and begged the members to reserve judgment until he could appear with complete information about the primary campaign. Vare's convenient illness brought the matter to a halt while the committee awaited further communication from him. He recovered sufficiently to journey to the Republican national convention in Kansas City early in the summer, but upon his return to his summer home in Atlantic City, New Jersey, Vare suffered a severe cerebral hemorrhage that left him paralyzed on the left side. From August to December 1928 he remained at his summer cottage under the care of a team of physicians.

On January 4, 1929, the special committee, clearly annoyed by Vare's long silences, convened one more time to permit the senator-elect to submit additional testimony, but Vare's attorney insisted that his client's fragile health demanded an indefinite postponement. The committee, its patience exhausted, complained that Vare was merely delaying the investigation and that there had been ample chance to respond during the period when he was well enough to participate actively in the national convention at Kansas City. Vare's counsel then submitted a written response to the charges, which the committee reviewed and decided contained no evidence to refute its findings regarding corruption in the general election.

With its principal duties at last ended, the committee unanimously reported to the Senate on February 22, 1929, that, in light of the evidence of fraud and corruption, William Vare was not entitled to his seat. Because of Vare's illness, the Senate took no action on the report, but it did vote on February 26 to retain the special committee and continue its authority into the Seventy-first Congress.

Full Senate

Progressive Republican George Norris of Nebraska, horrified at the reports of Vare's excessive expenditures in the primary, had actually campaigned against his fellow Republican in the 1926 Pennsylvania general election. Now, on September 9, 1929, armed with reports that Vare's health had improved, Norris introduced a resolution that cited Vare's vast expenditures as "harmful to the dignity and honor of the Senate" and called on members to deny the Pennsylvania senator-elect his seat among them. The Senate, however, decided to postpone consideration until the start of the regular session in December. At that time, the Committee on Privileges and Elections was expected to report the results of its two-year study, which rumors indicated might differ in its conclusions from those of the special committee.

On December 4, 1929, Vare was present in the Senate chamber and permitted to speak in his own behalf. Helped up the aisle by his physician, the infirm senator-elect sat and listened to Norris' charges before rising to speak. He defended his expenditures in the primary as necessary to build an organization across the state and described as simply clerical irregularities the special committee's evidence of fraud in the general election. The next day, the Committee on Privileges and Elections issued its report. Having reviewed the same evidence as the special committee, the majority reached a different conclusion, finding that, even when all questionable votes were eliminated, William Vare had received a plurality of legal votes and William Wilson had not sustained his allegations that Pennsylvania voting irregularities had robbed him of a plurality. A supplemental report from four committee members concurred that Wilson had no claim to the seat but disagreed that Vare had secured his victory through legal votes. These senators, greatly influenced by the evidence made available to them by the special committee, stated that the nearly $800,000 expenditure in the primary, the large expenditures for the general election, and fraud committed in his behalf tainted all aspects of Vare's election and that he was not entitled to a seat in the Senate.

After a floor debate that considered the reports of both committees, the Senate voted on December 6, 1929, in the case that had consumed three and one-half years of its time. The Senate ruled, 66 to 15, that William Wilson had not been elected, and it voted, 58 to 22, to deny Senator-elect William Vare a seat in the Senate.

Conclusion

Less than a week later, on December 12, 1929, the Senate seated Republican Joseph R. Grundy, appointed by Governor Fisher to fill the vacancy in the Pennsylvania seat. (See Case 113). A textile manufacturer, Grundy was also an influential backer of political campaigns, who had contributed heavily to Fisher's campaign.

In a related matter, Thomas W. Cunningham, a witness before the special committee, had challenged the committee's jurisdiction over the primary election and refused to answer any questions. At the direction of the Senate, Cunningham was arrested and remanded to the custody of the sergeant at arms. Cunningham's legal maneuvers, claiming the Senate had no power to arrest him, eventually reached the Supreme Court. In the case of *Barry* v. *United States ex rel. Cunningham,* decided in May 1929, the Court reaffirmed the authority of the Senate to adjudicate matters relevant to its own members and further held that, if in that process a member-elect is denied the oath of office during the investigation, the state involved is not losing its constitutional right to "equal suffrage in the Senate."

During the course of the investigation, the Senate's unusual decisions included: referring the case to a special committee rather than to Privileges and Elections, permitting a special committee to continue in force following the expiration of a Congress, using a resolution to extend a select committee between congresses, and asking the courts to clarify a legislative committee's investigative authority. The Vare case also resulted in the two landmark Supreme Court decisions discussed above.

Vare's biographer states flatly that the Senate refused to seat Vare "not for any illegal act, but for general reasons similar to those that closed the portals of the Union League to him: he was a ward politician without social background." It appears, however, that the ultimate disposition of the Vare election case was actually shaped by the irrefutable evidence of corrupt use of massive campaign expenditures. In rejecting William Vare, the Senate moved to check the growing public suspicion that millionaire candidates could buy a membership at will in the highest legislative body in the nation, demonstrating that, while Vare may have controlled Philadelphia, he could not do likewise with the United States Senate. Turned away from a seat in the Senate, the ailing Vare continued his political activities in Pennsylvania, although he gradually lost control over his Philadelphia organization. He died in 1934.

William B. Wilson spent the years until his death in 1934 involved in mining and agricultural pursuits in Pennsylvania.

Sources

U.S. Congress. Senate. *Congressional Record.* 69th Cong., 1st sess. (See pp. 9672–80, 9719, 9809, 10564, 11263–64, 11615, 12309, 12473–78.) 2d sess. (See pp. 119–20, 914, 987, 1260–61, 1333, 1338, 1413, 4307, 5513–22, 5529–31, 5895–96, 5914.)

———. *Congressional Record.* 70th Cong., 1st sess. (See pp. 4, 119–23, 166–76, 236–54, 295–338, 490, 782, 1496.) 2d sess. (See pp. 3167, 4007, 4211–18, 4331.)

———. *Congressional Record.* 71st Cong., 1st sess. (See pp. 3413, 3501–8, 3519–31.) 2d sess. (See pp. 37–48, 66, 69–94, 128–58, 188–98, 525–39.)

———. Senate Report No. 1197. 69th Cong., 2d sess., 1926.

———. Senate Report No. 1717. 69th Cong., 2d sess., 1927.

———. Senate Reports No. 603 and No. 1858. 70th Cong., 2d sess., 1929.

———. Senate Report No. 47. 71st Cong., 1st sess., 1929.

Astorino, Samuel J. "The Contested Senate Election of William Scott Vare." *Pennsylvania History* 28 (April 1961): 187–201.

Lowitt, Richard. *George W. Norris: The Persistence of a Progressive, 1913–1933.* Urbana, IL, 1971. (See pp. 386–93.)

Malone, Dumas, ed. *Dictionary of American Biography.* New York, 1946; reprint of 1935 edition. Vol. 19. (See pp. 223–24.) Vol. 20. (See pp. 348–49.)

McCusker, John J. *How Much Is That in Real Money? A Historical Price Index for Use as a Deflator of Money Values in the Economy of the United States.* Worcester, MA, 1992. (See pp. 330, 332.)

Salter, John T. *The People's Choice: Philadelphia's William S. Vare.* New York, 1971.

Case 110

Frank L. Smith

(1867–1950)

Illinois

Election Case
May 19, 1926 to January 19, 1928

Issues
Campaign financing; corruption

Result: Not Seated

Chronology:
Special committee created:
May 19, 1926
Referred to special committee:
May 19, 1926; Dec. 7, 1927
Committee reports: Dec. 16, 1926;
Feb. 12, 1927; Jan. 17, 1928
Credentials presented: Jan. 19, 1927
Referred to Privs. & Elects. Committee:
Jan. 20, 1927
Committee report: Mar. 4, 1927
Senate vote: Jan. 19, 1928

Background

President Warren G. Harding's unexpected support for American participation in the World Court had the unintended effect of intensifying party factionalism in Illinois state politics. In a free-wheeling April 1926 Senate primary contest, the Republican challenger, Frank L. Smith, seized on the World Court issue and in the process further split the already fragmented Cook County and Chicago Republican organizations, as he took his campaign to Chicago's immigrant and black neighborhoods. There he vigorously criticized incumbent Senator William B. McKinley's vote for Harding's resolution in favor of the World Court. Smith, chairman of the Illinois Commerce Commission, which regulated public utilities, and a former member of the U.S. House of Representatives, succeeded in defeating McKinley for the Republican nomination.

Statement of the Case

In the spring of 1926, allegations regarding excessive expenditures in the Pennsylvania primary prompted the Senate to convene a special five-man investigating committee to examine expenditures and possible corruption in that year's senatorial campaigns (See Case 109). Then, in late June, Arkansas Democrat Thaddeus H. Caraway delivered a speech in the Senate alleging the use of excessive expenditures, fraud, and corruption in the Illinois primary campaign. The charges included accusations that Frank Smith had spent $400,000 on the election and that Samuel Insull, the powerful owner of public utility corporations, contributed $125,000 to Smith's primary campaign fund while Smith was still chairing the commerce commission that oversaw such utilities.[1] Accepting such contributions in these circumstances represented a conflict of interest and was illegal under Illinois law. Newspaper reports of Caraway's charges drew national attention to the Illinois election, and the special committee, which had already been concerned about expenditures in that race, began focusing on the activities of Smith's campaign. Chaired by James A. Reed (D-MO), the committee conducted hearings in Chicago throughout the summer and fall of 1926, in addition to continuing its investigation of the Pennsylvania primary election.

Because these hearings were taking place during the general election campaign, some Illinois Republicans urged Smith to step aside and allow an untainted candidate to be nominated, but he refused and won the November election by more than 60,000 votes.

Then, in early December 1926, Senator William McKinley—who was not related to the late president of the same name—died, three months before his term was due to expire in March 1927. His death left a vacancy for the Illinois governor to fill, providing a new twist in a case that had already occupied the attention of the United States Senate for nearly six months. In the wake of McKinley's death, Senate Democrats moved quickly on December 9, 1926, to introduce a resolution that would disqualify Frank Smith based on the evidence gathered by the special committee. Their hasty action only two days after the death of the incumbent stemmed from reports that the Illinois governor planned to name Smith to the vacant seat until the full term began.

Response of the Senate

Special Committee

On December 16, 1926, the expectations of Senate Democrats materialized when the governor appointed Frank Smith to fill the remainder of McKinley's term. That same day, the special committee circulated a partial report on its investigation but made no recommendations to the Senate. The report explained that the committee had not yet obtained final contribution and expenditure figures. Because Illinois had no law restricting campaign expenditures, and the Supreme Court had ruled in the case of Truman Newberry (See Case 102) that the Federal Corrupt Practices Act could not constitutionally apply to primary elections, there was no requirement for candidates to file campaign finance information for those races with the Senate. In addition to direct contributions to specific candidates, other funds were contributed to and spent on behalf of groups of candidates for state and local offices who were allied with a senatorial candidate. From the information it could gather, the committee estimated that a total of more than $500,000 had been spent on behalf of McKinley and over $450,000 on behalf of Frank Smith.

---

[1] The outrage evoked by these expenditures becomes clearer if they are expressed in current dollars. In 1991 dollars, Smith's expenditures amount to more than $3 million and Insull's contribution becomes $965,000.

The special committee continued its investigation during February 1927, issuing two more partial reports about recalcitrant witnesses, including Samuel Insull, who refused to answer questions about their campaign contributions.

Privileges and Elections Committee

When Smith's credentials to fill the vacancy were presented on January 19, 1927, the Senate discussed whether Smith could be blocked from taking the oath for the appointive term if his credentials were in good order. Reed described the case as differing from earlier ones in which a senator-elect was seated while a committee reviewed the matter, because, at the time Smith arrived to take his seat, his primary election had already been under investigation for several months by a Senate committee that had found reason to believe that fraud and corruption had occurred. After prolonged debate, the Senate the next day refused to seat Smith until the Committee on Privileges and Elections reviewed the matter. That committee held hearings a few days later but recessed its deliberations when Smith became ill and returned to Illinois. When his credentials for the full term were presented on March 3, 1927, the Senate promptly referred them as well to the Committee on Privileges and Elections. The committee reported the next day, just before the end of the Sixty-ninth Congress, that Smith's election credentials appeared valid but the committee had been unable to take final action because of his illness. As a result, Congress adjourned with the matter unresolved.

During the ensuing months, Smith's supporters did not remain idle. They insisted that the charges that Smith knowingly abused his public office were irrelevant since the senator-designate satisfied all constitutional qualifications to serve in the Senate and thus had a right to take his oath.

Special Committee (continued)

When the Seventieth Congress opened on December 5, 1927, and Smith's credentials were again presented, the new Senate seemed no more willing to overlook the extravagant financial conduct of the senator-elect than had the previous body. Calling the Illinois election but one more example of a "battle royal of the millionaires," Republican George Norris (NE) introduced a resolution to deny Smith a seat in the Senate. Two days later, after considerable discussion, the Senate adopted a resolution to refer the matter back to the special committee, directing it to give Frank Smith a hearing and granting him the privilege of the Senate floor to plead his case. In the meantime, Smith was not seated.

The committee held a further hearing, at which Insull and other witnesses finally provided the information they had been withholding. Smith also appeared but offered no new evidence, simply contending that the Senate had no authority to rule on his right to a seat until after it had seated him as a senator. This argument was similar to one raised by Thomas W. Cunningham in connection with the special committee's review of the Vare case (Case 109).

That contention subsequently led to the Supreme Court's decision in *Barry* v. *U.S. ex rel. Cunningham* (1929), ruling that a member-elect falls under the Senate's constitutional right to judge the qualifications of its members.

On January 17, 1928, the committee issued its final report, together with a resolution declaring that Smith's election was tainted with blatant fraud and corruption. The committee based this conclusion on the generally undisputed evidence that public service corporations made excessive contributions to his campaign while he served as chairman of the Illinois Commerce Commission, empowered to regulate rates and conduct state utility business. Since Smith's acceptance of these contributions was "harmful to the dignity and honor of the Senate," the committee concluded that he should not be seated. After several days of debate, the Senate, unable to ignore the widespread and openly acknowledged transactions, voted 61 to 23 on January 19, 1928, that Frank Smith was not entitled to his seat in the United States Senate.

Conclusion

Three weeks later, Smith submitted his resignation to Governor Len Small. Small accepted the resignation, announced that a vacancy existed, and named Smith to fill it, although Smith took no action to claim the seat. When Small then scheduled a special election, Smith entered the spring primary. In April 1928 both Smith and Small were defeated by the forces of reform, marking the end of Smith's senatorial aspirations. Defeated for a seat in the House of Representatives in 1930, Smith remained active in Republican politics until his death in 1950.

Sources

U.S. Congress. Senate. *Congressional Record.* 69th Cong., 1st sess. (See pp. 9677–80, 9719, 9809, 12018.) 2d sess. (See pp. 119–20, 554–56, 558, 633, 987, 1039–49, 1489–1502, 1549–52, 1911–36, 1987–2014, 2058, 5531, 5914.)

———. *Congressional Record.* 70th Cong., 1st sess. (See pp. 3–5, 112, 119, 126–7, 155–63, 1219, 1581, 1597, 1665–72, 1703–18.)

———. Senate Report No. 1197. 69th Cong., 1st sess., 1926.

———. Senate Report No. 603. 70th Cong., 1st sess., 1927.

———. Senate Report No. 92. 70th Cong., 2d sess., 1928.

Garraty, John A., and Edward T. James, eds. *Dictionary of American Biography.* Supp. 4. New York, 1974. (See pp. 751–53.)

Lowitt, Richard. *George Norris: The Persistence of a Progressive, 1913–1933.* Urbana, IL, 1971. (See pp. 392–95.)

McCusker, John J. *How Much Is That in Real Money? A Historical Price Index for Use as a Deflator of Money Values in the Economy of the United States.* Worcester, MA, 1992. (See pp. 330, 332.)

Wooddy, Carroll Hill. *The Case of Frank L. Smith: A Study in Representative Government.* New York, 1974; reprint of 1931 edition.

Case 111

Arthur R. Gould

(1857–1946)

Maine

Censure Case
December 6, 1926 to Mar. 4, 1927

Issues
Charges of bribery; right of Senate to exclude a member-elect for actions long before election

Result: Not censured

Chronology:
Credentials presented: Dec. 6, 1926
Referred to committee: Dec. 7, 1926
Committee report: Mar. 4, 1927
No Senate action

Background

In 1911 Maine businessman Arthur R. Gould and his associates contracted with the Canadian government to build a railroad along the St. John River in New Brunswick. After more than two years of construction, the Canadian province terminated its agreement with the construction company. Charges regarding this contract were raised against Gould when Maine voters in 1926 elected him as a Republican to fill a U.S. Senate vacancy caused by the death of Bert M. Fernald.

Statement of the Case

On December 6, 1926, as Gould prepared to take his oath of office, Thomas J. Walsh (D-MT) charged that the Senate should not ignore allegations of bribery that a Canadian judge had leveled against the new senator in connection with the railroad contract. Despite these comments, the Senate seated Gould, but the next day the Montana Democrat again pressed his case. Walsh contended that the 1911 railroad contract was said to have been secured through a $100,000 bribe by Gould and his associates. Pointing to a recurring Senate problem, Walsh asked for a clear judgment regarding the Senate's right to exclude a member for actions taken long before that member's election to the Senate and unrelated to the primary or general election. He offered a resolution to refer the matter to the Committee on Privileges and Elections. Gould himself stated that he welcomed an investigation which he believed would exonerate him. He pointed out that the matter had been thoroughly discussed during the election campaign. After a brief debate, the Senate voted 70 to 7 to send the matter to the Committee on Privileges and Elections.

Response of the Senate

On March 4, 1927, the committee recommended that the Senate dismiss all charges against Arthur Gould based on testimony gathered during two weeks of hearings. Pointing out that the transaction under investigation had occurred more than fourteen years previously, the committee stated that there was no question regarding the legality of Gould's election.

In relation to the bribery charges, the committee learned that, when the Canadian province declared the American company to be in default and confiscated both the physical property and the company itself, the entrepreneurs, incensed at the loss of $400,000, demanded a hearing before a Canadian government arbitrator. That arbitrator ruled that the government was justified in abrogating the contract because, before the province signed the original contract, Gould had offered a $100,000 bribe to a provincial official to secure the deal. The committee, however, found that, although all participants agreed that money did change hands, Gould had vehemently opposed the payment of the "campaign contribution" that he considered to be a "hold up," but he had been outvoted by the other shareholders. The Senate committee therefore exonerated Gould, since he had not actually made the payment himself and had objected strenuously to the bribe, and because the Canadian official coerced the favor in return for the government contract.

The committee chose not to respond to Walsh's policy question beyond stating that "the committee believes that every case involving the exclusion of the senator-elect, or the expulsion of a member of the Senate for an offense alleged to have been committed prior to his election must depend upon the peculiar facts and circumstances of the particular case." Accepting the judgment of the committee, the Senate adopted the committee's report and took no further action in the case.

Conclusion

On April 30, 1928, the Senate agreed to reimburse Gould more than $10,000 for his expenses. Gould served in the Senate only until the end of the partial term in 1931. Declining to run for reelection, he returned to his business interests in Maine. He died in 1946.

Sources

U.S. Congress. Senate. *Congressional Record.* 69th Cong., 2d sess. (See pp. 8, 9, 38–44, 964, 5914.)

———. *Congressional Record.* 70th Cong., 1st sess. (See p. 7425.)

———. Senate Report No. 1715. 69th Cong., 2d sess., 1927.

Case 112

Hiram Bingham

(1875–1956)

Connecticut

Censure Case
October 17, 1929 to November 4, 1929

Issues
Hiring a lobbyist who was still being paid by a manufacturing organization

Result: Censured

Chronology:
Testimony to subcommittee: Oct. 17, 1929
Committee report: Oct. 26, 1929
Senate vote: Nov. 4, 1929

Background

Although Congress frequently debated lobbying regulation starting in 1911, it passed no legislation on the subject, and in the 1920s lobbyists' influence continued to concern members of Congress. In April 1929, Arkansas Senator Thaddeus H. Caraway (D) proposed creation of a committee to investigate the excesses of lobbyists. Persuaded by Caraway and Judiciary Committee Chairman George Norris (R-NE), the Senate authorized Norris to appoint a subcommittee of Judiciary to investigate lobbyists' activities.

On October 15, 1929, the subcommittee, chaired by Caraway, began its public hearings. Although Connecticut Senator Hiram Bingham's (R) name had not been mentioned in the investigation, he volunteered to appear before the panel on October 17, 1929, in order to defend his former staff member, Charles L. Eyanson. Newspaper stories had focused on the impropriety of Bingham using government funds to hire someone who was also an employee of the Manufacturers' Association of Connecticut, a well-known lobbying group.

Statement of the Case

Under Caraway's questioning, Bingham, a member of the Finance Committee who had served in the Senate since 1924, testified that he had asked the manufacturers' association to "loan" him Eyanson for his expertise during hearings on tariff legislation. The arrangement, he explained, was for the association to continue paying Eyanson's salary. When the Republican members of the Finance Committee began meeting in closed session to consider tariff proposals, Bingham had asked his principal clerk to formally resign his Senate post temporarily while continuing his duties and receiving his salary. Eyanson was then sworn in as an official Senate employee in the clerk's place, so that he could attend the closed sessions. He did not retain his Senate salary, however, but passed it along to the regular clerk. Bingham coolly defended this arrangement, asserting that he depended on Eyanson solely for professional advice and that he never considered him a lobbyist in the usual sense of the word, which Bingham defined as "going around visiting congressmen and senators and trying to get them to do something they did not want to do."

The investigating committee felt differently, and under persistent questioning by the members, Bingham acknowledged that he had perhaps made "a mistake" in hiring Eyanson and taking him into the closed meetings without telling the other senators that he was an employee of the Connecticut Manufacturers' Association. For his part, Charles Eyanson had difficulty giving a clear answer to repeated questions regarding whom he represented during the month he was on the payroll of both the U.S. Senate and the manufacturers' association. "Until I reported to Senator Bingham I would be a representative of the Manufacturers' Association," he explained, ". . . but actually I did not represent the association after I went with Senator Bingham. I represented Senator Bingham."

Citing "extraordinary circumstances," the committee issued a preliminary report dealing just with the Eyanson matter before it had completed its lobbying investigation. The report, dated October 26, 1929, questioned the propriety of Bingham taking Eyanson into the closed meetings. When the Manufacturers' Association of Connecticut obtained information about the secret committee proceedings, the implication, while not proved, was that the information could only have come from Eyanson. Although the committee's report condemned Bingham's arrangement with Eyanson, it presented no formal charges against the senator and made no recommendation for censure.

Response of the Senate

In submitting the report to the Senate on October 26, Caraway denounced the association between the senator and the lobbyist in stronger terms than were used in the report, but he still introduced no resolution for censure or other Senate action against Bingham. Two days later, however, Bingham, in defending his conduct, attacked the investigation as partisan and unfair. He claimed that Judiciary Committee Chairman George Norris, a progressive Republican, had stacked the special committee with opponents of the Hoover administration who disagreed with the Connecticut senator's support for administration policies. On November 1, calling Bingham's comments about the committee members "discourteous," Norris introduced a resolution to censure Bingham for behavior "contrary to good morals and senatorial ethics" that tended "to bring the Senate into dishonor and disrepute."

The floor debate took place on November 4, 1929. Bingham, who had had a distinguished career as an explorer and historian of South America before entering politics, once again boldly defended himself and Charles Eyanson, denying any intentional wrongdoing. The debate eventually concluded with

Norris expressing discouragement that the senator from Connecticut had "never yet grasped the fact that the action he took was injurious to the honor and dignity of the Senate, was injurious to public sentiment and to public opinion." Finally, after amending the resolution to state that Bingham had no corrupt motives, the Senate censured the Connecticut senator. In the 54-to-22 vote that broke along regional lines, twenty-two fellow Republicans from midwestern and western states abandoned their political colleague and voted with Democrats for censure, while northeastern Republicans supported Bingham.

Conclusion

Still unconvinced that he had done anything ethically wrong, Hiram Bingham, urbane and scholarly, returned to the Senate floor two days after the censure to take part in the tariff debate. He continued to serve in the Senate until March 1933, losing a bid for reelection in the 1932 Democratic landslide. Subsequently, Bingham continued his varied career and wide-ranging interests. Among other activities, he headed corporations, became an aviation lobbyist, wrote history books, and instructed naval officers during World War II. Bingham died in 1956.

Over the next decades, Congress continued to discuss ways to regulate lobbying, which proved difficult to accomplish because of the First Amendment right of citizens to petition their government. Focusing therefore on disclosure rather than on actual regulation of lobbyists' activities, Congress in the 1930s passed bills requiring registration by lobbyists for public utilities, shipping firms, and foreign agents. In 1946, as part of that year's Legislative Reorganization Act, it adopted the Federal Regulation of Lobbying Act, requiring that those hired to lobby register with Congress.

Sources

U.S. Congress. Senate. *Congressional Record.* 71st Cong., 1st sess. (See pp. 4046, 4922–27, 4947–57, 5063, 5113–32.)

———. Senate Report No. 43. Part 1, vol. C. 71st Cong., 1st sess., 1929.

———. *Lobby Investigation, Hearings before a Subcommittee of the Committee on the Judiciary.* Vol. 1 (October 15 to November 15, 1929), 71st Cong., 2d sess.

Garraty, John, ed. *Dictionary of American Biography.* Supp. 6. New York, 1980. (See pp. 58–60.)

Lowitt, Richard. *George W. Norris: The Persistence of a Progressive, 1913–1933.* Urbana, IL, 1971. (See pp. 422–23.)

Case 113

Joseph R. Grundy

(1863–1961)

Pennsylvania

Election Case (appointment)
December 12, 1929 to January 31, 1930

Issues
Campaign financing

Result: Seated

Chronology:
Credentials presented: Dec. 12, 1929
Referred to committee: Dec. 12, 1929
Committee report: Jan. 31, 1930
No Senate action

Background

On December 11, 1929, five days after the United States Senate denied William S. Vare his seat (See Case 109), Pennsylvania Governor John S. Fisher appointed Joseph R. Grundy, a wealthy woolen manufacturer, well-known lobbyist, and Republican party leader, to fill the vacancy. The names of both Governor Fisher and Senator-designate Grundy had been closely linked to the Vare investigation. Fisher and Grundy figured prominently in the Republican faction that opposed the ousted Vare, and the Senate investigation indicated that their enormous campaign expenditures had been equally reprehensible.

Statement of the Case

On December 12, 1929, Joseph Grundy's certificate of appointment was presented to the United States Senate. Gerald P. Nye (R-ND) immediately rose and asked that Grundy be denied his seat because of his connection to the recently decided William Vare corruption case. As a result of the Senate's intense review of the 1926 Pennsylvania primary, members already knew that Grundy, a spokesman for the state's manufacturing interests, had raised and contributed more than $400,000 to the campaign coffers of Governor Fisher. Nye fumed to his colleagues that they denied a place to "Half-million-dollar Vare" but faced the unsavory prospect of admitting a political crony of "Two-million-dollar Fisher."

Other senators shared Nye's distress that there seemed to be no end to the excessive expenditures involved in the Pennsylvania election but questioned the authority of the Senate to inquire into the legality of a gubernatorial contest. Nonetheless, members found it difficult to dismiss their recent consideration of the 1926 Pennsylvania election in which witnesses had reported that sums between $400,000 and $1,800,000 had been spent by various candidates and lobbyists. Although Grundy—commonly acknowledged to be one of the participants in the campaign transactions—was permitted to take his oath, the Senate referred his credentials to the Committee on Privileges and Elections.

Response of the Senate

On January 31, 1930, the committee returned a report stating that the appointment of Joseph Grundy complied with the constitutional requirements of the Seventeenth Amendment and therefore concluded that the Pennsylvania senator had a right to his seat. The report made no mention of Grundy's connection to the Vare scandal, his exorbitant campaign contributions, or the machine politics that had controlled the 1926 elections for governor and senator in Pennsylvania.

The Senate took no further action on this case. Apparently exhausted from the travail of the three-and-one-half-year Vare investigation, the senators did not pursue the matter.

Conclusion

Joseph Grundy filled the Pennsylvania seat that had been vacant since 1927. Defeated in the 1930 Republican primary, he served only one year in the Senate. In that time, he managed to articulate his conservative philosophy so effectively that the term "Grundyism" came to mean opposition to any change. Upon his return to Pennsylvania, Grundy continued to participate vigorously in politics and civic affairs. He died in 1961.

Sources

U.S. Congress. Senate. *Congressional Record.* 71st Cong., 2d sess. (See pp. 525–39, 2762.)

———. Senate Report No. 147. 71st Cong., 2d sess., 1930.

Garraty, John A., ed. *Dictionary of American Biography.* Supp. 7. New York, 1981. (See pp. 304–6.)

VIII. Pre- and Post-World War II: 1931–1949

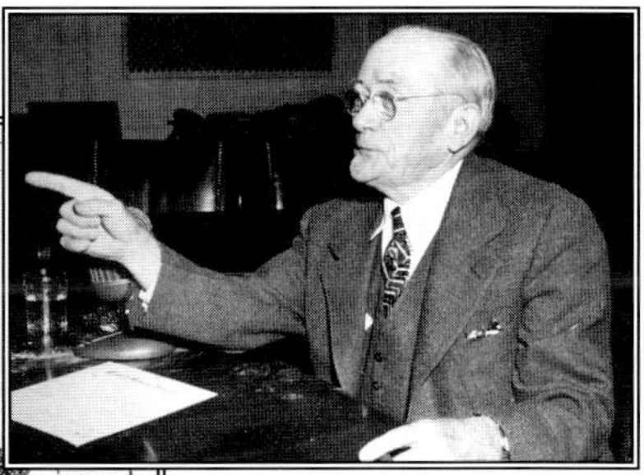

Theodore G. Bilbo
(Case 126)
U.S. Senate Historical Office

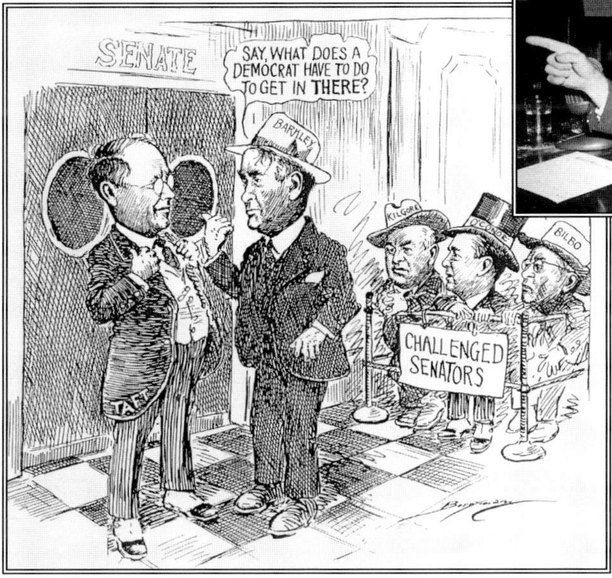

A cartoonist's view of contested election cases in 1947 *(Cases 126, 127, 128), The Berryman Collection, Center for Legislative Archives, National Archives*

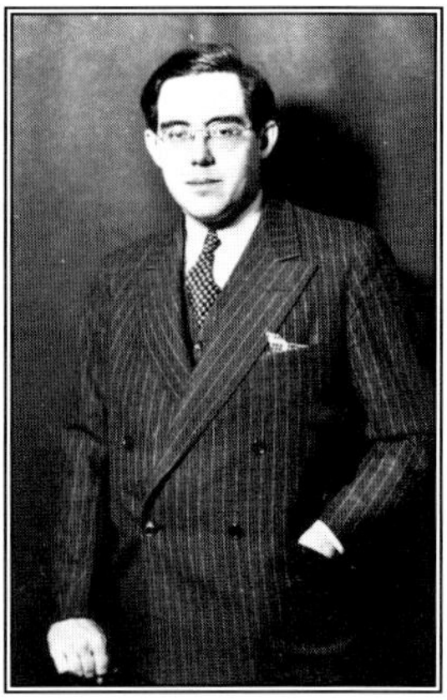

Rush D. Holt *(Case 119)*
U.S. Senate Historical Office

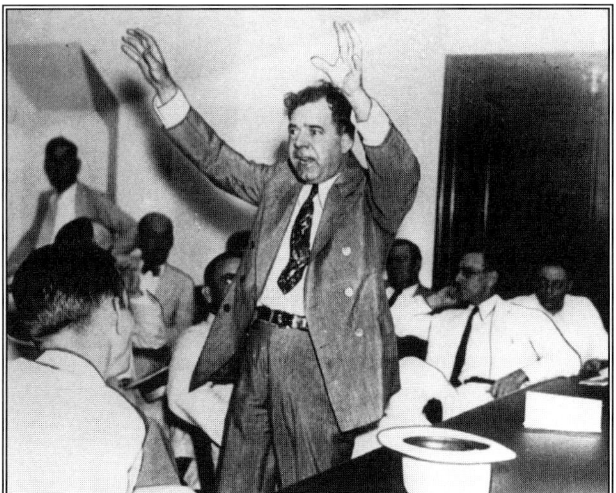

Huey P. Long *(Case 117)*
Martin Luther King Library

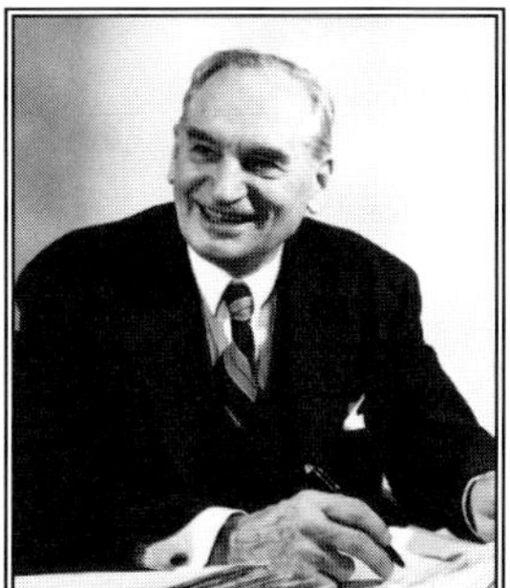

William Langer
(Case 123) U.S. Senate Historical Office

Case 114

J. Thomas Heflin v. John H. Bankhead II

(1869–1951) (1872–1946)

Alabama

Election Case
January 29, 1931 to April 28, 1932

Issues
Campaign irregularities; recount of disputed ballots

Result: Bankhead retained seat

Chronology:
Resolution introduced: Jan. 29, 1931
Referred to committee: Feb. 26, 1931
Committee report: April 18, 1932
Senate vote: April 28, 1932

Background

The 1923 Code of Alabama empowered state political organizations to establish qualifications for candidates, including mandatory disclosure of how an individual had voted in the most recent presidential election. Under this procedure, the Democratic state committee refused to allow incumbent Senator J. Thomas Heflin to run in the party's 1930 primary because he had backed Republican Herbert Hoover for president in 1928. With Heflin excluded from the race, John H. Bankhead II won the Democratic primary for the U.S. Senate. Heflin then abandoned the Democrats and joined the effort to launch a splinter party, the Jeffersonians or Independent party, which named him as its U.S. Senate candidate. In the general election, however, Democrat John Bankhead soundly defeated the two-term maverick senator.

Statement of the Case

When he returned to Washington in January 1931 for the final two months of his term, Thomas Heflin informed the Senate that he would contest the Alabama election and would request a recount. In a lengthy presentation, Heflin argued that he had "been defrauded of the right to run in the regular Democratic primary" and charged that Bankhead's election was invalid due to the misuse of voter lists and absentee ballots, irregularities in the tabulation and posting of returns, and payment of poll taxes for voters in arrears. By requesting an investigation of the election, Heflin clearly hoped to convince the Senate not to seat Bankhead when he appeared for the term that commenced on March 4, 1931. The Alabama legislature criticized Heflin's effort, adopting a resolution charging him with "poor sportsmanship in refusing to accept defeat like a man."

On February 26, 1931, the Senate acceded to Heflin's request and asked the Committee on Privileges and Elections to investigate the Alabama election. It authorized the committee to take possession of the ballots, poll lists, tabulation sheets, and all other records from the November 1930 senatorial contest. The members prudently attached an amendment that limited investigation expenses to $10,000, but before the tangled, intense case wound to its conclusion almost fifteen months later, the Senate had authorized and spent more than $100,000 on Heflin's challenge.

Response of the Senate

A subcommittee of three Republicans and two Democrats carried out a recount of the ballots and conducted hearings in both Alabama and Washington throughout 1931 and into the spring of the following year. Despite the continuing investigation, John Bankhead, armed with valid credentials, was seated when the Senate assembled for the first session of the Seventy-second Congress on December 7, 1931.

Once the massive volume of testimony had been gathered, Republican members of the subcommittee decided from the evidence that the Democratic primary had been invalid because it barred any candidate who had supported the Republican ticket in 1928. Additionally, they insisted that voting irregularities throughout Alabama had been so numerous and flagrant in the general election that the United States Senate should simply declare that no election occurred.

Democrats Walter George (GA) and Sam Bratton (NM) submitted a minority report that viewed the intricate political events somewhat differently. They argued that the Democratic state committee was within its legal rights in excluding Heflin from the primary. The Alabama statutes that permitted a party loyalty qualification did not conflict with federal legislation, because the federal government had not attempted to impose any jurisdiction over state primaries. They observed that Heflin had failed to question the state committee's regulations before the primary and had made no effort to block Bankhead's candidacy at the state level. Instead, Heflin had devoted his energies to organizing a new political party and did not formally protest the Democratic primary procedure until after he suffered defeat in the general election. Citing numerous legal precedents, George and Bratton asserted the overriding principle that, once the voters had chosen between two candidates, the manner of placing those candidates on the ballot was no longer relevant. They also stressed that, under Alabama law, an election could not be voided because of irregularities which were not shown to have changed the result of the election. The ballots thrown out in the recount still left Bankhead the winner by more than 34,000 votes. Bankhead himself had not been linked to any of the irregularities cited, nor were these found to be evidence of fraud.

George and Bratton succeeded in convincing the majority of the full Privileges and Elections Committee that Bankhead had been legally elected, and the committee adopted their report, which was presented to the Senate on April 18, 1932. Some committee members, however, continued to be troubled by such aspects of the Alabama election as broken ballot box seals and the occasional use of hat boxes for ballots, allowing ballots to be taken from the polling place and voted by individuals who were ill, and the failure to provide voting booths in some polling locations. As a result, three Republicans submitted a minority report. They acknowledged that Bankhead himself had not been revealed as personally corrupt, but they believed the widespread, blatant irregularities made it impossible to ensure that fraud did not occur. They therefore urged their colleagues to declare that no election had taken place.

During the floor debate, Heflin's friends arranged for him to address the Senate on April 26, 1932. Heflin used this opportunity to unleash his well-known passionate oratorical style in a dramatic appeal that his case should be properly investigated. The intensity of Heflin's rhetoric prompted such enthusiastic demonstrations of support from the galleries that the presiding officer finally ordered the spectators removed. In the face of Heflin's harangue, the previously silent Bankhead spoke in his own defense the next day, insisting that his election had been valid.

After a week of emotional debates, the Senate on April 28, 1932, agreed with John Bankhead and voted 64 to 18 that he had been duly elected and should retain his seat.

Conclusion

Heflin, who had been notorious during his Senate years for demagogic diatribes expressing his racial and religious bigotry, ran unsuccessfully for both the House and Senate in subsequent years. For several years, he served as a special representative of the Federal Housing Administration. Heflin died in 1951. John Bankhead remained in the Senate until his death in 1946, becoming influential in agriculture policy during the New Deal and World War II.

Sources

U.S. Congress. Senate. *Congressional Record.* 71st Cong., 3d sess. (See pp. 77, 3393, 3429–36, 3470–75, 5834–35, 6101, 6462–63.)

———. *Congressional Record.* 72d Cong., 1st sess. (See pp. 3–5, 923, 5356–57, 6448, 8349, 8555, 8586–90, 8660, 8673–94, 8765–79, 8864–77, 8918–45, 9020–39, 9110–23.)

———. Senate Report No. 568. 72d Cong., 1st sess., 1932.

Garraty, John A., ed. *Dictionary of American Biography.* Supp. 5. New York, 1977. (See pp. 290–91.)

Harper, Glenn T. "'Cotton Tom' Heflin and the Election of 1930: The Price of Party Disloyalty." *The Historian* 30 (May 1968): 389–411.

James, Edward T., ed. *Dictionary of American Biography.* Supp. 3. New York, 1973. (See pp. 49–51.)

Case 115

George M. Pritchard v. Josiah W. Bailey

(1886–1955) (1873–1946)

North Carolina

Election Case
March 3, 1931 to February 3, 1933

Issues
Campaign irregularities;
Senate refused recount

Result: Bailey retained seat

Chronology:
Petition filed: Mar. 3, 1931
Referred to committee: Mar. 3, 1931
Committee report: Feb. 3, 1933
Senate vote: Feb. 3, 1933

Background

North Carolina Democrats retained a powerful hold on the state's politics throughout the first third of the twentieth century. Only occasionally did Republicans manage to capture public office, as, for example, when Jeter C. Pritchard served in the United States Senate from 1893 to 1903 and George M. Pritchard, his son, won a seat in the United States House of Representatives in 1928. When George Pritchard declined to run for reelection to the House and instead sought a seat in the U.S. Senate in 1930, the Democratic candidate, Josiah W. Bailey, defeated him by more than 100,000 votes.

Statement of the Case

On March 3, 1931, the day before the term of Senator-elect Josiah Bailey began, his vanquished Republican opponent, George Pritchard, filed a petition contesting the North Carolina voting procedures, which the Senate referred to the Committee on Privileges and Elections. Pritchard charged that the state's election laws had been deliberately framed to give Democrats an unfair advantage. He specifically claimed that, because all 1,800 North Carolina voter registrars belonged to the Democratic party, they enjoyed an unchecked opportunity to manipulate and alter poll lists and registration books. This control resulted in such abuses as Democrats selecting all Republican representatives for state, county, and precinct boards; registrars applying the voter literacy test only to Republicans; Democratic poll judges forcing Republican watchers to stand where they could not see the ballot boxes; intimidation of voters; fraudulent use of absentee ballots; destruction of ballots after the election; and keeping polls open only during the hours when Democrats were available to vote.

On December 7, 1931, Josiah Bailey appeared in the Senate and took his oath of office. Republican Samuel Shortridge (CA) immediately announced that he would present a resolution to challenge Bailey's election. Ten days later, the Senate authorized the Committee on Privileges and Elections to investigate Pritchard's charges.

Response of the Senate

On January 13, 1932, Democratic Minority Leader Joseph T. Robinson (AR) protested a resolution that would allow the committee to spend $10,000 on the investigation, which the Arkansas Democrat deemed had no substantive basis. The Senate accepted Robinson's suggestion that it wait to pass the financial authorization until the full Committee on Privileges and Elections could meet to evaluate the significance of the allegations. Three days later, the committee gathered, reviewed George Pritchard's original petition, and received Josiah Bailey's spoken and written request to dismiss the charges. The committee decided to permit Pritchard to file an amended petition with more specific evidence of the election misconduct. In late January, Pritchard submitted a list of forty-two North Carolina counties, itemizing the nature of the election frauds that he anticipated could be proven in each through a full investigation.

In March 1932, Bailey replied confidently that all of Pritchard's accusations were of a "dragnet description" and founded on speculation rather than evidence. Denying all the allegations, Bailey asserted that no recount could possibly be justified, because even if all the votes in those forty-two counties were thrown out, he would still have won in the remaining fifty-eight unchallenged counties by a margin of 71,000 votes. He declared that the number of North Carolina Republican votes in 1930 were comparable to those in preceding elections and that Republicans enjoyed "full representation throughout the state election system." He added that Pritchard had made a public concession speech after the election and gave no indication until March 1931 that he planned to contest the result.

No further action occurred in the case until February 1933 when a subcommittee of Privileges and Elections issued a report recommending that the contest be dismissed. In a brief statement, the subcommittee declared that both the original and amended charges against Bailey had been so vague that they did not justify the time and expense of conducting a recount or a full investigation, especially since the margin of Bailey's victory had been so great. Without taking a recorded vote, the Senate agreed to the report and dismissed the contest.

Conclusion

On February 25, 1933, the Senate agreed to award Bailey $1,500, Pritchard, $4,000, and the state of North Carolina $500 for expenses incurred in the case. The payment to North Carolina covered the state's costs in impounding ballot boxes for the recount that did not materialize.

George Pritchard continued his law career in North Carolina and in 1948 made an unsuccessful try for the governorship. He died in 1955. Josiah Bailey served in the Senate until his death in 1946.

Sources

U.S. Congress. Senate. *Congressional Record.* 71st Cong., 3d sess. (See p. 7100.)

———. *Congressional Record.* 72d Cong., 1st sess. (See pp. 3–5, 278, 667, 1344, 1880–90, 8458, 12958, 13820.) 2d sess. (See pp. 3289, 3666, 5007–8.)

———. Senate Report No. 1151. 72d Cong., 2d sess., 1933.

Garraty, John A., and Edward T. James, eds. *Dictionary of American Biography.* Supp. 4. New York, 1974. (See pp. 42–43.)

Case 116

Einar Hoidale v. Thomas D. Schall

(1870–1952) (1878–1935)

Minnesota

Election Case
April 14, 1932 to February 7, 1933

Issues
Campaign irregularities

Result: Schall retained seat

Chronology:
Petition presented: Apr. 14, 1932
Referred to committee: Apr. 14, 1932
Committee report: Jan. 17, 1933
Senate vote: Feb. 7, 1933

Background

Minnesota Republican Thomas D. Schall, whose election to the Senate in 1926 had been contested by his defeated opponent (See Case 106) faced a second such challenge after his reelection in 1930. In the latter campaign, Schall bested his Democratic opponent, Einar Hoidale, by more than 11,000 votes in a multi-candidate race.

Statement of the Case

On December 7, 1931, Thomas Schall appeared in the Senate and took his seat for a second term without protest.

On April 14, 1932, Einar Hoidale filed a petition charging that the Republican senator secured his election through illegal methods and fraud. Hoidale alleged that Schall violated state and federal corrupt practices laws by filing false financial reports, illegally promising patronage positions in return for political support, failing to itemize names of campaign contributors and those receiving disbursements, accepting large contributions from bootleggers, and misusing franking privileges to distribute campaign literature. The Senate referred the petition to the Committee on Privileges and Elections.

The next day, Thomas Schall responded, insisting that the charges, "a mass of generalities, insinuations, and falsehoods . . . are groundless and they will fall of their own weight."

Response of the Senate

On July 16, 1932, the committee notified Hoidale that, unless he submitted an amended petition that included more detailed information, his case would be dismissed. On August 30, shortly before the committee's deadline, Hoidale submitted a revised petition. In it, he detailed large unreported expenditures made by Schall's campaign and named individuals he said had been promised patronage positions in return for campaign support, as well as postmasters who had allegedly been pressured to contribute money to retire

Schall's campaign debt. In response, Schall presented several affidavits from Minnesota citizens, all of whom swore the senator had not engaged in any illegal activities during the primary or general elections. Postmasters insisted they had received their commissions without paying the senator a penny and that all their campaign contributions had been voluntary and not connected to the distribution of patronage.

The committee reported on January 17, 1933, recommending that the contest be dismissed. It argued that Hoidale had failed to contest the election in Minnesota or to initiate legal action in the Minnesota courts regarding Schall's alleged state offenses within the deadline set by law. The allegations regarding contributions from postmasters had all been contradicted by sworn affidavits from the individuals involved and were therefore dismissed by the committee. The panel determined that, even if Hoidale had accurate information concerning the misuse of franking privileges, the sum involved could not have exceeded $100, an amount the committee deemed insignificant. In general, the committee concluded that Hoidale's charges were too vague and indefinite to warrant further investigation.

The Senate appeared willing to accept the committee's view that Schall had responded satisfactorily to the more serious charges and that the others were too minor to require attention. Without debate, the Senate on February 7, 1933, agreed by voice vote that Schall had been duly elected and should retain his seat.

Conclusion

Thomas Schall, who was permanently blinded at the age of twenty-nine, was a self-made man whose zeal and determined spirit won the admiration of even his political opponents. He served in the Senate until his death in 1935 from injuries sustained when he was struck by an automobile outside the Senate office building.

Einar Hoidale served in the U.S. House of Representatives from 1933–1935 and was again an unsuccessful candidate for the Senate in 1934. He died in 1952.

Sources

U.S. Congress. Senate. *Congressional Record.* 72d Cong., 1st sess. (See pp. 5, 3177, 8346, 8745, 15664–69.) 2d sess. (See pp. 1932, 2957, 3544.)

———. Senate Report No. 1066. 72d Cong., 2d sess., 1933.

Starr, Harris E., ed. *Dictionary of American Biography.* Supp. 1. New York, 1946. (See pp. 649–50.)

Case 117

Huey P. Long and John H. Overton

(1893–1935) (1875–1948)

Louisiana

Election Case/Expulsion Case
September 21, 1932 to June 16, 1934

Issues
Campaign irregularities

Result: Long and Overton retained seats/Not expelled

Chronology:
Request for investigation:
Sept. 21, 1932
Referred to committee:
Sept. 21, 1932 (Special)
April 14, 1933 (Judiciary)
Jan. 10, 1934 (Privs. & Elects.)
Committee reports:
Jan. 16, 1934 (Special)
Mar. 19, 1934 (Judiciary)
June 16, 1934 (Privs. & Elections)
Senate vote: June 16, 1934

Background

When the Louisiana voters in 1930 elected Huey Long to the United States Senate, the thirty-seven-year-old dynamo already exercised a tight grip over state politics, built up during his years as governor. Unwilling to relinquish the reins of state power to an unfriendly lieutenant governor, Long delayed claiming his Senate seat until January 1932. The next summer, he employed his charismatic eloquence on behalf of both presidential candidate Franklin D. Roosevelt and his personal choice for the second Louisiana Senate seat, U. S. Representative John H. Overton. Long's strength in Louisiana had no equal, and in the September 13, 1932, primary, John Overton easily defeated incumbent Senator Edwin Broussard for the Democratic nomination, a prelude to an unopposed victory in the general election.

Statement of the Case

On September 21, 1932, soon after his defeat in the primary, Edwin Broussard wrote to the chairman of a Special Committee to Investigate Campaign Expenditures in the 1932 election, which had been established in July 1932, requesting that the Senate investigate instances of corruption in the Louisiana election. He specifically charged that, for several weeks prior to the election, the state administration—under the control of the Long machine—brought in a horde of campaign workers drawn from employees of such state agencies as the highway commission, the board of health, the tax commission, and the insane asylums. State employees were also forced to make financial contributions to Overton's campaign. Broussard further contended that state officials promised the families of penitentiary inmates that their relatives would be freed in return for supporting Overton at the polls. Broussard did not claim that he himself had been elected but charged that there had been so much corruption in the election that Overton should be denied his seat.

Based on Broussard's complaint and others received from Louisiana citizens' groups, the special committee established a subcommittee to look into the matter. Meanwhile, on March 4, 1933, John Overton arrived in the Senate and was seated without challenge.

Response of the Senate

Select Committee

Between October 1932 and December 1933, the subcommittee, chaired by Robert B. Howell (R-NE), conducted three lengthy investigations in Louisiana. Although the public assumed that Huey Long's 1930 election represented the true focus of the inquiry, the committee was authorized only to examine elections that took place in 1932. During the period of the investigation, the subcommittee faced a variety of obstacles, as the chairman died in March 1933, one committee member resigned from the Senate, and a shift in party control of the Senate from Republicans to Democrats caused a reorganization of the committee. This change did not help Long, however, because the new chairman, Democrat Tom Connally of Texas, who had chaired the subcommittee through many of the hearings, disliked Huey Long and found Louisiana politics distasteful.

In the course of the hearings, the Long lieutenants who had directed Overton's campaign testified that they had kept no record of either contributions or expenditures, had dealt entirely in cash using no bank accounts, and had no idea how much money had been spent on the primary race. None of this was illegal, for Louisiana had no law limiting or requiring reports of campaign expenditures. While Long's opponents continued to raise charges of corruption, the committee members chided them for producing little hard evidence related to fraud in Overton's primary. The proceedings became increasingly rowdy as the anti-Long forces decided the committee was not seriously pursuing the investigation and turned their efforts to disruption, with shouted harangues and crowds of noisy onlookers at the public hearings.

On January 16, 1934, an exhausted and frustrated special committee reported that, in a "maelstrom of political passion and bitter factional controversy," it had great difficulty unraveling the truth about the events surrounding the 1932 primary. In the course of its lengthy Louisiana investigation, the committee had spent the entire $25,000 allocated to it for examining Senate campaign expenditures in the whole country. Decrying "the deplorable and distressing political conditions" in Louisiana, the committee concluded that Huey Long's organization "in 1932 absolutely dominated the politics of the state" and that Long had used state government employees in the Overton campaign. The committee also deplored the Long organization's "practice of coercing officeholders to contribute to political campaigns." On the other hand, any fraud that occurred had not affected the outcome of the election and there was no indication that Overton himself had been aware of any such fraud.

The committee did express concern about Broussard's charge that Long's operation was able to influence the selection of election commissioners in the precincts by recruiting "dummy candidates" to file for election to local offices. Long's organization paid the filing fees for these candidates, who had no actual intention of running. Since election commissioners were chosen by lot and every local candidate (but not candidates for statewide office) could submit a name for the pool from which the five commissioners for a precinct would be drawn, the committee noted that the use of dummies by one Senate candidate could place so many friendly names in the pool that all the commissioners chosen in a precinct could well turn out to be supporters of that candidate. In New Orleans, for example, there were more than 1,000 Overton commissioners compared to only 60 for Broussard. The committee strongly condemned the use of dummies, which it said had affected about a third of the precincts in the state, because, even though such a situation was not in itself proof of fraud, it provided the opportunity for fraud. The committee, however, found no evidence that John Overton was personally aware of the use of dummies.

Since no contested election was involved, the committee merely submitted its findings without recommendations. Overton therefore promptly declared that he was absolved of any wrongdoing, and Huey Long introduced a resolution demanding an investigation into the sources of the "libel" and "propaganda" used against him. The Senate referred this resolution to the Committee on Privileges and Elections, which took no action on the matter. Long also took the floor on January 30 to defend the practices of Louisiana and his organization, including the use of dummy candidates, which he asserted was common in other states as well.

Judiciary Committee

Meanwhile, the Senate struggled with a continuing stream of petitions from Louisiana citizens calling for Long's expulsion because of irregularities in his 1930 election. In April 1933 Long, upset because the newspapers had published many of the allegations, asked that the Senate refer these papers and petitions to the Judiciary Committee in order to resolve the legal question whether they were privileged from actions for libel and whether they should have been received by the Senate. The committee eventually reported in March 1934 that the petitions were "scurrilous and defamatory... and fail to give any detail or facts... such as to justify action on the part of the Senate." The committee added that, if the Senate had realized their vague nature, it should probably never have agreed to receive these petitions, but once they had been received they were "clothed with a limited privilege."

Privileges and Elections Committee

In January 1934 the Senate also referred the multitude of petitions seeking the expulsion of both Long and Overton to the Committee on Privileges and Elections to consider the substantive issues raised. After the ruling by the Judiciary Committee, Privileges and Elections held yet another series of public hearings in May 1934. On June 16, 1934, that committee, too, concluded that the evidence did not warrant further Senate action, and the Senate agreed on a voice vote. Huey Long and John Overton thus retained their seats.

Conclusion

Throughout 1934 and 1935, Huey Long moved aggressively into national politics and became an increasingly vehement anti-Roosevelt spokesman. He served in the Senate until his death in 1935 at the hands of an assassin in the Louisiana state capitol. John Overton remained in the Senate until his death in 1948.

Sources

U.S. Congress. Senate. *Congressional Record.* 72d Cong., 1st sess. (See pp. 4988, 8458, 9018, 14990.) 2d sess. (See pp. 1719, 4299, 4690, 4787.)

———. *Congressional Record.* 73d Cong., 1st sess. (See pp. 4, 1618, 1712–14.) 2d sess. (See pp. 307–8, 672, 674, 699–714, 1545, 1552–67, 1818, 1836–38, 1996–97, 4758, 12015–16.)

———. Senate Report No. 191. 73d Cong., 2d sess., 1934.

———. Senate Report No. 499. 73d Cong., 2d sess., 1934.

Hair, William Ivy. *The Kingfish and His Realm: The Life and Times of Huey Long.* Baton Rouge, LA, 1991.

Williams, T. Harry. *Huey Long.* New York, 1969.

Case 118

Dennis Chavez v. Bronson M. Cutting

(1888–1962) (1888–1935)

New Mexico

Election Case
February 23, 1935 to June 4, 1935

Issues
Campaign irregularities

Result: Cutting died; contest dismissed; Chavez appointed to seat

Chronology:
Petition filed: Feb. 23, 1935
Referred to committee: Feb. 25, 1935
Committee report: June 4, 1935
Senate vote: June 5, 1935

Background

The New Mexico senatorial election campaign of 1934, pitting Republican incumbent Bronson M. Cutting against Democratic House member Dennis Chavez, proved to be one of the closest and most bitter in that state's turbulent political history. With 30 percent of the state's residents on relief as a consequence of the deepening economic crisis, both contestants ran on similar platforms, stressing aid to farmers and small businessmen. Yet their personalities and background could not have been more dissimilar.

Bronson Cutting, born to great wealth and educated at Groton and Harvard, moved to New Mexico in 1910 at the age of twenty-two to be cured of tuberculosis. A classmate and friend of Franklin D. Roosevelt, Cutting established his political base as owner of the influential *Santa Fe New Mexican*. The dynamic Anglo politician emerged as a progressive reformer who developed a strong following among the state's large Hispanic voting bloc and the growing population of laborers in New Mexico's eastern oil fields. Appointed to the Senate in 1927 to fill a vacancy, Cutting won election to a full term in 1928.

In contrast to Cutting, Chavez spent his early years struggling against the political barriers of poverty and the prejudice of the state's political elite against his Hispanic origins. During the 1920s, he tirelessly worked his way into the confidence of New Mexico's Democratic hierarchy and in 1930 was rewarded for his services and party loyalty with the nomination to New Mexico's only seat in the House of Representatives. Chavez easily defeated his Republican opponent, and won reelection two years later by a wide margin. As a result, by 1934 Chavez had become his party's most potent political force in New Mexico.

Meanwhile, the progressive Bronson Cutting had endorsed Roosevelt in 1932 and supported the New Deal. In doing so, he severed his ties with the

Republican party's old-guard conservative power structure and built a potent coalition of Hispanic Americans and dispossessed Anglos. During the 1934 campaign, however, Chavez as the Democratic candidate gained both the endorsement of President Roosevelt and the support of the national Democratic party, which supplied money and prominent speakers. Cutting, for his part, portrayed Chavez as representing the conservative, monied power structure in the state.

Statement of the Case

Although Chavez ran a strong race, Cutting's personal popularity carried him to a narrow 1,261-vote victory. When the state canvassing board met in December 1934, Chavez filed a formal complaint charging voting irregularities in five of the state's thirty-one counties. In San Miguel County, according to Chavez, many votes had been cast by persons who were unregistered, underage, repeat voters, convicts, aliens, or insane. He requested that all the returns be thrown out in precincts where unregistered voters had participated. Cutting responded that the state canvassing board had no authority to throw out any votes. When the board agreed and prepared to declare Cutting the winner, Chavez petitioned the state supreme court to force the board to exclude the unregistered votes. The court, however, consisting of four Democrats and one Republican, voted 3 to 2 to support the board's action, and, finally, on December 31, 1934, Cutting received a certificate of election. On January 3, 1935, he presented his certificate to the Senate and took his oath for a second term.

Seven weeks later, on February 23, 1935, Dennis Chavez filed a petition with the Senate, disputing the validity of Cutting's election and requesting a recount. He apparently hoped that the overwhelming Democratic majority in the Senate would vote to unseat Cutting. The petition alleged "undue influence, deception, and intimidation of voters, and the unlawful use of money... and of fraudulent, wrongful, and unlawful conduct of various and sundry persons who were election judges, clerks, and counting judges, challengers, and party workers in and about said general election." Specifically, Chavez charged that illegal votes had been counted for Cutting, while many legal votes for the challenger were not counted. The Senate referred the matter to the Committee on Privileges and Elections.

On March 25, 1935, Cutting formally moved to dismiss the challenge, complaining that the charges were untrue, the petition was deceptive and ambiguous, the contest was a "fishing expedition," and Chavez had failed to exhaust his remedy in the state courts. Back in New Mexico, the legislature created a committee of Democrats to investigate the election, while Cutting's lawyers were busily seeking evidence on his behalf, as well as any indications of voting fraud by the Democrats. In February, the legislative investigating committee reported that it had found a number of irregularities in the election and recommended some changes in the state's election code to prevent such violations. The committee, however, took no position on the outcome of the Cutting-Chavez race.

Response of the Senate

On April 10, 1935, the Senate Committee on Privileges and Elections held a hearing on Cutting's dismissal motion and decided to drop Chavez's charges of illegal use of money and unlawful expenditures. The committee directed Cutting to prepare a formal response to the allegations of conspiring to have illegal votes counted for him and legal votes not counted for Chavez. Cutting therefore flew back to New Mexico to determine the accuracy of the disputed voting lists. On his return trip to Washington on May 6, 1935, the senator was killed when his plane crashed in a dense fog at Atlanta, Missouri. Less than a week later, New Mexico's Democratic governor appointed Dennis Chavez to fill the vacant seat.

The Committee on Privileges and Elections met again on June 4. Chavez notified the committee that he wished to dismiss the challenge, but Cutting's friends urged the committee to take formal action to rule on the allegations so that his name could be cleared. Cutting's counsel presented the late senator's formal response, specifically refuting the charges, based on the lawyers' detailed research. Among other points, the response explained that most of the individuals listed as unregistered were actually properly registered with some slight variation in the spelling or form of the name—such as a woman being registered under her given name and voting under her husband's name. As a result, the committee voted unanimously to dismiss the contest, with the declaration that "no evidence has been adduced, and there is nothing in the record which, in any way, reflects, either directly or indirectly, upon the honor or integrity" of Cutting. The Senate on June 5, 1935, agreed by voice vote to the committee's recommendation, and the matter was dropped.

Conclusion

In the months before Bronson Cutting's death, many people had considered him a possible contender for his party's 1936 presidential nomination. His death shattered the Republican party in New Mexico; not until 1972 did the state again elect a Republican to the U.S. Senate.

Dennis Chavez went on to win a special election in 1936 with 55 percent of the vote and was reelected for four subsequent terms, serving until his death in November 1962. He, too, was subjected to an election contest when his defeated opponent in the 1952 race charged him with election fraud (See Case 132).

Sources

U.S. Congress. Senate. *Congressional Record*. 74th Cong., 1st sess. (See pp. 7, 291, 538, 2513, 6999, 8663.)

———. Senate Report No. 793. 74th Cong., 1st sess., 1935.

———. Committee on Privileges and Elections. *Senator From New Mexico.* Hearings. April 10 and June 4, 1935.

Garraty, John A., ed. *Dictionary of American Biography.* Supp. 7. New York, 1981. (See pp. 121–22.)

Lowitt, Richard. *Bronson M. Cutting: Progressive Politician.* Albuquerque, NM, 1992.

Pickens, William H. "Bronson Cutting vs. Dennis Chavez: Battle of the Patrones in New Mexico, 1934." *New Mexico Historical Review* 46 (January 1971): 5–36.

Pickens, William H. "Cutting vs. Chavez: A Reply to Wolf's Comments." *New Mexico Historical Review* 47 (October 1972): 337–59.

Seligmann, G. L., Jr. "The Purge That Failed: The 1934 Senatorial Election in New Mexico: Yet Another View." *New Mexico Historical Review* 47 (October 1972): 361–81.

Wolf, T. Phillip. "Cutting vs. Chavez Re-Examined: A Commentary on Pickens' Analysis." *New Mexico Historical Review* 47 (October 1972): 317–36.

Case 119

Henry D. Hatfield v. Rush D. Holt

(1875–1962) (1905–1955)

West Virginia

Election Case
April 19, 1935 to June 21, 1935

Issues
Qualifications: age; runner-up ruled ineligible even if winner fails to qualify

Chronology:
Petition received: April 19, 1935
Referred to committee: April 19, 1935
Committee report: June 19, 1935
Senate vote: June 21, 1935

Result: Holt retained seat

Background

The 1934 West Virginia senatorial campaign of Rush D. Holt centered on the candidate's youthfulness, a topic widely discussed in the press and at state political gatherings. Holt had not yet reached the constitutionally mandated age of thirty when he sought and won the Democratic nomination in the primary and went on to victory in the general election. Although Holt placed his credentials on file with the Senate on January 3, 1935, he did not present himself in the chamber nor attempt to take the oath of office, reaffirming his campaign promise to claim his seat on June 19, 1935, his thirtieth birthday.

Statement of the Case

On April 18, 1935, Holt's defeated Republican opponent, the incumbent Senator Henry D. Hatfield, filed a petition with the Senate charging that Holt's failure to meet the constitutional age requirement invalidated his election. Hatfield therefore asked that he be declared senator, having received the next highest number of votes. The former senator further alleged that Holt had violated the West Virginia primary election laws by submitting a fraudulent eligibility certificate. Not only did the certificate, according to Hatfield, falsely state that Holt was eligible to serve in the Senate, it had been filed in a county other than the one recorded on the document. In May a West Virginia citizens' group petitioned the Senate to declare the seat vacant so that the governor could appoint a qualified person to serve until the next regular election. The citizens' memorial and Hatfield's charges were referred to the Committee on Privileges and Elections.

Response of the Senate

On June 19, 1935, Rush Holt arrived in the Senate to take the oath of office. At the request of the Privileges and Elections Committee, however, he agreed to stand aside until it could present its report. A majority of the committee submitted a report favorable to Rush Holt. It dismissed as insignificant the irregularities in the eligibility certificate, noting that Holt had made his sworn statement before a legitimate officer of the state and that no complaints had been raised against the certificate prior to either the primary or general election. Holt had told the committee that in swearing he was eligible he was under the impression that, since the Senate had seated Henry Clay in 1806 when he was less than thirty years old, a precedent had been set. The committee majority found the charge that Holt tried to mislead the voters about his age unsupported by the evidence, since he had made no secret that he was twenty-nine years old, and the issue had been thoroughly discussed during the campaign. The majority believed that the constitutional provision would not apply until the time Holt actually took the oath of office, and Holt had announced that he would wait to do so until his thirtieth birthday. The report also dismissed Hatfield's claim to the seat by restating a well-established Senate rule that the ineligibility of the winning candidate gives no title to the candidate receiving the next highest number of votes.

A minority report argued that Hatfield's challenge raised the question of whether the constitutional age requirement applied on the day of the election, the day on which the term commenced, or the day on which the senator-elect took his seat. The minority believed the Constitution required a senator to be thirty years old when his term began. They pointed out that an act of Congress provided that even a senator-elect who had not yet been sworn in would be placed on the payroll at the beginning of his term if his credentials were in order. The committee minority therefore thought the election was void because Holt was not qualified when his term began. They also considered that the presentation of Holt's credentials on January 3, 1935, the addition of his name to the payroll, and his appointment of secretaries and clerks constituted an illegal attempt to claim his seat before he became eligible. Both the minority report and a separate report by Hiram W. Johnson (R-CA) expressed concern that seating Holt would violate Senate precedents set in the earlier cases of Albert Gallatin and James Shields (See Cases 1 and 21). In each of these cases the Senate had voided the election because the winning candidate had not been a citizen for the requisite nine years. Johnson objected that the Constitution could hardly intend that "a senator should have attained the age of thirty years sometime within the six years of his term."

The committee reports sparked a lengthy debate on June 20 and 21. Those who supported seating Holt stressed that a new member was a senator-elect at the beginning of his term but did not become a senator until he took the oath of office. Walter George (D-GA), the chairman of the Privileges and Elections Committee, observed that the Gallatin and Shields cases differed from that of Holt because neither of them had been a citizen for nine years either at the beginning of his term or at the time he took the oath of office. In this case, Holt had waited to be sworn in until his thirtieth birthday. Asking, "if one is ineligible at the time the term begins, does that bar him from later on becoming eligible?" Huey Long (D-LA) reminded the Senate that it had seated without question a number of members who had been state governors when elected and had chosen to wait beyond the beginning of the term before resigning the governorship and being sworn in as senators. Several had waited a number of months; Robert M. La Follette, Sr. had waited a year; and Long himself had waited a year and three months before taking the oath of office. He added that a federal court had ruled that an individual did not become a senator until being sworn in. The Senate, he insisted, should only be concerned with qualifications at the time the person arrived to take the seat, and in this case Rush Holt was qualified.

Finally, on June 21, the Senate voted, 62 to 17, to adopt the committee majority's resolution permitting the senator-elect to take his oath, and Rush Holt came forward to be seated.

Conclusion

In this case, the Senate set two precedents. It ruled that the constitutional age qualification did not apply until a senator-elect was actually sworn in, and it reaffirmed that even if a winning candidate was ruled ineligible, the runner-up in the election would not be declared elected.

In June 1937 the Senate refused to grant Henry Hatfield's request for compensation for his attorneys' fees. Hatfield, who had left a distinguished career as a physician to serve in a variety of political offices, returned to the practice of medicine. He died in 1962.

Rush Holt failed to be renominated in 1940 and remained in the Senate for only one term. After 1941 he served in the state legislature and devoted himself to research, an outgrowth of his early career as an instructor in the state teachers' college. He was unsuccessful in later attempts to win statewide office when he ran for the West Virginia governorship and the U.S. Senate. Holt died in 1955.

Sources

U.S. Congress. Senate. *Congressional Record.* 74th Cong., 1st sess. (See pp. 4, 5915–16, 7547, 9650–51, 9750–78, 9824–42.)

———. Senate Report No. 904. 74th Cong., 1st sess., 1935.

———. *Riddick's Senate Procedure,* by Floyd M. Riddick and Alan S. Frumin. S. Doc. 101–28. 101st Cong., 2d sess., 1992. (See p. 701.)

Case 120

George L. Berry

(1882–1948)

Tennessee

Election Case (appointment)
May 11, 1937 to June 14, 1937

Issues
Charges related to actions before Senate; ruling on termination date of appointment

Result: Retained seat

Chronology:
Petition received: May 11, 1937
Referred to committee: May 11, 1937
Committee report: June 14, 1937
Senate vote: June 14, 1937

Background

As a young man, George Berry took a job as a pressman. For the remainder of his life he was closely associated with the interests of workers. In 1907 Berry became president of the International Printing Pressmen and Assistants' Union of America, an organization that dominated his professional life for the next forty years. A Democrat who had run unsuccessfully for governor and U.S. senator and who actively supported President Franklin D. Roosevelt's reelection campaign in 1936, Berry was appointed by the Tennessee governor in May 1937 to fill the unexpired term of recently deceased Senator Nathan L. Bachman.

Statement of the Case

On May 10, 1937, George Berry presented his credentials and took his oath of office. The following day H. C. Lowry, a citizen of Tennessee, filed a petition with the Senate asking for an investigation of Berry's right to the seat. Lowry charged Berry with numerous irregularities in connection with various business and union activities. He claimed that Berry had been involved in a lawsuit regarding misuse of union funds, had failed to pay his taxes, and had engaged in "chiseling" business tactics. He also contended that someone representing President Roosevelt had urged the governor to appoint Berry. The Senate referred the petition to the Committee on Privileges and Elections.

Response of the Senate

George Berry immediately fired off a letter to the committee in which he denied Lowry's allegations. He explained that the episode over union monies had involved a 1917 lawsuit against the board of directors of the International Printing Pressmen and Assistants' Union at the time Berry was actually with the U.S. forces in France. Ultimately, that legal action had been withdrawn and the costs assigned to the plaintiffs. Berry denied the charges regarding his business practices and insisted that he only negotiated collective bargaining agreements through recognized labor organizations. He scoffed at the idea that he had not paid his taxes and called "ridiculous" the suggestion that a friend of President Roosevelt had pressured the Tennessee governor to make the senatorial appointment.

On June 14, 1937, the committee unanimously reported that it found the allegations insufficient to warrant Senate action. The Senate agreed by voice vote that same day, and George Berry retained his seat.

Conclusion

George Berry served until November 8, 1938, when a successor, Tom Stewart, was elected to fill the remainder of the term. Stewart, a district attorney general in Tennessee, did not take his seat until January 16, 1939, thus raising the question of the exact date on which Berry's term ended and prompting a subcommittee of the Judiciary Committee to hold hearings on the matter. The committee reported that, although a Tennessee law stated that an appointed senator held office until a successor was elected and qualified, the Seventeenth Amendment to the Constitution took precedence over any state law. That amendment decreed that states could empower governors to fill vacancies by appointment until a successor was elected. In addition, the committee pointed out that Congress had passed a law in 1935 stating that the pay of an individual chosen in a special election to fill a vacancy would begin on the day after the election. On February 2, 1939, the Senate agreed to the committee's recommendation that Berry's term had ended on the day of Stewart's election, November 8, 1938. On February 6, Berry—who apparently still wanted clarification regarding possible additional salary due him—asked the Senate to reconsider the decision. Although his petition was referred to the Judiciary Committee, no further action was taken.

George Berry, who maintained interests as a banker and a farmer, resumed his post as president of the International Printing Pressmen and Assistants' Union of North America and continued in that capacity until his death in 1948.

Sources

U.S. Congress. Senate. *Congressional Record.* 75th Cong., 1st sess. (See pp. 4257, 4318, 5633.)

———. *Congressional Record.* 76th Cong., 1st sess. (See pp. 5, 990–98, 1058, 1142.)

———. Senate Report No. 710. 75th Cong., 1st sess., 1937.

———. Senate Report No. 16. 76th Cong., 1st sess., 1939.

———. *Riddick's Senate Procedure,* by Floyd M. Riddick and Alan S. Frumin. S. Doc. 101–28. 101st Cong., 2d sess., 1992. (See pp. 1251–53.)

Garraty, John A., and Edward T. James, eds. *Dictionary of American Biography.* Supp. 4. New York, 1974. (See pp. 74–75.)

Case 121

John R. Neal v. A.T. (Tom) Stewart

(dates unknown) (1892–1972)

Tennessee

Election Case
January 16, 1939 to March 31, 1939

Issues
Campaign financing; campaign irregularities

Result: Stewart retained seat

Chronology:
Petition filed: Jan. 16, 1939
Referred to committee: Jan. 16, 1939
Committee report: Mar. 31, 1939
Senate vote: Mar. 31, 1939

Background

In 1938, as Tennessee Democrats competed fiercely for that party's nomination in a special election to fill the unexpired term of the recently deceased Nathan L. Bachman, the United States Senate received complaints from one contestant about irregularities in the primary campaign. The Senate dutifully referred the petition to a select committee charged with investigating campaign expenditures in the 1938 senatorial elections. The committee investigated the charges of John R. Neal, who, after his defeat in the primary, ran as an independent in the general election. In that race, Neal succeeded in attracting only 9,100 votes, while his opponent, Tom Stewart, won a decisive plurality of almost 195,000. Stewart's victory was made even more secure by a report from the select committee on January 3, 1939, that dismissed Neal's allegations about the conduct of the primary and added that there should be no question of Stewart's right to his seat.

Statement of the Case

Tom Stewart appeared and was seated on January 16, 1939. On that same day, John Neal filed a second petition with the Senate in which he charged that Stewart procured his seat through fraudulent procedures that violated the laws of Tennessee and the United States. He therefore asked that Stewart be disqualified and that he himself be seated instead. Neal specifically alleged that Stewart spent more than $250,000 in the primary and general elections, seriously exceeding the state campaign expenditures limit of $20,000 for the two elections. He further charged that on election day foremen of the Works Progress Administration "herded" employees to the polls and forced them to vote for Stewart, after earlier coercing campaign contributions from many federal workers. The Senate referred these charges to the Committee on Privileges and Elections.

An amended petition submitted on February 17, 1939, largely reiterated Neal's original claims of excessive expenditures; illegal use of poll-tax receipts; irregular use of absentee ballots; registration of persons who were actually deceased, aliens, or minors; and unlawful campaign assessments of federal employees. Neal further stated that Stewart's coalition, under the guise of building farm-to-market roads, constructed hundreds of private thoroughfares and driveways to elicit voter support in the general election.

Response of the Senate

On March 31, 1939, the committee returned a report favorable to Tom Stewart. Although Neal's allegations echoed those of other election contests of the era, the committee noted that he was in a singularly weak position as a candidate. Stewart's margin of victory was so great that the investigation could not possibly throw out enough votes to make Neal the winner in the race. The committee therefore saw no need to carry the investigation further. It also reminded the Senate that the select committee had previously determined that Neal could in no way claim to have won the primary nomination. The committee therefore proposed a resolution to dismiss the contest against Tom Stewart. The Senate agreed by voice vote that same day and dismissed the contest.

Conclusion

Stewart, who had served as the district attorney general in Tennessee for sixteen years, remained in the Senate for ten years. In 1942 he faced another election challenge from John Neal (See Case 125), but the Senate also dismissed that contest. Stewart returned to the practice of law in 1949 and died in 1972.

Sources

U.S. Congress. Senate. *Congressional Record.* 76th Cong., 1st sess. (See pp. 4, 8, 350, 369–70, 1535, 3611–12.)

———. Senate Report No. 242. 76th Cong., 1st sess., 1939.

Raymond E. Willis v. Frederick Van Nuys

(1875–1956) (1874–1944)

Indiana

Election Case
March 13, 1939 to April 13, 1939

Issues
Campaign irregularities; Senate refused recount

Result: Van Nuys retained seat

Chronology:
Petition received: Mar. 13, 1939
Referred to committee: Mar. 13, 1939
Committee report: April 13, 1939
Senate vote: April 13, 1939

Background

As Senator Frederick Van Nuys (D) faced his Republican challenger, Raymond E. Willis, in the 1938 Indiana senatorial contest, the incumbent found it necessary to disavow any connection with a Democratic political organization of unsavory repute, the Two Per Cent Club. During his campaign, Van Nuys denounced the organization, stating, "I could not have accepted aid from the Two Per Cent Club...for the simple reason that I regard that organization as violative of both the Federal and State Corrupt Practices Act." After Van Nuys won the general election by 5,100 votes, this uncompromising pronouncement proved helpful when the defeated Willis decided to request a recount.

Statement of the Case

On January 3, 1939, Van Nuys presented his credentials and took his oath of office. On March 13, Raymond Willis submitted a petition alleging that serious irregularities—such as tampering with voting machines and allowing improperly registered persons to vote—had occurred during the Indiana election. Willis also charged that recipients of Works Progress Administration jobs and relief were told that they would not receive future assistance if they failed to vote for the Democrats, and he complained about the infamous Two Per Cent Club, which was said to have violated the corrupt practices acts by collecting and disbursing thousands of dollars for the senatorial election without keeping appropriate records. In calling for a recount, Willis made clear that Van Nuys had not known about or participated in the election misconduct. The Senate referred the matter to the Committee on Privileges and Elections.

Response of the Senate

It took the committee only a month to return a report favorable to Van Nuys. The committee called the allegations vague and doubtful, noting that, even if some irregularities could be proven, the number of votes affected totalled only about 120, not sufficient to alter the outcome of the election. The committee added that it was already aware of some voting abuses connected with federal relief programs and the promises of "jobs, food, and favoritism" in return for votes. It had recently reported to the Senate a bill designed "to protect persons on relief in the freedom and sanctity of their voting rights." No allegations connected Van Nuys with any of the violations, and he had explicitly dissociated himself from the activities of the Two Percent Club.

On April 13, 1939, the committee recommended that Willis' petition for an investigation and recount be dismissed. Without debate, the Senate immediately agreed by voice vote, and Frederick Van Nuys retained his seat without further challenge.

Conclusion

Raymond Willis, unsuccessful candidate in 1938, won a seat in the Senate in 1940. He served one term and then returned to the publishing business in Indiana. He died in 1956. Frederick Van Nuys remained in the Senate until his death in 1944.

Sources

U.S. Congress. Senate. *Congressional Record*. 76th Cong., 1st sess. (See pp. 7, 2610, 4183.)

———. Senate Report No. 281. 76th Cong., 1st sess., 1939.

Case 123

William Langer

(1886–1959)

North Dakota

Exclusion/Expulsion Case
January 3, 1941 to March 27, 1942

Issues
Right of Senate to exclude or expel a member-elect for actions before election

Result: Retained seat/Not expelled

Chronology:
Petition received: Jan. 3, 1941
Referred to committee: Jan. 3, 1941
Committee report: Jan. 29, 1942
Senate vote: Mar. 27, 1942

Background

North Dakota Republican William Langer had a colorful political career for decades before he entered the United States Senate. From 1916 to 1920, he served as the state's attorney general, fiercely enforcing Prohibition. During those years, he had led a posse against illegal liquor stores, commandeered telephone lines during a vice raid, censured 275 North Dakota schools for failing to display the American flag, been blamed for the suicide of a former attorney general, and escaped impeachment by one vote. His unorthodox methods, Langer conceded, "tended to make feelings rather bitter." A vigorous champion of the North Dakota farmers, Langer enjoyed immense popularity and in 1932 won the governorship. In 1934, following conviction on charges of political corruption, he was removed from office, but after a reversal on appeal and two new trials, he was exonerated and again elected governor. In 1940 Langer won a seat in the United States Senate.

Statement of the Case

On January 3, 1941, William Langer appeared to take his oath of office. Before he could do so, Senate Majority Leader Alben Barkley (D-KY) informed the Senate that several North Dakota citizens had that day filed a petition of protest against Langer. This complaint accused the senator-elect of bribery in the leasing of government property, receiving kickbacks, collecting fees for fictitious services, and converting proceeds from litigation settlements. Barkley asked that Langer be seated without prejudice and that the matter be referred to the Committee on Privileges and Elections. In the debate that followed, the chair indicated that seating without prejudice meant that the Senate could later rule on Langer's fitness for office by a majority vote, rather than by the two-thirds vote required to expel a senator. Langer took his oath of office, and the protest documents went to the committee. A subcommittee held hearings over the next two weeks, followed by full committee hearings in November 1941.

Response of the Senate

On January 29, 1942, the committee returned a majority report recommending that William Langer was not entitled to his seat. While acknowledging that Langer fulfilled the constitutional requirements of age, citizenship, and residence, and that he had not been charged with any disorderly behavior during his membership in the Senate that would justify expulsion, the report questioned his "moral fitness to be a senator" and recommended that he be excluded by a majority vote.

An extraordinary assortment of testimony, both from witnesses and from Langer himself, led the committee majority to its negative conclusions. The report cited the North Dakota senator for his "moral turpitude" as a public official and charged that he never permitted the law to stand between himself and his personal desires, ambitions, and greed. Allegations detailed a chain of unethical episodes that included jury tampering, attempting to influence the federal judge in his corruption case, accepting $56,000 in return for approving questionable bond transactions, subornation of perjury, inciting a riot, and accepting $25,000 to lower taxes for the Great Northern Railway Company. In one particularly outrageous occurrence, witnesses recounted a 1932 occasion when Langer as a private attorney kidnapped his own client from a local jail, transported the man and his ex-wife across the state line, and convinced the woman to agree to a marriage ceremony. Langer did not deny that he concocted this bizarre scheme to prevent the wife—the only eyewitness to a sordid murder—from testifying against her husband. In exchange for her cooperation, Langer promised to arrange a second divorce without fees right after the trial. The woman subsequently married someone else on Langer's assurance that she was free to do so, only to learn nine years later that he had in fact neglected to arrange her divorce.

Clearly shocked by these outlandish events, the members of the majority concluded that the gross improprieties, "lawlessness, shot-gun law enforcement, jail-breaking," and general obstruction of the administration of justice throughout Langer's career, as well as instances of lying to the committee, demanded his removal from the Senate. In the majority's view, Langer's behavior demonstrated "a continuous, contemptuous, and shameful disregard for the high concepts of public duty." The voters of North Dakota, they contended, were not fully informed about such activities when they voted to send Langer to Washington, and he should therefore be denied his seat.

A vigorous minority report objected to the tone of the majority report and the conduct of the investigation, noting that never in Senate history had such a sweeping review been made of a member's past. This report criticized the process used to gather evidence, the lack of stated rules by which evidence was admitted, and the general suppression of Langer's rights. It called the "evidence" little more than gossip and hearsay and questioned the reliability of witnesses. The lengthy report itemized and refuted in detail each of the charges against Langer and pointed out that, despite his colorful career,

Langer had always been vindicated. In fact, these senators declared, all of the complaints against Langer were well known in North Dakota and had been widely discussed during the campaign, yet the voters had selected him anyway. Matters of the character and behavior of a senator, they believed, "are best determined by the members of the community" in which the challenged individual resides. These committee members therefore expressed reluctance to judge a colleague in the absence of "the most clear and convincing proof that such step is necessary." They were particularly concerned about the danger of establishing the precedent that the Senate could be used by a member's political opponents to overturn the will of a state's citizens as expressed at the polls. Referring to the majority report, the authors of the minority report, Ellison D. Smith (D-SC) and Abe Murdock (D-UT), warned the Senate, "We cannot think of a better illustration of the danger of being swept away by a barrage of slander." Tom Connally (D-TX) concurred in the conclusion that there was insufficient evidence to warrant expelling or excluding Langer.

With the distribution of the reports, the floor debate opened on March 9, 1942, and continued over a period of two weeks. Langer himself was present to hear his detractors hammer away at his "moral turpitude," while his supporters repeatedly stressed that new qualifications for a Senate seat could not be added to those set by the Constitution. In the end the constitutional arguments won out. On March 27, 1942, the Senate rejected the first part of the committee's resolution, which stated that Langer could be denied his seat by a simple majority vote. This meant that the case would be considered an expulsion and would require a two-thirds vote. Ignoring the recommendation of the majority report, the Senate then refused by a vote of 30 yeas to 52 nays to deny Langer his seat.

Conclusion

On September 17, 1942, the Senate voted to pay $16,500 in attorney's fees for Langer's defense of his seat, after defeating an amendment to reduce the amount to $10,000.

William Langer served in the Senate until his death in 1959. Throughout the post-World War II era he clung steadfastly to his isolationist principles, being one of only two senators to vote against the United Nations Charter.

Sources

U.S. Congress. Senate. *Congressional Record.* 77th Cong., 1st sess. (See pp. 3–4, 34, 460.) 2d sess. (See pp. 822, 828, 1253, 2077–2110, 2165–80, 2239–63, 2328–44, 2382–2406, 2412, 2472–94, 2564, 2630–52, 2699–2720, 2759–67, 2791–2806, 2842–55, 2858–63, 2914–23, 2959–70, 2972–78, 2989, 3038–65, 5668, 6684–85, 7170–75.)

———. Senate Report No. 1010. Parts 1 and 2. 77th Cong., 2d sess., 1942.

Garraty, John A., ed. *Dictionary of American Biography.* Supp. 6. New York, 1980. (See pp. 360–62.)

Larsen, Lawrence H. "United States v. Langer, et al.: The U.S. District Attorney's Files." *North Dakota History* 51(Spring 1984): 4–13.

Case 124

Clarence E. Martin v. Joseph Rosier

(1880–date unknown) (1870–1951)

West Virginia

Election Case (appointment)
January 14, 1941 to May 13, 1941

Issues
Challenge to governor's authority to appoint

Result: Rosier seated

Chronology:
Credentials presented: Jan. 14, 1941
Referred to committee: Jan. 14, 1941
Committee report: April 29, 1941
Senate vote: May 13, 1941

Background

Matthew M. Neely (D), patron of West Virginia coal interests, played a dominant role in the state's local and national fortunes for more than thirty-five years. Neely, a strong supporter of President Franklin D. Roosevelt and the New Deal, served in the U.S. Senate for ten years. Then, in November 1940, he ran for governor and was elected for a term beginning January 13, 1941, with two years still left to run in his Senate term. Because Neely and the outgoing governor each sought to appoint Neely's Senate successor, that body was forced to grapple with the exact time the Senate seat became vacant and the time at which Neely became governor.

Statement of the Case

On January 10, 1941, outgoing West Virginia Governor Homer A. Holt, who belonged to a more conservative faction of the Democratic party than Neely, appointed the equally conservative Clarence E. Martin to the vacancy that would be created when Matthew Neely resigned. On the same day, Neely sent Holt a notice, which the governor received at 1:30 p.m. on January 11, stating that he intended to resign from the Senate at midnight on January 12. In an effort to deflect controversy over the question of when the Senate seat and the governorship had become vacant, Holt repeated his appointment of Martin on January 11, to take effect once Neely resigned. Then, in the first moments of January 13, right after Neely's resignation took effect at midnight, creating an actual Senate vacancy, Holt once again appointed Martin to the Senate. The former governor later testified that he had signed that third appointment "just as the second hand of the Naval Observatory time as recorded in the office of the Western Union Telegraph Co. in Charleston passed 12 o'clock, at midnight."

Matthew Neely, equally aware that the issue hung on the timing of his resignation, took great precautions to ensure his authority to appoint his own successor. To this end, Neely took the preliminary qualifying oaths required by West Virginia law at 11:35 p.m. and 11:45 p.m. on January 12. His resignation became effective at the stroke of midnight on January 12, and he took the oath of office as governor of West Virginia one second later on January 13. Then, having ensured that he, not Holt, was governor the very moment the Senate vacancy occurred, Neely later that day appointed Fairmont State College President Joseph Rosier (D) to the Senate vacancy. The certificate of Neely's oath as governor was filed with the West Virginia secretary of state at 12:50 a.m. on the thirteenth. Certificates of the preliminary oaths were filed on January 25.

The U. S. Senate, confronted with credentials for Clarence Martin and Joseph Rosier each validated by a different governor, as well as by the presence of both claimants in the chamber on January 14, 1941, referred the matter to the Committee on Privileges and Elections.

Response of the Senate

On April 29, 1941, a closely divided committee announced that all members agreed the issue centered on which man had been governor of West Virginia at the time the Senate vacancy occurred. Committee members, however, differed regarding whether that individual had been Homer Holt or Matthew Neely. The interpretation of the case came to rest upon West Virginia law and the clock.

The majority report was signed by nine Democratic committee members, including West Virginia's other senator, Harley M. Kilgore (D), a Neely-Rosier supporter. This report argued that Neely signed his West Virginia qualifying oaths on January 12 merely to fulfill a state law but that he did not commence his gubernatorial duties until he took the oath of office at "the first moment of January 13, 1941." Thus, he had not vacated his Senate seat on the twelfth, nor did he hold conflicting offices. The majority maintained that Neely became governor when he took the oath of office, not when the certificate was filed some fifty minutes later. All of Homer Holt's attempts to name Clarence Martin had been illegal, the report continued, because the governor had acted either before a Senate vacancy existed or after his own gubernatorial authority had expired.

An emphatic minority report of May 6, 1941, signed by eight Republican and southern Democratic committee members, asserted that the appointments of Martin made by Homer Holt on January 11 and 13 were both valid. Citing the 1891 case of Horace Chilton (See Case 81) as a Senate precedent, they defended the right of a governor to make an anticipatory appointment before a vacancy occurs. These members further argued that the appointment Holt made on January 13 had occurred prior to the start of Neely's gubernatorial term, which could not commence until Neely had both taken the oath of office and filed his certificate of oath with the secretary of state. In addition, they declared that Neely could not legally take the qualifying oaths on January 12 while he was still a U.S. senator. The report concluded that Clarence Martin had been properly appointed and should be seated.

Despite the minority report's passionate appeal to "rules of fitness and ethics," the senators were swayed by the majority report's argument that, in previous cases of anticipatory appointment like the Chilton case, there had been no element of "midnight certificates," for the governors had not made those appointments just as they were leaving office. In addition, the voters had known when they elected Matthew Neely governor that he intended to name his Senate successor, since he had made his plan clear during the campaign. On May 13, 1941, after several days of debate, the Senate narrowly defeated an amendment to seat Martin, by a vote of 38 to 40, and then accepted the majority report by voice vote. The following day Joseph Rosier took his oath of office.

Conclusion

Joseph Rosier completed the remainder of Matthew Neely's term. Upon his departure from the Senate, he returned to his earlier profession as an educator. A former teacher and superintendent of schools, Rosier resumed the presidency of Fairmont State College, a post he had first accepted in 1915. Rosier died in 1951.

After his term as governor, Matthew Neely sought and won election to the U.S. House of Representatives. In 1949, he returned to the U.S. Senate, where he remained until his death in 1958.

Sources

U.S. Congress. Senate. *Congressional Record.* 77th Cong., 1st sess. (See pp. 140–42, 3378–82, 3605, 3745–55, 3764–66, 3814–16, 3822–40, 3888–3909, 3952–77, 4017.)

———. Senate Report No. 223. Parts 1 and 2. 77th Cong., 1st sess., 1941.

Maddox, Robert Franklin. "The Martin-Rosier Affair." *Capitol Studies* 5 (Spring 1977): 57–69.

Case 125

John R. Neal v. A.T. (Tom) Stewart

(dates unknown) (1892–1972)

Tennessee

Election Case
February 4, 1943 to February 25, 1943

Issues
Campaign financing; campaign irregularities

Result: Stewart retained seat

Chronology:
Petition received: Feb. 4, 1943
Referred to committee: Feb. 4, 1943
Committee report: Feb. 25, 1943
Senate vote: Feb. 25, 1943

Background

Democrat Tom Stewart first came to the United States Senate in 1939 to fill the unexpired term of the recently deceased Tennessee Senator Nathan L. Bachman. Stewart's opponent in that contest, John R. Neal, had filed an unsuccessful petition of contest with the United States Senate (See Case 121). The 1942 Tennessee senatorial election pitted the two against each other for a second time, with Neal opposing Stewart in the Democratic primary and after his defeat running as an Independent in the general election. Once again Tom Stewart claimed the victory and came to Washington to assume his Senate duties.

Statement of the Case

Tom Stewart appeared and was seated on January 6, 1943. On February 4, John Neal filed a petition challenging Stewart's election. While John Neal conceded that Stewart's nomination in the August 6, 1942, Democratic primary had been proper and legal, he based his protest on the charge that his right to run as an independent candidate had been systematically hampered by the planned efforts of Stewart and other Democrats running for state offices. Neal alleged that Stewart and the Democratic candidates for governor and state commissioner for public utilities supported one another's election and that they had illegally spent more than $200,000. Neal also charged that this Democratic team raised money by assessments on federal employees living in the state and obtained votes by threatening relief recipients with the loss of their aid. In some regions of the state, Neal claimed, his own name had been deliberately omitted from the ballot. The challenger therefore asked the Senate to disqualify Stewart and declare that Neal had been elected. The Senate referred the petition to the Committee on Privileges and Elections.

Response of the Senate

On February 25, 1943, after reviewing Neal's allegations, the committee returned a brief report favorable to Tom Stewart. None of the charges had convinced the committee to recommend a formal investigation into the Tennessee election, and the committee unanimously voted to dismiss Neal's petition. The Senate agreed to this action by voice vote the same day.

Conclusion

Tom Stewart served in the Senate until 1949. Not renominated in 1948, he returned to Tennessee and practiced law. He died in 1972.

Sources

U.S. Congress. Senate. *Congressional Record.* 78th Cong., 1st sess. (See pp. 3, 567, 1286.)

———. Senate Report No. 63. 78th Cong., 1st sess., 1943.

Case 126

Theodore G. Bilbo

(1877–1947)

Mississippi

Election Case
September 19, 1946 to January 4, 1947

Issues
Campaign irregularities; voter intimidation; corruption

Result: Bilbo died before Senate could act

Chronology:
Petition received: Sept. 19, 1946
Referred to committee: Sept. 19, 1946
Committee reports:
Jan. 2, 1947 (Defense investigation)
Jan. 3, 1947 (Campaign expenditures)
No Senate action

Background

Theodore G. Bilbo, a vocal presence in Mississippi politics for forty years, served in the state legislature and was twice elected governor before winning a seat in the United States Senate in 1935. In his second term, Bilbo began to escalate his rhetoric of white supremacy in unrestrained speeches that increasingly dismayed many of his Senate colleagues and brought him to the attention of the national press. This behavior reached a climax in his 1946 reelection campaign.

Statement of the Case

On April 1, 1946, the Senate established a special committee to investigate election practices in that year's senatorial contests. Mississippi held its Democratic primary in July 1946, and on September 19 the special committee received a petition filed by a group of black Mississippi residents protesting the tactics employed by Bilbo in the state's primary election. The petitioners charged that Bilbo "conducted an aggressive and ruthless campaign ... with the purpose ... to effectively deprive and deny the duly qualified Negro electors ... of their constitutional rights ... to register and vote." According to the petition, Bilbo's "inflammatory appeals" to the white population exacerbated racial tensions and led to many incidents of violence against black voters, discouraging enough blacks from voting to affect the outcome of the primary. Naming Bilbo as a member of the Ku Klux Klan, which conducted a "reign of terror" using force and violence to win, the petitioners therefore asked the Senate to void Bilbo's election and refuse to seat him in the new Congress. This request did not come as a total surprise to the Senate. Less than three months before, on June 26, 1946, Glen H. Taylor (D-ID), a strong supporter of civil rights, had asked the Committee on Privileges and Elections to investigate Bilbo's campaign speeches.

Response of the Senate

Campaign Expenditures Committee

The Special Committee to Investigate Senatorial Campaign Expenditures sent three investigators to Mississippi, where they conducted a preliminary inquiry. The findings of the initial investigation came before the committee in Washington on November 16, 1946. Chairman Allen Ellender (D-LA), a self-confessed white supremacist, defended the local restrictions against black voters and recommended dismissing the charges against Bilbo. Republican Bourke Hickenlooper (IA), however, dissented and asked that additional hearings be conducted in Mississippi. When no serious objection was voiced to Hickenlooper's proposal, the committee agreed to travel to Jackson, Mississippi.

Early in December 1946, the committee convened for four days of hearings, during which it heard testimony from more than one hundred witnesses—two-thirds of them black—who outlined local election practices that systematically restricted black registration and voting. The committee learned that Mississippi's Democratic primaries had traditionally been viewed as for whites only. A 1944 Supreme Court decision in a Texas case (*Smith* v. *Allwright*, 321 U.S. 649) had invalidated similar restrictions on the primary there, leading a number of civil rights organizations to encourage African American citizens of Mississippi to participate in the July 1946 primary. In addition, the Mississippi legislature that spring had exempted all veterans, black and white, from paying poll taxes for the past two years if they were in the service. These factors, coupled with the recent return to the state of 65,000 to 70,000 black veterans who, after their service in World War II, were anxious to exercise the right to vote, had made the Democratic primary a focus of considerable interest. During the hearings, Bilbo basked in the limelight, smiling broadly for the cameras and winking at committee members. His buoyancy and Ellender's premise that Mississippi tradition rather than Bilbo's virulent rhetoric kept blacks from the polls, were no match, however, for the orderly and chilling recitations by civil rights leaders.

On January 3, 1947, the campaign expenditures committee, specifying that Bilbo's financial conduct was in no way an issue, filed a majority report that found Bilbo guilty of nothing more than crude and tasteless campaign oratory. These senators attributed the intensity of Bilbo's 1946 antiblack campaign to his concern about the "outside agitators," such as the national press and media, he thought were interfering in the internal affairs of Mississippi. They therefore recommended that Bilbo be permitted to take his seat in the Senate when the Eightieth Congress convened.

Republicans Styles Bridges (NH) and Bourke Hickenlooper submitted a minority report charging that Bilbo had violated federal laws against intimidating citizens who were exercising their rights under the Constitution. Particularly damaging were complaints that he had "advocated the use of any means" to prevent blacks from registering and voting. In the campaign, these senators wrote, Bilbo had used "vile, contemptible, inflammatory, and dangerous language" that they called "a corrupt and flagrant abuse of the right of free speech." The minority report thus concluded that, in the primary campaign, Theodore Bilbo had violated the U. S. "Constitution, the Federal Criminal Code, and the Hatch Act" and had vigorously urged the officials of his state to do the same.

National Defense Committee

The review of Bilbo's campaign practices represented only one of his problems. In November 1946, almost at the same time that the campaign expenditures committee agreed to the Mississippi hearings, the Senate Special Committee to Investigate the National Defense Program launched its own probe into Theodore Bilbo's association with war contractors. The inquiry developed out of reports that Bilbo had accepted financial gifts and real estate improvements from certain Mississippi companies.

The tone of these hearings, held in Washington, D.C. from December 12–19, 1946, differed markedly from the circus-like atmosphere of the campaign committee's. The Senate panel made little effort to conceal its personal distaste for Bilbo, who dropped the posturing and grinning he had engaged in at the earlier hearing. The defection of a Bilbo associate aided greatly in substantiating charges that the senator improperly accepted "gifts, services, and political contributions" from construction firms he had helped to gain government contracts. These illegal gifts included: a new Cadillac, a swimming pool, excavation of a lake to create an island for his home, construction of a private roadway, painting of his "Dream House No. 1," and furnishings for his "Dream House No. 2." The estimated value of these benefits, together with contributions made to the senatorial campaign of a Bilbo protégé in 1942, totalled between $57,000 and $88,000. Questionable donations, in response to Bilbo's solicitation, had also been made to build a parsonage for his Juniper Grove Baptist Church. By the time the hearings ended, the committee had gathered sufficient evidence to report to the Senate that Bilbo used his Senate office for his own personal gain. The report, signed by six of the nine members of the national defense program committee, went to the Senate on January 2, 1947.

Full Senate

The Eightieth Congress, in which the Republicans took over control of the Senate for the first time since 1933, opened on January 3, 1947, the day the Senate received the report from the civil rights investigation. Armed with the findings of the two inquiries, Bilbo's opponents, led by Glen Taylor, asked that Bilbo be denied his seat until the Committee on Rules and Administration could review the matter. Taylor emphasized that both the press and the public were seriously concerned about the information gathered by the committees and that many speculated that the Senate would not have the courage to act against Bilbo. The Idaho senator pointed out that precedent existed for asking a senator to stand aside when a Senate committee had already found evidence of corruption (See Cases 109 and 110). The Senate, however, voted 38 to 20 to table Taylor's resolution. Southern senators then began a brief filibuster that blocked efforts to elect Senate leadership and organize the body for the new Congress. The impasse was broken the next day when Minority Leader Alben Barkley (D-KY) announced that Bilbo needed to return to Mississippi for urgent surgery and wished his credentials to remain on the table without action until he could recover and return to Washington. Under the agreement reached, the Mississippi senator would continue to receive his Senate salary in the meantime.

In the next few months, Theodore Bilbo, who was suffering from cancer of the mouth, underwent a series of unsuccessful operations. He died on August 21, 1947, and the Senate took no further action on his case.

Conclusion

Theodore Bilbo's virulent rhetoric during 1946 knew no restraint, as he vilified the North, the press, black citizens, Clare Boothe Luce, and Eleanor Roosevelt. Yet, at the time he passed from the political scene, the conclusion of World War II and the return of black veterans to southern states were encouraging the emergence of an early national concern for civil rights.

Sources

U.S. Congress. Senate. *Congressional Record.* 79th Cong., 2d sess. (See p. 2866.)

———. *Congressional Record.* 80th Cong., 1st sess. (See pp. 3–33, 76, 83–85, 91–94, 108–9, 171–72.)

———. Senate Report No. 110. Part 8. 79th Cong., 2d sess., 1947.

———. Senate Report No. 1. Parts 1 and 2. 80th Cong., 1st sess., 1947.

———. *Riddick's Senate Procedure,* by Floyd M. Riddick and Alan S. Frumin. S. Doc. 101–28. 101st Cong., 2d sess., 1992. (See p. 708.)

Ethridge, Richard C. "The Fall of the Man: The United State Senate's Probe of Theodore G. Bilbo in December 1946." *The Journal of Mississippi History* 38 (August 1976): 241–62.

Peterson, F. Ross. "Glen H. Taylor and the Bilbo Case." *Phylon* 31 (1970) 4: 344–50.

Case 127

D. John Markey v. Herbert R. O'Conor

(dates unknown) (1896–1960)

Maryland

Election Case
December 10, 1946 to May 20, 1948

Issues
Recount of ballots

Result: O'Conor retained seat

Chronology:
Petitions received:
Dec. 10, Dec. 31, 1946
Referred to committee:
Dec. 10, 1946 (Campaign)
Jan. 6, 1947 (Rules)
Committee report:
Jan. 31, 1947 (Campaign)
May 13, 1948 (Rules)
Senate vote: May 20, 1948

Background

Democrat Herbert O'Conor rose through the ranks of Maryland politics from state's attorney to attorney general and governor, before seeking a seat in the United States Senate. On November 5, 1946, O'Conor defeated his Republican opponent, D. John Markey, by a surprisingly narrow margin of only 2,232 votes out of more than 470,000 cast.

Statement of the Case

On December 10, 1946, John Markey turned to the Special Committee to Investigate Senatorial Campaign Expenditures (1946) that had been established in April 1946 and asked for a prompt recount in Baltimore City and Montgomery County. Markey stressed that the matter was urgent because Maryland had no mechanism for an official recount and the two districts he named used voting machines, which officials were permitted to clear within weeks after the election. He also alleged that O'Conor's campaign had committed a number of campaign financing violations. The committee acceded to Markey's request only because the state was not in a position to carry out its own recount. It reviewed the votes in the two jurisdictions mentioned but found just the slightest variance from the official tally, affecting about 400 votes. The committee then indicated to Markey its willingness to survey an additional five counties that he designated as most likely to reveal tally irregularities. Markey selected Anne Arundel, Baltimore, Prince George's, St. Mary's, and Howard Counties.

Before the committee could proceed with this phase of the recount, the Eightieth Congress convened, and Herbert O'Conor presented his credentials. A Senate debate over the seating of Mississippi Senator Theodore G. Bilbo (See Case 126) briefly delayed O'Conor's seating, but on January 4, 1947, he came forward and took his oath of office.

The previous day, January 3, 1947, John Markey filed a new petition requesting a full recount of the November Maryland election. Because the Committee on Privileges and Elections, which had handled previous contested election cases, was terminated at the beginning of the new Congress and its functions transferred to the Committee on Rules and Administration, the Senate on January 6, 1947, referred Markey's new petition, and with it the responsibility for further investigations into the Maryland election, to the Committee on Rules and Administration. The newly formed Subcommittee on Privileges and Elections set to work on a recount of the ballots from the five counties selected by Markey. Meanwhile, the special campaign expenditure committee concluded its portion of the investigation by filing a report on January 31, 1947.

Response of the Senate

Between January and April 1947, Markey continued to press the committee to conduct the recount quickly. His petitions implied that at any moment all the physical evidence of the 1946 election might vanish. By the end of May 1947, the committee had completed the recount in the five designated counties. In the tedious process, the ballot boxes and seals were examined for signs of tampering, the boxes opened, the ballots evaluated, recounted, and the results tabulated—precinct by precinct.

At the conclusion of the recount, O'Conor still held a lead of 1,465 votes. Markey protested, complaining about the Democratic state machine that had been entrenched since 1864, the failure of law enforcement personnel to halt abuses at the polls, and the O'Conor control over all state government. He appealed to the Senate to expand the recount to include the whole state, an approach he believed would be approved by the people of Maryland. The committee began recounting ballots from the remainder of the state in early June and finished its work in January 1948, finding that O'Conor retained a 1,624-vote majority.

On May 13, 1948, the Committee on Rules and Administration submitted a report prepared by its Subcommittee on Privileges and Elections. This report declared that Herbert O'Conor had been properly elected. On May 20, 1948, the Senate unanimously agreed that O'Conor should retain his seat.

Conclusion

Herbert O'Conor, a prominent and popular public figure in Maryland, remained in the Senate until 1953 and then returned to the practice of law. He died in 1960.

Sources

U.S. Congress. Senate. *Congressional Record.* 80th Cong., 1st sess. (See p. 119.) 2d sess. (See pp. 5757, 6160.)

———. Senate Report No. 1. Part 2. 80th Cong., 1st sess., 1947.

———. Senate Report No. 1284. 80th Cong., 2d sess., 1947.

Kirwin, Harry W. *The Inevitable Success: Herbert R. O'Conor*. Westminster, MD, 1962.

Case 128

Tom Sweeney v. Harley M. Kilgore

(dates unknown) (1893–1956)

West Virginia

Election Case
January 4, 1947 to July 28, 1949

Issues
Campaign irregularities;
Senate refused recount

Result: Kilgore retained seat

Chronology:
Petition received: Jan. 3, 1947
Referred to committee: Jan. 6, 1947
Committee report: July 28, 1949
Senate vote: July 28, 1949

Background

A precinct in which intoxicated polling officials menacingly brandished firearms to intimidate voters was but one of the election irregularities charged by unsuccessful Republican candidate Tom Sweeney after his failure to oust incumbent Democrat Harley M. Kilgore in the 1946 West Virginia senatorial contest. Sweeney also asserted that Democrats bought votes at the polls and that Republican ballots had been stolen before they could be tallied. At the conclusion of this hectic election, the disappointed Sweeney fell short of victory by fewer than 4,000 votes.

Statement of the Case

On January 4, 1947, Harley Kilgore presented his credentials and was seated for a second term in the United States Senate. The day before, Tom Sweeney had filed a petition contesting the West Virginia election and itemizing numerous abuses in twelve West Virginia counties. Charging that the "errors, irregularities, illegalities, and fraud" were sufficient to have affected the outcome and that he, not Kilgore, had been legally elected, Sweeney asked the Senate to investigate. The Senate referred his petition to the Committee on Rules and Administration, which forwarded the matter to its Subcommittee on Privileges and Elections.

The subcommittee conducted a preliminary investigation in two counties cited by Sweeney and decided on July 9, 1947, to recommend a full investigation in all twelve counties.

Response of the Senate

On July 15, 1947, Harley Kilgore asked the committee to dismiss the charges against him, insisting that Sweeney had shown only that the opportunity for wrongdoing existed in some counties. The senator called the claim that county commissioners were biased "a reflection by inference and innuendo" upon the honor of West Virginia officials. The Rules Committee, however, on July 16 rejected Kilgore's request and instead agreed to the subcommittee's call for an investigation into the records of the twelve counties in question. If that inquiry showed Sweeney rather than Kilgore in the lead, the committee would then extend the probe to the remaining counties in the state.

Emphasizing that its sole purpose was to check voting irregularities, the committee denied the request to recount all the ballots statewide. A few days earlier, on July 9, the subcommittee had decided not to carry out a recount, consistent with its policy that the Senate should not undertake recounts when they could be conducted under state law. Because Sweeney had originally asked West Virginia for recounts in several counties but had abandoned the effort before any had been completed, thus failing to "pursue this remedy available under state law," the full committee saw no need for the Senate to act.

A year later, on July 28, 1949, the committee reported that a team of twenty-two field investigators had taken eighteen months to compile the needed information about the West Virginia election. In a number of counties, the investigators found poorly kept voting registers in which recorders failed to delete a citizen's name upon a death or family move, but in only two of those precincts did they uncover evidence of fraud, and that affected a total of only 274 votes divided between both candidates. In three counties evidence did show that "a substantial amount of money was paid to individual voters" by representatives of both parties. The committee noted, however, that it was impossible to determine the actual number of votes affected, since it appeared that the Democrats generally paid people who would have voted for the party's candidates anyway while the Republicans gave money to their own supporters. Thus, the payments were "more in the nature of a subsidy for the physical act of voting" than for choosing a particular candidate. A long-standing family feud turned out to be the cause of the single incident of drunken election officials, one of whom had brandished a pistol. No evidence was found of excessive campaign expenditures by either Senate candidate. In one county, 2,300 ballots had been stolen, but since they had already been officially counted, the loss did not affect the final tally. The committee did recommend throwing out all the votes from three precincts where evidence was found of substantial and blatantly fraudulent voting. Eliminating these ballots still left Kilgore the victor by a margin of more than 2,900 votes.

A mountain of evidence had led the committee to conclude that "neither the Democrats nor Republicans appear to have had a monopoly" on the rampant illegalities, to which there was no identifiable general pattern. For this reason, the committee informed the Senate that it saw no point in expanding the investigation to the entire state. The committee therefore recommended that Harley Kilgore be declared duly elected and entitled to retain his seat. That same day, the Senate agreed by voice vote.

Conclusion

Harley Kilgore, the first West Virginia senator elected to three consecutive terms since direct election in 1914, served in the Senate until his death in 1956.

Sources

U.S. Congress. Senate. *Congressional Record.* 80th Cong., 1st sess. (See pp. 109–10, 119, 8870.)

———. *Congressional Record.* 81st Cong., 1st sess. (See pp. 10321–22, 10652.)

———. Senate Report No. 802. 81st Cong., 1st sess., 1949.

Garraty, John A., ed. *Dictionary of American Biography.* Supp. 6. New York, 1980. (See pp. 335–36.)

Maddox, Robert Franklin. *The Senatorial Career of Harley Martin Kilgore.* New York, 1981. (See Chapter IX.)

Frank E. Hook v. Homer Ferguson

(1893–1982) (1889–1982)

Michigan

Election Case
January 5, 1949 to July 28, 1949

Issues
Campaign irregularities;
Senate reread some voting machines

Result: Ferguson retained seat

Chronology:
Petition received: Jan. 5, 1949
Referred to committee: Jan. 5, 1949
Committee report: July 28, 1949
Senate vote: July 28, 1949

Background

In 1948 Democrat Frank E. Hook, former coal miner, woodsman, and lawyer, decided after ten years in the United States House of Representatives to make a bid for the Senate seat of Michigan Republican incumbent Homer Ferguson. General disorder at the polls, coupled with confusion on the part of some Michigan citizens who remained devoted to the Progressive party—which fielded no candidate in the senatorial election—resulted in an election day marred by rancor and charges of fraud. In this climate of dissension, Homer Ferguson won by more than 44,000 votes and returned to Washington for his second term in the United States Senate.

Statement of the Case

On January 3, 1949, Homer Ferguson presented his credentials and was sworn in without objection. Two days later, a petition submitted on behalf of the defeated Democrat, Frank Hook, asked the Senate to investigate charges of fraud in the Michigan election. This petition, referred by the Senate to the Rules Committee's Subcommittee on Privileges and Elections, alleged multiple violations by Michigan Republicans. Among his grievances Hook charged that towns with Republican majorities refused to appoint bipartisan inspection committees, denied the credentials of Democratic poll workers, and returned tally counts that exceeded the total number of registered voters for a community. A separate allegation stated that the collection of hundreds of thousands of dollars in campaign contributions from Michigan Ford, Lincoln, and Mercury automobile dealerships represented a violation of election finance laws.

Response of the Senate

On July 28, 1949, the subcommittee returned a report favorable to Homer Ferguson. Committee investigators had traveled to Michigan in

January and February to read voting machines in the disputed counties but found only minor discrepancies with the earlier official count. These investigators did, however, uncover evidence to support some of the other complaints. For example, they discovered that local election boards were not always bipartisan as required by state law. In a number of areas election inspectors acknowledged that they had failed to count for Hook split ballots in which the Progressive party was checked in general and an "x" placed beside Hook's name as the Democratic Senate candidate, in the absence of any Progressive party candidate for the seat. In several Michigan counties frustrated voters had tried until two in the morning to gain admittance to polling places where disorganization and chaos had especially "militated against the class of people attempting to vote after the completion of their day's work." In several precincts the lack of sufficient checkers added to the confusion and made the final counts highly questionable. Despite the ample evidence of misconduct at many Michigan polling places, the subcommittee failed to find that the unruly state of affairs had been intended to undermine the outcome for either candidate.

The subcommittee noted that the courts had already handled the Michigan Automobile Dealers Association's connection to illegal contributions. Under the Federal Corrupt Practices Act, several corporate figures had been indicted, pleaded nolo contendere, and been sentenced for their action. The Senate committee found nothing to link Ferguson to the fundraising by automobile dealerships throughout the state.

The subcommittee chastised Michigan election officials for permitting the circus atmosphere on election day that had, perhaps unintentionally, deprived citizens of their civil right to vote, deplored the decision to discard those ballots that voted for both the Progressive party and Frank Hook, and decried the methods of raising campaign funds. At the same time, it exonerated Homer Ferguson of knowledge or involvement in any of these matters. The subcommittee therefore recommended that no further investigation be conducted and that Ferguson be declared duly elected.

The Senate on July 28, 1949, accepted the committee's recommendation by voice vote, and Homer Ferguson retained his seat.

Conclusion

The unsuccessful contestant, Frank Hook, abandoned political life and practiced law in Michigan and Wisconsin until his death in 1982.

Defeated for reelection in 1954, Homer Ferguson served as ambassador to the Philippines from 1955 to 1956 before becoming a judge on the United States Court of Military Appeals. He died in 1982.

Sources

U.S. Congress. Senate. *Congressional Record.* 81st Cong., 1st sess. (See pp. 3, 34, 10321.)

———. Senate Report No. 801. 81st Cong., 1st sess., 1949.

IX. McCarthy Era: 1950–1954

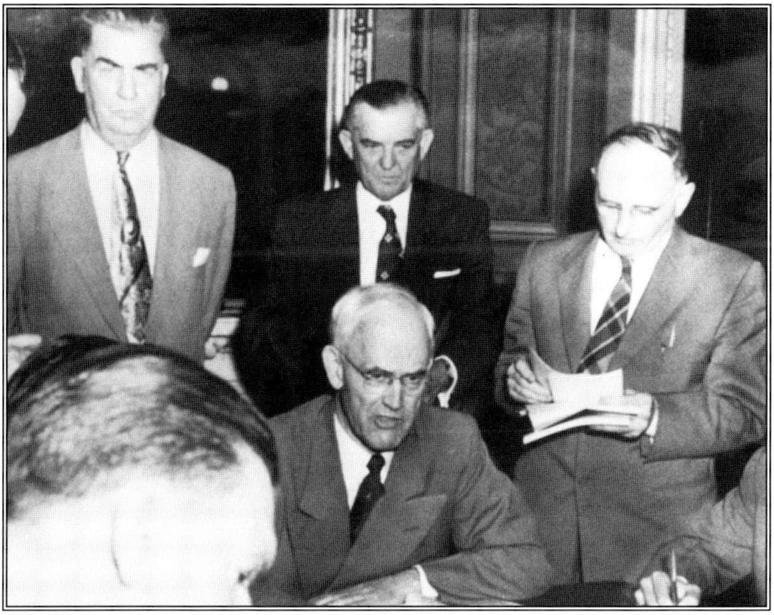

Members of the Select Committee to Study Censure Charges Against Senator McCarthy
(Left to right, rear, Edwin Johnson, John Stennis, Francis Case; front, Arthur Watkins, chairman.)
U.S. Senate Historical Office

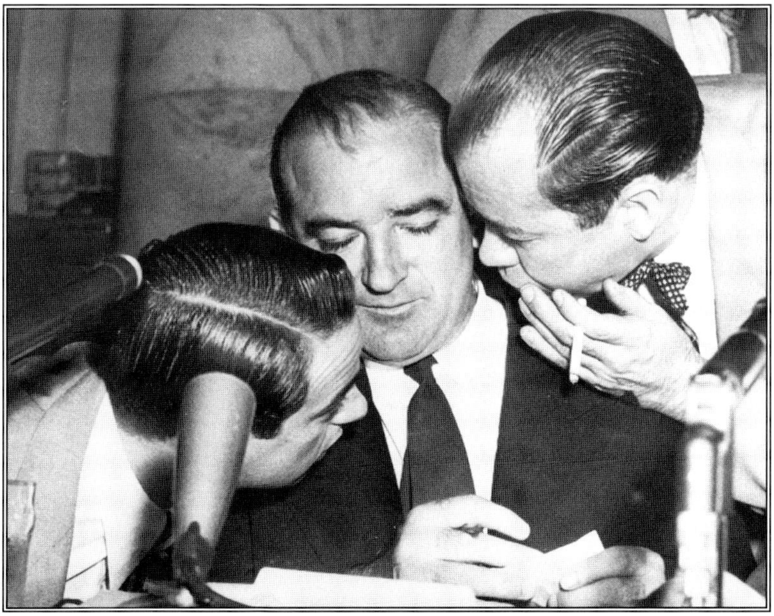

Joseph R. McCarthy and staff of Permanent Investigations Subcommittee, Government Operations Committee
Martin Luther King Library

Case 130

Millard Tydings v. John Marshall Butler

(1890–1961) (1897–1978)

Maryland

Election Case
November 7, 1950 to August 20, 1951

Issues
Campaign irregularities

Chronology:
Complaint received by committee: Dec. 1950
Committee report: Aug. 20, 1951
No Senate action

Result: Butler retained seat

Background

In November 1950 incumbent Senator Millard Tydings (D-MD), a veteran of twenty-four years in the Senate, had every expectation of chalking up yet another Maryland political victory. The conservative Democratic senator, however, had underestimated the bitter grudge held against him by his Senate colleague Joseph R. McCarthy (R-WI). Earlier that year, when Tydings had chaired a subcommittee investigating the Wisconsin senator's charges that Communists had infiltrated the State Department, his report described the allegations as "a fraud and a hoax." In retaliation, McCarthy entered the Maryland campaign on behalf of the Republican challenger, John Marshall Butler, and, after a vicious contest, Butler upset Tydings on November 7 by more than 43,000 votes.

Statement of the Case

In mid-December Millard Tydings complained to the Rules Committee's Subcommittee on Privileges and Elections that he believed unfair campaign practices, as well as violations of federal and state election laws, had affected the outcome of the November vote. On January 3, 1951, the Senate permitted John M. Butler to be seated "without prejudice," while authorizing the subcommittee to continue its inquiry into the Maryland campaign.

After a preliminary investigation, the subcommittee on February 3, 1951, agreed to hold public hearings on the Butler campaign. Although Tydings was not officially contesting the election, the subcommittee recognized that results of the investigation might lead to efforts to unseat John Butler. The complaints centered on reports of excessive campaign expenditures, massive out-of-state contributions unlisted in the required financial reports, and attempts to eradicate records of questionable expenses. A highly visible campaign activity involved the distribution of cheap tabloids, published under false statements of sponsorship and filled with half-truths and doctored photographs, that smeared the patriotism and loyalty of Millard Tydings.

Response of the Senate

From February 20 to April 11, 1951, a special bipartisan group of four senators conducted public hearings on behalf of the subcommittee. They accorded Butler every courtesy, allowing him to appear and make his own observations about the campaign.

Among the questionable aspects of the senator's campaign had been the role played by Jon M. Jonkel, a Chicago public relations director, whose reckless management of the financial records had resulted in his indictment and conviction in the Maryland courts. Testimony conclusively revealed that the strategy for the Butler campaign had been mapped out not only by Jonkel, but also with aggressive assistance from Joseph McCarthy and his staff. They organized a massive publicity crusade designed to convince the public that Tydings bore the responsibility for the Korean War and had generally undermined American defenses against foreign enemies. In one particularly egregious example, they created a composite photograph to make it appear that Tydings hobnobbed with former Communist party head Earl Browder and then circulated 300,000 copies of the tabloid containing the manufactured photo.

After the hearings ended, the subcommittee delayed for four months before issuing its report in August 1951. When the report finally appeared, it criticized McCarthy for his role in the Maryland election. Decrying the dual nature of the political race—Butler's "dignified 'front street'" speeches contrasted with the "despicable 'back street' campaign" conducted by outsiders—the report faulted Butler for failing adequately to oversee his campaign. Yet, despite the subcommittee's clear recognition that John Butler had willingly permitted McCarthy to infiltrate the Maryland election with illegal financial transactions and the use of falsehoods and smear tactics, the report found there was insufficient basis to urge that Butler be unseated. The subcommittee members believed that it would be unfair to take action against him in the absence of an existing specific standard of campaign conduct. Instead, they urged the Rules Committee to establish guidelines for the future that would make "acts of defamation, slander, and libel sufficient grounds" for "declaring a Senate seat vacant." The report also encouraged the national political parties to adopt a set of fair campaign standards.

Although the subcommittee had invited McCarthy to testify, he declined to appear. He did, however, ask for and receive permission to include as part of the committee's report a lengthy statement of his individual views about the Maryland election. His rhetoric attacking Tydings and the subcommittee's inquiry proved too much for William Benton (D-CT) who, after reading the report, bravely introduced a resolution calling for McCarthy's expulsion from the Senate and in the meantime demanded that he should resign. (For the Senate's action on this resolution, see Case 131.)

The full Rules and Administration Committee accepted the subcommittee's report. Since it did not call for measures against Butler, no Senate action was required.

Conclusion

That John Marshall Butler retained his Senate seat was in part a reflection of Joseph McCarthy's power at that stage in his career. Although the Butler and Tydings case came to an end, Senate concerns about McCarthy's conduct would continue for more than three years longer.

Millard Tydings retained a keen desire to recapture the Senate seat he felt had been unjustly wrested from him. He came close in 1956, until illness forced him to relinquish the party's nomination. He died in 1961. John Marshall Butler served in the Senate until 1963. He died in 1978.

Sources

U.S. Congress. Senate. *Congressional Record.* 82d Cong., 1st sess. (See pp. 3, 1655–64, 1670–73, 10304–8, 10319–37.)

———. Senate Report No. 647. 82d Cong., 1st sess., 1951.

Keith, Caroline H. *"For Hell and a Brown Mule": The Biography of Senator Millard Tydings.* Lanham, MD, 1991. (See pp. 417–26.)

Oshinsky, David M. *A Conspiracy So Immense: The World of Joe McCarthy.* New York, 1983. (See pp. 214–16.)

Case 131

Joseph R. McCarthy and William Benton

(1908–1957) (1900–1973)

(Wisconsin) (Connecticut)

Expulsion Case
August 6, 1951 to January 2, 1953

Issues
Allegations of corruption

Result: McCarthy not expelled

Chronology:
Resolution introduced: Aug. 6, 1951
Referred to committee: Aug. 6, 1951
Committee report: Jan. 2, 1953
No Senate action

Background

When Joseph R. McCarthy (R-WI) launched his famous 1950s crusade against communism in the United States government, he found supporters among both Democrats and Republicans. As his methods took on characteristics of libel and sensationalism, however, other senators increasingly became uneasy about his free-wheeling allegations and lack of regard for congressional decorum. McCarthy's undeniable influence in the election defeat of Maryland Senator Millard E. Tydings in 1950 deeply disturbed other members uncertain as to how to control their unorthodox colleague.

Statement of the Case

On August 6, 1951, at the close of the investigation into McCarthy's association with the campaign of Maryland's John Marshall Butler (R) (See Case 130), Connecticut Democrat William Benton introduced a resolution calling for an inquiry and the possible expulsion of the vitriolic Wisconsin senator. Benton, a former advertising executive and State Department official, deplored McCarthy's involvement in the smear tactics used in the Maryland election but also charged the senator with fraud, deceit, perjury, and lack of fitness to hold the office of senator. Benton, who had entered the Senate in 1949 to fill a vacancy, had been particularly outraged by McCarthy's recent attack on General George C. Marshall as a traitor "steeped in falsehood."

Benton's strongly worded resolution caught more experienced senators by surprise, and none rose to offer supporting speeches. The Senate referred the resolution to the Committee on Rules and Administration, which passed it on to the Subcommittee on Privileges and Elections. Many senators believed that calling for censure, which only required a simple majority vote, would have been a more sensible approach; the Senate had rarely mustered the two-thirds vote needed for expulsion and then only in cases of actual disloyalty to the nation.

Response of the Senate

On September 17, 1951, before the subcommittee had formally decided whether to hold hearings, Joseph McCarthy assumed the offensive by sending a letter to subcommittee chairman Guy Gillette (D-IA), declaring that the hearings planned in response to the Benton resolution were intended to punish him for exposing Communists in the American government. McCarthy demanded the right to cross-examine witnesses, a request the committee denied on September 24 when it voted to hold hearings. Anxious to placate McCarthy and to grant appropriate courtesies to a fellow senator, the committee invited him to appear and testify on September 28 and October 1, 1951. McCarthy refused, calling Benton's charges against him the type routinely found in the *Daily Worker,* the newspaper of the American Communist party.

In addition to Chairman Gillette, the subcommittee consisted of Mike Monroney (D-OK), Thomas C. Hennings (D-MO), Margaret Chase Smith (R-ME), who had already spoken out against McCarthy in her June 1950 "Declaration of Conscience" speech; and Robert C. Hendrickson (R-NJ), who had also signed the Declaration of Conscience.

Benton testified on September 28, charging McCarthy with perjury for denying under oath that in his February 1950 speech in Wheeling, West Virginia, he had claimed there were 205 Communists in the State Department. Benton also asserted that the Wisconsin senator had accepted an illegal $10,000 contribution from the Lustron Corp. and had made false and deceitful statements about fellow senators. Not eager to take on McCarthy, the subcommittee delayed opening an investigation into Benton's charges. Then, in November and December 1951, McCarthy unleashed an all-out attack against the subcommittee. He questioned the jurisdiction of the panel and obtained personnel files of committee staffers which, he said, confirmed their Communist connections. The ferocity of his barrage forced the committee to postpone conclusive action. McCarthy's supporters pressured Margaret Chase Smith to leave the subcommittee and replaced her with his staunch ally, Herman Welker (R-ID).

Finally, when nothing seemed to abate the Wisconsin senator's overwhelming verbal assault, the panel turned to the full Senate for support and on March 6, 1952, asked for a vote of confidence in its investigation. With the agreement of the full Rules and Administration Committee, Chairman Carl Hayden (D-AZ) on April 8, asked the Senate to discharge the subcommittee from further consideration of the question of Joseph McCarthy's conduct. Senators responded in anger when they realized that the ability of a Senate committee to act had been thoroughly impeded by a single senator's intimidating tactics. On April 10, after a torrent of heated debate, the Senate voted unanimously against discharging the subcommittee from the investigation. The 60 to 0 vote upheld the jurisdiction of the committee, affirmed the honesty and integrity of its membership, and approved the continued investigation of Joseph McCarthy. The decision was not as clearcut as it seemed, however, for once again McCarthy had succeeded in muddying the issue, this time by announcing that, in spite of his lack of confidence in the subcommittee, he would vote against ending its investigation. Still, the vote of confidence enabled the subcommittee to move ahead and hold hearings in May 1952 on McCarthy's acceptance of the $10,000 from Lustron Corporation, a manufacturer of prefabricated houses, which depended on money from the government's Reconstruction Finance Corporation (RFC). McCarthy had served on a subcommittee overseeing the RFC at the time he had accepted the money from Lustron.

Always ready to take the offensive, McCarthy struck back on April 10, 1952, the day of the Senate's vote of confidence in the subcommittee, by introducing a resolution that charged William Benton with failing to report certain campaign expenditures. This request for an investigation of Benton was also referred to the Subcommittee on Privileges and Elections. On July 3, 1952, McCarthy testified at a public hearing that, during Benton's tenure at the State Department, he had been a Communist in disguise. He waved Benton's tax records, which he had secured through questionable means. Benton, the object of McCarthy's attacks for almost a year, began to buckle, and the subcommittee itself fell into disarray. Not only had Margaret Chase Smith been replaced in late 1951, but both Chairman Gillett and the chief counsel, overwhelmed by the constant barrage of verbal assaults, left the subcommittee in September 1952 after McCarthy won renomination in the Wisconsin primary. Also in September 1952, McCarthy supporter Herman Welker, who had taken Smith's place, resigned after publicly attacking the subcommittee's approach.

Under the chairmanship of Thomas Hennings, the remaining three members sought to complete the investigation. Both McCarthy and Benton were invited to testify during late November 1952, but only Benton appeared. The subcommittee chose not to subpoena McCarthy because it considered the inquiry to be an internal Senate matter and believed that it had given the Wisconsin senator ample opportunity to appear and refute the charges if he had wished to do so. Instead, he had "deliberately set out to thwart any investigation of him" by making repeated attacks upon the subcommittee and its members. The inquiry trickled to an unsatisfactory end as the senators prepared the long-awaited report covering both McCarthy and Benton. If the document was not to appear partisan, it needed the approval of the lone Republican remaining on the subcommittee, Robert Hendrickson, who was also feeling pressure from McCarthy. Thus, while the report finally filed on January 2, 1953, dealt principally with the Wisconsin senator, it also mildly criticized Benton for an unreported campaign contribution.

By describing at length the process of the investigation, the report made clear the extreme difficulties under which the subcommittee had operated, as McCarthy blocked its efforts at every turn. His actions, the report declared, reflected "a disdain and contempt for the rules and wishes of the entire Senate body, as well as the membership of the Subcommittee on Privileges and Elections." The report discussed at length the evidence supporting six questions it had asked McCarthy in a November 1952 letter, to which he had responded tersely, "The answer to the six insulting questions... is 'No.'" The questions concerned whether it was proper for McCarthy to have accepted the $10,000 fee from Lustron, the possible personal use of funds donated to fight communism, the propriety of other financial transactions, his activities on behalf of special interest groups, possible violations of the tax and banking laws, and possible campaign financing violations. The report called McCarthy's acceptance of the Lustron fee "highly improper" but otherwise concluded simply that "the record should speak for itself." The subcommittee urged action by the entire Senate, although it made no specific recommendations.

But the Senate did not act. The report had been filed the day before the new Republican Congress convened on January 3, 1953. In the November 1952 Republican landslide, McCarthy had won election to a new six-year term, although he collected significantly fewer votes in his state than President Dwight D. Eisenhower and other Wisconsin Republicans. Still, he appeared untouchable, while William Benton, the sole senator to challenge his conduct openly, had been soundly defeated in the election.

Conclusion

When the Senate failed to act, the subcommittee sent its report and files to the Justice Department, asking it to conduct an inquiry into McCarthy's financial dealings. This approach proved no more effective, however, for in October 1953, the attorney general of the United States announced that the department's investigation had failed to discover any evidence of fraud and corruption. The subcommittee's report did become something of a bestseller, as a magazine sold 150,000 copies of a condensed version and more than 7,000 privately reprinted copies were distributed.

At the height of the Benton-McCarthy clash, Benton had offered to waive his senatorial immunity if McCarthy chose to take the matter to the civil courts. In March 1952 McCarthy brought a $2 million libel suit against Benton but withdrew it two years later.

Joseph McCarthy's intense political career soon moved on to another phase, in which his intransigent behavior to the subcommittee played a role (See Case 133). William Benton, a courtly, genial liberal, served as the United Nations UNESCO ambassador in Paris from 1963 to 1968. He died in 1973.

Sources

U.S. Congress. Senate. *Congressional Record.* 82d Cong., 1st sess. (See pp. 1221, 9498–9501, 9871–72, 11855–58.) 2d sess. (See pp. 2441–42, 2444–45, 3701, 3833–3934, 3935–54, 8910–11, 9544.)

———. *Congressional Record.* 83d Cong., 1st sess. (See pp. 8619, 9185, 9346–47, 9352–54.)

———. Report of the Subcommittee on Privileges and Elections to the Committee on Rules and Administration, "Investigation of Senators Joseph R. McCarthy and William Benton." 82d Cong., 2d sess., 1953.

Griffith, Robert. *The Politics of Fear.* Lexington, KY, 1970. (See pp. 152–84.)

Keith, Caroline H. *"For Hell and a Brown Mule": The Biography of Senator Millard E. Tydings.* Lanham, MD, 1991. (See pp. 430–38.)

Oshinsky, David M. A *Conspiracy So Immense: The World of Joe McCarthy.* New York, 1983. (See pp. 217–25, 247–50.)

Case 132

Patrick J. Hurley v. Dennis Chavez

(1883–1963) (1888–1962)

New Mexico

Election Case
December 30, 1952 to March 23, 1954

Issues
Campaign irregularities;
recount of ballots

Result: Chavez retained seat

Chronology:
Petition filed: Dec. 30, 1952
Referred to committee: Jan. 7, 1953
Committee report: Mar. 16, 1954
Senate vote: Mar. 23, 1954

Background

Thanks to his outstanding strategic abilities, Senator Dennis Chavez (D-NM) had won three senatorial elections in New Mexico's tumultuous political climate by 1952. After a narrow defeat by Bronson Cutting in his first senatorial race in 1934, Chavez contested the election results (See Case 118). When Cutting died in a 1935 plane crash, the New Mexico governor appointed Dennis Chavez to fill the unexpired term. Chavez won a special election in 1936 and was reelected in 1940 and 1946. In 1952, his Republican opponent for a third complete term was retired Major General Patrick J. Hurley, whom he had defeated in the 1946 election and who had run again unsuccessfully for the Senate in 1948.

Having served as secretary of war in Herbert Hoover's administration and ambassador to China under Franklin D. Roosevelt, Patrick Hurley persistently sought a Senate seat as a forum for his anticommunist views. In the 1952 election, Chavez, who was viewed as a New Deal liberal, faced the problems of increasing public disillusionment with liberalism and a Republican ticket headed by two popular figures, presidential candidate Dwight D. Eisenhower and incumbent Governor Edwin L. Mechem. When the votes in the close Senate race were were finally tallied, Chavez, the Democrat, had narrowly won reelection by 5,071 votes, in spite of easy victories in the state by Eisenhower and Mechem.

The day after the election, November 5, 1952, Hurley challenged the results, but on November 29, the New Mexico state canvassing board certified that Chavez had been elected. Hurley then demanded a recount which, when completed in December, resulted in increasing the incumbent's majority by 304 votes. Having exhausted his remedies in the state, Hurley filed a petition of contest with the United States Senate on December 30, 1952.

Statement of the Case

When the Eighty-third Congress convened on January 3, 1953, the Senate permitted Dennis Chavez to take the oath of office subject to a request by Robert A. Taft (R-OH) that he be seated "without prejudice to the right of anyone contesting the seat to proceed with the contest." On January 7, the Senate referred Patrick Hurley's petition to the Subcommittee on Privileges and Elections of the Committee on Rules and Administration. The complaint alleged numerous irregularities in the conduct of the 1952 New Mexico election, particularly violations of ballot secrecy.

After a preliminary staff investigation, the Committee on Rules and Administration decided on April 17, 1953, to conduct a full inquiry, including a recount of all ballots, examination of voter registration records, a field investigation, and hearings. The committee submitted two separate resolutions to the Senate seeking funds for the investigation and eventually spent almost $229,000. The subcommittee, consisting of Chairman Frank A. Barrett (R-WY), Charles E. Potter (R-MI), and Thomas C. Hennings, Jr. (D-MO) devoted considerable effort to developing a set of written procedures prior to the field investigation. Still, the committee's work soon assumed a highly partisan tone, to the degree that Hennings, the minority member of the subcommittee, found himself virtually excluded from the investigation, as it continued throughout 1953 and into early 1954.

The partisanship was understandable. More than the single Senate seat was at stake, since transfer of that seat from a Democrat to a Republican could affect party control of the Senate. When the Eighty-third Congress was organized, the Republicans had a clear majority of 49 seats to the Democrats' 47. In July 1953, however, Robert Taft had died and a Democrat was appointed to replace him. Also during 1953, Wayne Morse of Oregon, originally elected as a Republican, declared himself an Independent. As a result of these changes, the Democrats could claim a bare majority of 48 to 47, although the Republicans retained the leadership positions within the Senate. If Hurley were seated instead of Chavez, the Republicans would again have a clear majority. Because of the pivotal nature of the case, it often received front-page coverage in major national newspapers.

Response of the Senate

When the subcommittee had still not released its report by March 1954, Democratic senators became increasingly concerned that the Republican-dominated committee would defer action until after the fall elections, when their party might hold the majority with sufficient votes to unseat Chavez easily. Senate Democrats therefore pressed the issue on March 9 by challenging the committee to issue a report within one week or face a Democratic effort to remove the issue from the committee. Two days later, the Privileges and Elections Subcommittee filed its report with the full Rules

Committee, which quickly adopted it on March 16 by a party-line vote of 5 to 4. A resolution accompanying the report stated that no one had been elected to the Senate from New Mexico and that a vacancy existed. If the resolution were adopted, Governor Mechem, a Republican, could appoint a temporary replacement for Chavez.

The report contended that the New Mexico election "revealed the deplorable spectacle of exploitation and breakdown of an electoral system through irresponsible and ineffective administration." Specifically, the investigation discovered that at least 55,000 citizens were deprived of a secret ballot; assistance to 4,000 disabled voters was improperly provided; and ballots were fraudulently altered in 33 precincts, making all 17,000 votes cast in those precincts suspect. After an intense investigation, the subcommittee found that in 21 counties no voting booths were provided, so that voters had to "mark their ballots in an open room" in full view of election officials. In a number of other counties, booths were provided but violations of secrecy still occurred. Other problems uncovered included difficulties with the registration system, permitting aliens to vote, and illegal, premature destruction of ballots in three counties. The majority therefore concluded that all votes tainted by such irregularities should be eliminated and that the Senate should declare that no one had been elected to the Senate from New Mexico in 1952.

Thomas Hennings, the lone Democratic member of the subcommittee, filed a minority report, deploring the subcommittee's failure to conduct an objective and nonpartisan inquiry. He complained that he had not been consulted by the other members regarding either their deliberations or the final report. Stating that the majority report contained no evidence either of corruption or fraud by Dennis Chavez or that the vote for Chavez was increased as a result of the irregularities, Hennings charged that the Senate would set an unfortunate precedent if it disfranchised New Mexico's voters and unseated Chavez simply because the state's election officials failed to comply with the election code. He then refuted the majority's findings point by point and concluded that the Senate should find Dennis Chavez to be the legally elected senator.

As the Senate began to debate the committee's resolution on March 22, newspapers both in New Mexico and across the country expressed opposition to voiding the results of an election that had chosen a decidedly bipartisan ticket. Many pointed out the irony that such a decision would place the power to appoint a temporary successor in the hands of a Republican governor chosen in the same supposedly flawed election.

Soon after the debate began, Guy Cordon (R-OR) introduced an amendment significantly altering the resolution. It stated, "And that it is the sense of the Senate that said vacancy should be filled only by election held pursuant to the laws of the State of New Mexico." The amendment was intended to deflect Democratic arguments and relieve concerns about having a Republican chosen in the same flawed election appoint a replacement to fill the vacated Senate seat. During the debate, Republican speakers, such as Subcommittee Chairman Frank Barrett, focused on the irregularities in the 1952 election, primarily the failure of election officials to provide voting booths. The Democrats argued that Cordon's amendment violated the Seventeenth Amendment to the Constitution, which delegates the power to fill a vacancy to the governor until an election can be held. Hennings led the opposition, joined by such powerful fellow Democrats as Walter George (GA), Carl Hayden (AZ), and Allen J. Ellender (LA). George reiterated Hennings' view that there was no historical precedent for the Senate to deprive citizens of their votes based on the misconduct of election officials. In general, the Democratic senators stressed that, because the lengthy and expensive investigation had failed to find fraud or wrongdoing by Dennis Chavez, he was entitled to retain his seat.

On March 23, Minority Leader Lyndon B. Johnson (D-TX) submitted a unanimous consent agreement, which the Senate agreed to, limiting the debate and setting a time for the final vote later that afternoon. When the roll-call votes on the amendment and the resolution took place, with Major General Hurley and his family observing from the gallery, Vice President Richard Nixon presided over the Senate. After voting down the Cordon amendment, 36 to 53, the Senate defeated the committee's resolution declaring a vacancy, again by a 36 to 53 vote. On each vote, 5 Republicans joined 47 Democrats in supporting Chavez, although not exactly the same 5 crossed party lines in each case. Although Chavez was present for the debate, he refrained from voting. The *New York Times* observed that the Democrats stood "in a solidarity they had not exhibited on a major issue in many years" and further noted that Lyndon Johnson had worked for weeks to make certain that none of his party colleagues would be absent on this critical day.

Conclusion

Of his vindication, Dennis Chavez commented that "truth and decency were on trial and as always in the end, they too prevailed." He was reelected to a fifth complete term in 1958 but died after a long illness on November 18, 1962.

Patrick Hurley had also filed complaints with the U.S. attorney of New Mexico and the Federal Bureau of Investigation (FBI). After listening to the FBI's report on September 24, 1954, a grand jury in Albuquerque found that Chavez had won an honest victory. It concluded that most of the allegations made by Hurley and others were politically motivated. Hurley returned to New Mexico, where he died in 1963.

The Chavez case exemplifies one of the dilemmas associated with Senate election cases. Most of the Senate agreed that reforms were needed in New Mexico's election procedures, but many senators clearly felt uncomfortable about directing the way a state should conduct its elections. While the New Mexico press defended the practice of voting at open tables if there were long lines at voting booths, newspapers in other parts of the country condemned this approach, though they agreed that Chavez had not been responsible for these conditions and should retain his seat.

Sources

U.S. Congress. Senate. *Congressional Record.* 83d Cong., 1st sess. (See pp. 7, 147.) 2d sess. (See pp. 3610–11, 3613–29, 3630–43, 3696–3733.)

———. Senate Report No. 1081. Parts 1 and 2. 83d Cong., 2d sess., 1954.

Garraty, John A., ed. *Dictionary of American Biography.* Supp. 7. New York, 1981. (See pp. 121–22, 376–77.)

Lowitt, Richard. "Two-Star General, Three-Time Loser: Patrick Hurley Seeks a Senate Seat in New Mexico." *In Politics in the Postwar American West,* ed. Richard Lowitt. Norman, OK, 1995. (See pp. 162–73.)

Case 133

Joseph R. McCarthy

(1908–1957)

Wisconsin

Censure Case
July 30, 1954 to December 2, 1954

Issues
Abuse of a Senate committee

Result: Censured

Chronology:
Resolution introduced: July 30, 1954
Referred to committee: Aug. 2, 1954
Committee report: Nov. 8, 1954
Senate vote: Dec. 2, 1954

Background

On April 22, 1954, the Permanent Subcommittee on Investigations of the Senate Government Operations Committee chaired by Joseph R. McCarthy (R-WI) opened hearings into aspects of security in the United States Army. McCarthy temporarily stepped aside as committee chairman after the army charged him with seeking special treatment for a former staff member, and the committee decided to look into that complaint as well. Still, the Wisconsin senator continued to play an active role in the hearings, with power to cross-examine witnesses. The Army-McCarthy hearings, fully covered on national television, showed McCarthy in an increasingly unattractive light, as he badgered witnesses while ignoring parliamentary procedures and the rules of common courtesy. By the time the hearings ended in June, he had greatly damaged his image with the American people.

Joseph McCarthy, who had appeared invincible when investigated by a Senate subcommittee in 1952 (See Case 131), had finally gone too far, convincing his Senate colleagues that his power must be curtailed.

Statement of the Case

On July 30, 1954, Ralph Flanders (R-VT) introduced a resolution calling for the censure of the colleague who had dominated the American press and the United States Senate for the past four years. Flanders declared that Joseph McCarthy's conduct as chairman of the Senate's Permanent Subcommittee on Investigations ran "contrary to senatorial traditions" and brought the whole body into disrepute. He therefore called on his colleagues to condemn McCarthy's behavior. Earlier, on June 11, Flanders had offered a resolution to strip McCarthy of his chairmanships, but consultation with other senators had indicated that censure would be easier to achieve, since many members objected to undercutting the seniority system of choosing committee chairmen.

In discussing the Flanders resolution the Senate demonstrated that, although weary of McCarthy's embarrassing antics, it wished to conduct the inquiry in an orderly fashion. In general, McCarthy's party colleagues did not attempt to defend his actions but focused instead on procedural concerns, as senators added forty-six specific charges of misconduct to the original censure resolution. On August 2, the Senate decided to refer the matter to a bipartisan select committee, whose members were notable for their impeccable reputations and legal expertise, and asked for a report before the end of the Eighty-third Congress in late 1954. The group of three Republicans and three Democrats, led by Chairman Arthur V. Watkins (R-UT), included three former judges and two former governors. Only Joseph McCarthy complained about the composition of the panel.

Response of the Senate

The select committee recognized that the few previous censure cases had dealt with specific incidents of unacceptable action, rather than a whole pattern of behavior over a period of years as in the McCarthy case. Therefore, the committee, anxious to restore the sense of dignity so sorely absent in the recent army hearings, plotted each move with care. It agreed to exclude television cameras from the hearings, in order to foster a judicial atmosphere and avoid a repetition of the unseemly show presented to the public by the recent debacle with McCarthy and the military. Because the hearings would be judicial in form rather than adversarial, the committee would not call Flanders and other supporters of censure as witnesses, thus offering McCarthy no targets for personal attacks. He would, however, have the right to be present and be represented by counsel, although only one individual—either McCarthy or his attorney—would be permitted to conduct questioning or cross-examination on a given subject. McCarthy was also allowed to make an opening statement.

After reviewing the forty-six counts of misconduct, the committee reduced the charges to five categories: "contempt of the Senate or a senatorial committee"; encouraging federal government employees to violate the law by providing him with classified materials; "receipt or use of confidential or classified document"; abuse of Senate colleagues; and abuse of Brigadier General Ralph W. Zwicker during the army hearings. Because each of these charges was based on the massive collection of documents already at the committee's disposal, including the material from the 1952 investigation by the Subcommittee on Privileges and Elections, very few witnesses needed to be called.

The hearings were held after the Senate recessed to allow members to campaign for the November election, opening on August 31, 1954, and continuing through September 13. The committee soon felt the full thrust of McCarthy's oratorical attack, but Chairman Watkins exercised strict control and ruled many of McCarthy's interruptions and diversions out of order. Unmoved by the Wisconsin senator's objections, the committee completed the hearings and set about drafting its report, which it released to the press on September 27 (although it was not officially printed until the Senate reconvened on November 8).

The select committee unanimously recommended that Joseph McCarthy be censured for his actions in two of the five categories: (1) his refusal to appear before the Subcommittee on Privileges and Elections to answer questions about his personal character, and his general obstruction to the work of the panel during its investigation of him in 1951 and 1952 (See Case 131); and (2) his conduct on February 18, 1954, when he publicly abused and defamed General Zwicker during his appearance before the army hearings. The committee also strongly deplored McCarthy's actions in the other three categories as "improper" and irresponsible but determined that they did not "constitute a basis for censure."

On November 8, 1954, as the Senate convened in a rare post-election session to deal with the McCarthy case, a lengthy and tangled debate developed. McCarthy attacked the individual members of the committee and its work so fiercely that each senator found it necessary to counter his assault with legal arguments. To keep the discussion as nonpartisan as possible, Minority Leader Lyndon B. Johnson (D-TX) urged Democratic liberals to remain quiet and allow moderate and conservative Republicans to carry the fight against McCarthy.

Those who defended Joseph McCarthy and sought to defeat the recommendation argued that censure would impose an unwise code of conduct for the future—that McCarthy should not be censured for his behavior in a previous Congress, and that a censure vote would interfere with the guarantees of free speech. As he warmed to the fight, McCarthy labeled the select committee the "unwitting handmaiden of the Communist Party," attacked Arthur Watkins as "cowardly," and referred to the entire proceeding as a "lynch party." Chairman Watkins responded with an emotional speech about the dignity of the Senate that brought cheers from the galleries.

When McCarthy entered the hospital with an elbow injury, the Senate recessed for ten days until he could again be present. Finally, on December 2, 1954, after three more days of debate, the Senate concluded the case and adjourned for the year. Exchanging the count relating to General Zwicker for one regarding his behavior to the Watkins committee, the Senate, on a vote of 67 to 22, censured Joseph McCarthy "for his non-cooperation with and abuse of the Subcommittee on Privileges and Elections . . . in 1952" and "for abuse of the Select Committee to Study Censure" of 1954.

After four years of nearly unchallengeable political power, Joseph McCarthy fell before the demand of the Senate that its members conform to the body's rules of comity and civility.

Conclusion

Many observers believed that the Watkins committee really wanted to avoid the unpleasantness of censure and had taken every measure possible to accommodate McCarthy, but his raucous demeanor and attacks on the committee members finally pressed them too far. Even so, the committee based its recommendations on McCarthy's violation of Senate behavioral norms and took no position on his anticommunist crusade.

McCarthy tried to appear unaffected by the censure, but it became apparent that the Senate vote had robbed him of his power and status. As his political fortunes waned, so did his health. He died in 1957.

Sources

U.S. Congress. Senate. *Congressional Record.* 83d Cong., 2d sess. (See pp. 5298–5301, 8032–33, 8116, 8240, 8444, 8519, 8521, 12729, 12893, 12902, 12919, 12938–13001, 13394, 15716, 15851, 15911, 15921–32, 15935, 15940, 15954, 15959, 15966, 15986, 15990, 16006, 16011, 16018, 16030, 16038, 16052, 16056, 16076, 16083, 16090, 16112, 16149, 16156, 16169, 16186, 16195, 16268, 16279, 16344, 16353.)

———. Senate Report No. 2508. 83d Congress, 2d sess., 1954.

Griffith, Robert. *The Politics of Fear.* Lexington, KY, 1970. (See pp. 280–317.)

Oshinsky, David M. *A Conspiracy So Immense: The World of Joe McCarthy.* New York, 1983. (See pp. 472–94.)

X. Modern Era: 1964–1990

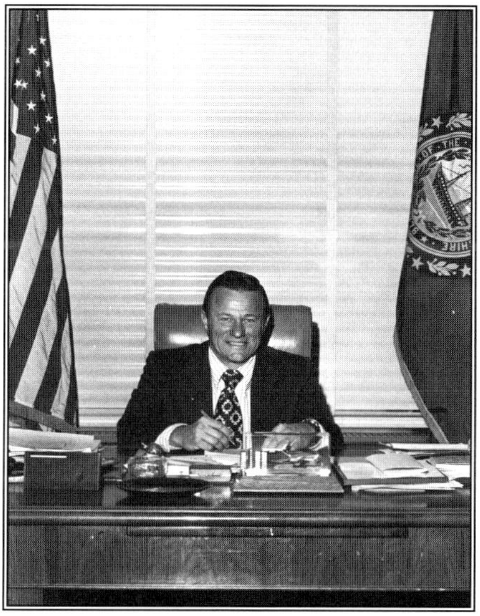

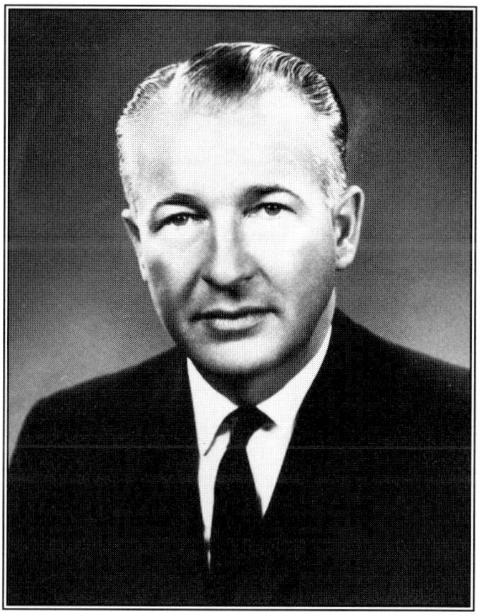

John Durkin, Louis C. Wyman *(Case 137)*

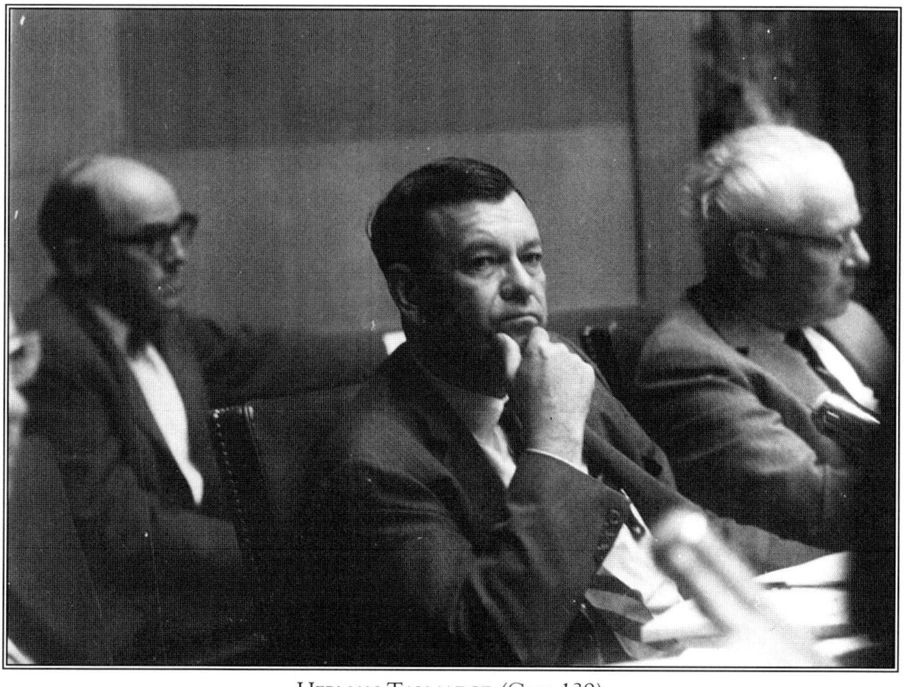

Herman Talmadge *(Case 139)*
U.S. Senate Historical Office

Case 134

Pierre E.G. Salinger

(1925–)

California

Election Case (appointment)
August 5, 1964 to August 13, 1964

Issues
Qualifications: residency

Result: Retained seat

Chronology:
Credentials presented: Aug. 5, 1964
Referred to committee: Aug. 5, 1964
Committee report: Aug. 12, 1964
Senate vote: Aug. 13, 1964

Background

On August 5, 1964, Senate Majority Leader Mike Mansfield (D-MT) presented the credentials of Pierre E.G. Salinger, appointed by California Governor Edmund G. Brown to fill a vacancy caused by the death of Senator Clair Engle. Salinger's credentials clearly indicated his appointment was temporary—to continue only until the California voters, by special election, chose Engle's permanent replacement. Salinger, who had served as press secretary to President John F. Kennedy and his successor Lyndon B. Johnson, had resigned from that position in March 1964 to run for the U.S. Senate.

Statement of the Case

Before Salinger could be sworn in, Republican Leader Everett Dirksen (IL) announced that many California citizens protested the legality of the appointment. One of those objecting was George Murphy, the Republican candidate in the race to fill Engle's seat. Dirksen hastened to add that the challenge, "in no way involves the acceptability or character of the appointee. this . . . goes clearly to the . . . appointment by the governor of California." California Republicans based their charges upon a state constitutional requirement that the governor could only appoint a "state elector" to a Senate vacancy. A state elector was defined as a person resident in California for at least one year. Salinger, formerly of Virginia, had lived in California less than the mandatory twelve months.

Mike Mansfield responded immediately to the protest, with the traditional argument that the only valid qualifications for a United States senator are those listed in the U.S. Constitution. Mansfield informed his Republican colleagues that the challenge was meaningless because "the Constitution of the United States sets forth in crystal clear language . . . that states cannot impose additional qualifications."

As the discussion unfolded, members turned more and more to constitutional wizard Sam Ervin (D-NC) for an analysis of the fine points involved.

In his homey way Ervin advised the Senate that the distinction between an elected and an appointed senator was not "as wide as the distinction between tweedle-dum and tweedle-dee . . . those . . . are the qualifications . . . which must be possessed by any Senator . . . whether he comes to the Senate by election or by appointment."

At the conclusion of these exchanges, the Senate voted 59 to 29 to seat Salinger, without prejudice, and referred his credentials for investigation to the Committee on Rules and Administration's Subcommittee on Privileges and Elections.

Response of the Senate

On August 12, 1964, the committee returned a report favorable to Pierre Salinger. The committee agreed with those who, in the earlier debate, had insisted that the laws of an individual state had no bearing on the Senate's right to judge the qualifications of its members. In essence, the committee found that a state constitution transgressed the law by adding qualifications for a United States senator and that a state executive was within his rights to ignore such restrictions.

Although the debate assumed a highly partisan tone, members could not ignore the declaration by Republican Milton Young (ND) that he intended to support Salinger because his own 1945 Senate appointment had been in direct violation of the North Dakota constitution. Young observed that no one in North Dakota had questioned the governor's action, because it was widely recognized that the United States Senate would be the sole judge of his qualifications. A minority group led by Carl Curtis (R-NE) insisted that Salinger did not meet California requirements, but the Senate upheld its traditional view and resisted any encroachment by a state into the area of Senate qualifications. On August 13, 1964, the Senate voted that Pierre Salinger was entitled to retain his seat.

Conclusion

In November 1964, Pierre Salinger failed to be elected to fill the remainder of Engle's term. He served in the Senate only until the end of that year. He subsequently pursued a varied career in private ventures and became widely known for his journalism and television reporting.

Sources

U.S. Congress. Senate. *Congressional Record.* 88th Cong., 2d sess. (See pp. 18107–20, 19396–413, 19416, 19421–22, 21411.)

———. Senate Report No. 1381. 88th Cong., 2d sess., 1964.

Case 135

Thomas J. Dodd

(1907–1971)

Connecticut

Censure Case
February 23, 1966 to June 23, 1967

Issues
Personal use of campaign funds; standards of conduct for senators

Result: Censured

Chronology:
Request for committee investigation: Feb. 23, 1966
Committee report: Apr. 27, 1967
Senate vote: June 23, 1967

Background

The Thomas J. Dodd (D-CT) censure case represents the first modern-era Senate ethics case. Its conduct reflected a growing impetus for reform in the wake of the Bobby Baker and Representative Adam Clayton Powell (D-NY) scandals.

Bobby Baker was a senior Senate aide accused of personally profiting from his public position. The Senate Rules and Administration Committee's investigation of his case produced an extraordinary level of partisan rancor. In response to the Baker investigation, the Senate in 1964 established the bipartisan Select Committee on Standards and Conduct but rejected a proposal providing for routine disclosure of members' income. The committee was charged with developing a Senate code of ethics but set this work aside to pursue its investigation of Dodd.

Statement of the Case

Journalists Drew Pearson and Jack Anderson published a series of syndicated newspaper columns in January 1966, describing Thomas Dodd's association with Julius Klein, a public relations consultant for several West German clients. Additional articles appeared detailing alleged fundraising improprieties and other financial wrongdoing by the senator.

In the authorizing resolution creating the select committee, the Senate outlined only a set of mandated tasks, allowing the new committee to design its specific procedures. Well aware of the precedent-setting nature of its work, the committee carefully reviewed its authority to conduct investigations of misconduct and in April 1966 retained former Supreme Court Justice Charles E. Whittaker as consulting counsel. Because there were no procedures for misconduct proceedings, the committee began by adopting rules prior to its first hearings.

The committee divided its work into two parts. Part 1 addressed Dodd's relationship with Julius Klein, and Part 2 investigated such allegations of financial misconduct as the conversion of campaign funds to personal use. The second part of the investigation, which the committee considered more serious, ultimately resulted in the recommendation for censure. Separate hearings were held for each part, although the committee issued only one report.

Part 1

On February 2, 1966, the committee's staff began looking into the revelations about the senator's relationship with publicist Julius Klein that were made in the first Pearson and Anderson articles. On February 23, 1966, after the staff prepared a preliminary report, Thomas Dodd requested a full inquiry by the committee. In late June 1966 the committee held both public and closed hearings.

Rather than reporting at the time, the committee discussed its findings on Part 1 in the final report filed on April 27, 1967. There, the committee noted that, after Senate Foreign Relations Committee hearings in 1963 had criticized Julius Klein's activities, he had lost some of his West German clients. Klein then pressed Dodd, a member of the Foreign Relations Committee, to travel to West Germany and meet with officials there on his behalf. Dodd did indeed go to West Germany in April 1964, ostensibly on Senate Judiciary Committee business, but it appeared that his purpose was influenced by Klein's requests. The committee did not pursue its concern that the senator had directly intervened with West German officials because it had difficulty in obtaining evidence from a sovereign foreign government. Although the committee failed to find enough evidence of wrongdoing to warrant further Senate action, it noted that Dodd's behavior towards Klein was "indiscreet" and "beyond the responsibilities of a Senator to any citizen." Although the committee heard allegations that Dodd had received a number of favors from Klein, the only firm evidence indicated that Dodd had repeatedly used the lobbyist's suite in the Essex House hotel in Manhattan.

Part 2

While the committee was investigating the senator's relationship with publicist Klein, additional newspaper coverage raised questions about his political and official financial ties to contributors and businessmen. In response to these articles, the committee formally began an investigation in April 1966, which uncovered additional evidence. The committee then requested a complete financial report from Thomas Dodd and when he refused advised him on June 15, 1966, that it would hold public hearings. Because of several legal challenges brought by the senator's attorney, as well as the need to reassemble complex, detailed financial data, the hearings were not held until mid-March 1967.

Thomas Dodd's legal challenges to the committee's Part 2 inquiry began almost immediately. His attorneys argued that the committee had no jurisdiction over the senator's finances and that these financial matters were essentially tax related. The committee responded that it had a responsibility to examine the ethical implications of his conduct. Later challenges claimed that the hearings would prejudice future determinations by the Internal Revenue Service (IRS), which was conducting an investigation of income Dodd had derived from political events. The senator's attorneys formally raised these arguments several times, and eventually the committee granted a special hearing for Dodd's lawyers. When hearings on the full case were completed, the committee met a final time on the issue of jurisdiction and determined that the evidence "related directly to Senator Dodd's conduct as a sitting Senator and was within the jurisdiction of the Committee." On three separate occasions, the committee formally ruled that it had jurisdiction.

A major problem arose concerning the nature of the committee's initial evidence. The revelations that appeared in the Pearson and Anderson articles were based on approximately four thousand documents that staff members had stolen from Dodd's office. To maintain the integrity of the case, the committee decided to use none of these documents but instead painstakingly reassembled back records and other materials.

The committee's final report, issued on April 27, 1967, concluded that Dodd and his staff had organized seven fundraising events between 1961 and 1965. These events were represented to the public as testimonials or campaign fundraisers, but Dodd had used a significant portion of the monies raised for his own benefit. Dodd contended that the contributors knew the purpose of these occasions was to raise money for his personal expenses, and he obtained four hundred affidavits stating that the donations were gifts rather than political contributions. The select committee considered the affidavits but did not accept them as testimony, because the events' invitations and press coverage demonstrated that they had been represented to the public as political fundraisers or testimonials. The committee members believed that, since the senator and his staff were directly involved in planning these events, he must have been aware that they were essentially political. Contributions received totalled at least $203,983. In addition, Dodd received at least $246,290 in support of his 1964 campaign, for a combined total of $450,273. Of this amount, according to the committee report, Dodd had used $116,083 for personal purposes, such as income taxes, home improvements, and payments to family members. He also received $8,000 in cash from the International Latex Corporation, allegedly in exchange for an ambassadorship.

The funds raised from one of the events had been placed in Thomas Dodd's personal bank account and used to pay his personal expenses. The proceeds of the other gatherings were deposited in a "testimonial for Senator Dodd" account and comingled with campaign contributions. Nearly $95,000 was later transferred from this account to Dodd's personal bank account and used for personal purposes. The remaining money in the testimonial account was used by Dodd for both personal and political expenses, according to the committee's findings.

The committee also determined that on seven occasions Dodd had accepted reimbursement for the same travel from both the Senate and private groups. In addition, he had accepted gifts of automobiles that he used for both political and personal travel between 1964 and 1965.

In conclusion, the committee declared that the senator had used the power of his office to raise campaign funds and that he spent a portion of these funds, as well as money from the 1964 campaign, for personal purposes. Also, he had accepted double reimbursement. It was on these grounds that the select committee recommended censuring Dodd. The committee also referred its findings on some of the improprieties to the U.S. attorney general as possible violations of law.

Response of the Senate

The full Senate began discussing the Dodd censure resolution on June 13, 1967, and the issue dominated Senate business until the final vote on June 23. The committee had proved that a bipartisan group could conduct a dignified investigation, but the floor debate at times degenerated into a turbulent display of anger and frustration. Senators discussed in great detail the fundamental concepts of the emerging reforms in governmental ethics, such as the need for written standards of behavior and standards for evaluating evidence, as well as the nature of the process used to investigate and discipline members. Since Thomas Dodd's lawyers were not permitted to speak on the Senate floor, Russell B. Long (D-LA) assumed the role of Dodd's chief advocate. He and Dodd presented evidence in the form of charts, documents, and briefs. Select Committee Chairman John C. Stennis (D-MS) struggled valiantly to restrict the debate to the committee's work and the draft resolution. He cogently identified the real issue, "If we pass up this matter, then sometime, somewhere, in some way, something big will slip out of this Chamber, and a lesser standard or lesser role or lesser conduct will have to be accepted."

The lack of formal standards for senatorial behavior caused difficulty in the Dodd case. At that time, there was not yet a federal ethics law, and campaign financing was still regulated by the 1925 Corrupt Practices Act. The committee was therefore in the awkward position of first articulating a set of standards and then evaluating Dodd's past actions against them. Dodd argued that this approach subjected him to ex post facto justice and that the committee's procedures had denied him due process. Nevertheless, a consensus emerged that, while Thomas Dodd's conversion of campaign funds to personal use did not break any laws, the Senate had to decide whether this activity should be condoned. Stephen M. Young (D-OH) transcended these arguments over standards with a simple clarity: "In my considered judgment, honesty is easy to define. Surely, it is not difficult to define. Neither is dishonesty difficult to define."

The debate reflected a lack of agreement about the nature of the censure process. In defending Dodd, Russell Long argued that the senators were being asked to function as prosecutors. Others, like committee member Eugene J. McCarthy (D-MN), stated that the Senate was simply applying certain broad standards of conduct. Others raised the question that, if the Senate was conducting a judicial trial proceeding, then what type of standard should be applied to the evidence, criminal or civil?

By the second week of the debate, tempers grew short, Thomas Dodd was shaken and exhausted, and the press coverage became increasingly negative. The Senate was aware that the nation was watching and, in Norris H. Cotton's (R-NH) words, "entitled to some affirmative action." As the debate inched towards closure, senators began raising concerns about the use of the word "censure" in the resolution. Eugene McCarthy said that the dictionary contained seven or eight definitions among which members should choose. Long offered an alternative resolution that essentially eviscerated the censure motion, which the Senate rejected by a vote of 92 to 2. John Tower (R-TX) proposed the term "reprimand." But John Stennis stood firm, pointing out that the word "censure" had been used in all previous Senate cases. "The facts are all in," he declared. "The case is known. And anything short of the word 'censure' will not meet the situation."

Stating that he did not wish to embarrass his colleagues, Dodd requested and obtained permission to be absent during the vote. Allen J. Ellender (D) of Louisiana, unconvinced that an adequate case had been made against Dodd on the charge of double-billing for travel expenses, moved to delete that point from the resolution. The Ellender amendment passed by a roll-call vote of 51 to 45. Immediately afterward, the Senate voted 92 to 5 to adopt the revised resolution censuring Thomas Dodd for converting campaign funds to personal use. The resolution stated that Dodd had used his office as a United States senator "to obtain and use for his personal benefit, funds from the public through political testimonials and a political campaign." It further stated that this conduct was "contrary to accepted morals, derogates from the public trust expected of a Senator, and tends to bring the Senate into dishonor and disrepute." In the final minutes of the session, Thomas Dodd rose and stated, "I believe now, I shall continue to believe, that history will justify my conduct and my character."

Conclusion

In handling its first censure case, the newly created Select Committee on Standards and Conduct demonstrated an awareness of the precedent-setting nature of its work and sought to operate in a nonpartisan manner in order to ensure a fair hearing based on federal judicial procedure. In a substantial change from the previous practice in which the full Senate had referred allegations of corruption to a committee, the Standards and Conduct Committee had the power to initiate its own inquiries without referral by the Senate.

When the Democratic party denied Thomas Dodd the nomination for a third term in 1970, he left the party and ran as an Independent, seeking vindication from the voters of Connecticut. The voters did not comply, and Dodd finished third in the race that elected Republican Lowell P. Weicker to the Senate. Less than a year later, Dodd died suddenly from a heart attack. Newspaper obituaries mentioned the impact of the Senate censure vote on his career while noting that both throughout the proceedings and until his death the senator had steadfastly claimed that he was innocent.

The Senate's censure of Thomas Dodd was only the seventh time in almost two hundred years that the body had censured one of its members. It was the first such case that focused solely on a senator's finances, reflecting changing mores within both society and the Senate. Media attention devoted to the Bobby Baker, Adam Clayton Powell, and Thomas Dodd cases led the public to demand more accountability from its elected officials. For the Senate, the case demonstrated the need to adopt formal rules of conduct and to enforce its standards of behavior. In 1968, prompted by concerns over ethical problems, the Senate adopted four new rules of ethical conduct, including a form of financial disclosure. The 1970s would bring additional significant reforms.

Sources

U.S. Congress. Senate. *Congressional Record.* 90th Cong., 1st sess. (See pp. 15421–22, 15663–706, 15735–50, 15773, 15998–16030, 16104–135, 16348–75, 16561–87, 16976–17000, 17005–73.)

———. Senate Report No. 193. 90th Cong., 1st sess., 1967.

Amer, Mildred. "History of Congressional Ethics Enforcement." *CRS Report for Congress.* 93–239 Gov., February 18, 1993.

Baker, Richard Allan. "The History of Congressional Ethics." In *Representation and Responsibility: Exploring Legislative Ethics,* ed. Bruce Jennings and Daniel Callahan. New York, 1985. (See Chapter 1.)

Jennings, Bruce. "The Institutionalization of Ethics in the U.S. Senate." The Hastings Center Report, 1981.

Case 136

Richard L. Roudebush v. R. Vance Hartke

(1918–1995) (1919–)

Indiana

Election Case
November 17, 1970 to July 24, 1972

Issues
Contested election:
Indiana recount of ballots

Result: Hartke retained seat

Chronology:
Request for recount: Nov. 17, 1970
Hartke seated: Jan. 21, 1971
Supreme Court decision: Feb. 23, 1972
Recount completed: July 24, 1972

Background

In 1970 Democrat R. Vance Hartke of Indiana received his party's nomination for a third term in the United States Senate. His Republican opponent was five-term Representative Richard Roudebush. Roudebush had agreed to President Richard M. Nixon's request that he give up a safe House seat to challenge Hartke, a persistent critic of the administration's Vietnam War policies. The ensuing race was described as "one of the most acrimonious and bitterly fought Senate campaigns in recent American history." Roudebush attempted to portray his opponent as sympathetic to Communist countries in general and North Vietnam in particular. He condemned Hartke's acceptance of a $30,000 campaign contribution from a Chicago mail order firm shortly before his appointment to the Senate Post Office and Civil Service Committee. Hartke, for his part, attacked the administration's military and economic policies, and his supporters suggested that Roudebush had not fully recovered from a head injury suffered in a plane crash two years earlier. On election day, Hartke received a slim plurality of 4,500 votes out of 1.7 million votes cast.

Statement of the Case

Richard Roudebush exercised his right under Indiana law to demand a recount, claiming irregularities in eleven counties. Vance Hartke successfully blocked his opponent's petition before a United States District Court, based on the argument that a recount would interfere with the Senate's constitutional right to judge the elections and qualifications of its members. Roudebush appealed this decision to the United States Supreme Court. Pending this appeal, the Senate seated Hartke on January 21, 1971, "without prejudice to the outcome" of the court case. Hartke then moved to dismiss Roudebush's appeal as moot, a claim that the Supreme Court rejected.

Conclusion

A year passed before the Supreme Court ruled on February 24, 1972. In the case of Roudebush v. Hartke (495 U.S. 15), the Court decided that Indiana officials were within their rights to conduct a recount, but that the Senate was not bound by the results and could arrive at an independent determination. The subsequent recount reduced Hartke's plurality by only 48 votes; and on June 12, 1972, Roudebush acted to terminate the recount. On July 24, Howard W. Cannon (D-NV), chairman of the Senate Subcommittee on Privileges and Elections, announced that "Vance Hartke is the duly elected Senator from the State of Indiana and is entitled without reservation or qualification to his seat in the Senate."

In 1971 President Nixon had appointed Roudebush to a high-ranking post in the Veterans' Administration. In 1974, President Gerald R. Ford nominated him as that agency's administrator. The Senate Committee on Veterans' Affairs, chaired by Vance Hartke, recommended confirmation, which occurred on October 1, 1974. Roudebush served in that position until the start of the Carter administration in 1977. He died in 1995.

Hartke lost his 1976 reelection bid to Republican Richard Lugar.

Sources

U.S. Congress. Senate. *Congressional Record.* 92d Cong., 1st sess. (See pp. 7–9.) 2d sess. (See pp. 25022–23.)

Roudebush v. Hartke. 405 U.S. 15 (1972).

American Bar Association *Journal* (58) May 1972, 514.

Current Biography. "Richard Lowell Roudebush" (1976). (See pp. 352–55.)

Case 137

John A. Durkin v. Louis C. Wyman

(1936–) (1917–)

New Hampshire

Election Case
December 27, 1974 to July 30, 1975

Issues
Contested election:
recount of disputed ballots

Result: Seat declared vacant; new election held

Chronology:
Petition of contest filed: Dec. 27, 1974
Referred to committee: Dec. 30, 1974
Committee report: Jan. 13, 1974
Referred back to committee: Jan. 28, 1975
Committee report: May 22, 1975
Senate vote: July 30, 1975

Background

In 1973 Norris H. Cotton's (R-NH) announcement of his plans to retire from the Senate the next year thrust New Hampshire politicians into a vigorous contest for the seat. The fall campaign of 1974 pitted the youthful Democrat John A. Durkin, who had served as the state's insurance commissioner, against the conservative, widely known Republican representative, Louis C. Wyman. With a solid record of public service and good political connections, Wyman anticipated an easy victory in his traditionally Republican state. Surprisingly, on November 5, the expected Republican landslide failed to materialize as Wyman's lead dwindled to a mere 355 votes out of more than 200,000 cast. Durkin charged voting irregularities, demanded a recount, and declared, "it's still a horse race."

On November 27, after completing the recount, the secretary of state named John Durkin the winner by ten votes, and the governor issued him a conditional certificate of election. Louis Wyman promptly appealed to the New Hampshire State Ballot Law Commission, a move Durkin tried to check by legal maneuvers that eventually involved all levels of the New Hampshire courts. Durkin's attorney also sought an injunction in federal court to send the matter directly to the U.S. Senate, but on December 18 a federal district court denied the request. The ballot commission therefore conducted its own partial recount and announced on December 24 that Wyman was the victor by two votes. Republican Governor Meldrim Thomson, Jr., therefore issued a certificate of election to Louis Wyman on December 27 and rescinded Durkin's credentials, explaining that he had issued them prematurely. Wyman himself, however, still urged a new election as the best solution. With Durkin stripped of his credentials and a distressed public calling for a new election, it became increasingly clear that the stalemate would be taken to the United States Senate for resolution.

Statement of the Case

Based on the constitutional provision that each house of Congress is the final arbiter of its elections, John Durkin on December 27, 1974, filed a petition of contest with the U. S. Senate, which referred the matter to the Rules and Administration Committee's Subcommittee on Privileges and Elections. Durkin challenged Wyman's right to the seat and defended the validity of the first recount. On January 5, 1975, Wyman filed a response requesting that the Durkin challenge be dismissed and that he be seated. Meanwhile, because Norris Cotton had resigned, effective December 31, Governor Thomson appointed Wyman to fill the vacancy for the last few days of Cotton's term. Wyman thus became a senator for that brief period, although Congress was not in session at the time.

The subcommittee began by holding a hearing but, after a day of acrimonious testimony, passed the matter to the full Committee on Rules and Administration. When the full committee, made up of 5 Democrats and 3 Republicans, considered the matter on January 13, it deadlocked 4 to 4, first on a motion to seat Wyman without prejudice and then on one to ask both Durkin and Wyman to stand aside pending a review of the case. Democrat James Allen of Alabama, who believed strongly that Wyman should be seated provisionally because he presented valid credentials, voted with the Republicans both times to create the deadlock. The committee then unanimously decided that the contest should be brought before the full Senate.

Response of the Senate

When the Senate of the Ninety-fourth Congress convened on January 14, 1975, with Democrats holding an overwhelming majority, John Durkin and Louis Wyman sat at separate tables at the back of the chamber as they listened to a floor debate rooted in party divisions. Pointing out that the New Hampshire courts had sustained the recall of Durkin's credentials, Republicans insisted that, since only Wyman possessed legitimate credentials issued by the governor, he should be seated without prejudice while the Rules Committee considered the matter. In the other contested election case facing the Senate at the time, they observed, the body did in fact seat Henry Bellmon (R-OK) while referring the issue to the Rules Committee (See Case 138). Democrats retorted that, although there were no allegations of fraud against Wyman, there were charges of error in the recount, and there was ample precedent for asking both claimants to step aside. Under existing New Hampshire law, a new election could only be held in the case of a tie, and on January 6, 1975, the supreme court of New Hampshire had ruled that the state courts were not empowered to review a contested federal election. Since Durkin had exhausted the New Hampshire state procedures, it was now up to the U. S. Senate to resolve the conflict.

Action was postponed for two weeks, after both sides agreed to delay a vote on the issue until January 28. In the meantime, the New Hampshire legislature on January 22 adopted a measure providing for a new election if the Senate declared that a vacancy existed, and Governor Thomson himself carried the new state law to Washington. Wyman then asked the Senate to rule the New Hampshire seat vacant so that state officials would be free to order the new election. When January 28 arrived, however, the Senate, with Democrats voting in the majority, first refused either to seat Wyman provisionally or to declare the seat vacant and then voted 58 to 34 to send the disputed New Hampshire election back to the Rules Committee. As James Allen complained on the Senate floor, refusing to seat a duly certified senator-elect was contrary to Senate precedent in cases where there were no allegations of fraud. "This is a matter that should not be decided on the basis of party lines," he declared.

After an additional three weeks of discussion, the Rules Committee on February 19 agreed to a procedure for recounting 3,500 disputed ballots. In attempting to weed out those that were not clearly controversial, the eight senators depended on a complicated system of, wherever possible, "masking" candidates' names and party affiliations on the ballots as they sought to interpret the confusing marks made by some voters. A special three-member auditing panel, consisting of the Democratic and Republican subcommittee counsels and Senate Parliamentarian Emeritus Dr. Floyd M. Riddick, was to review any remaining disputed ballots. The committee adopted rules requiring this panel to reach unanimous agreement on any questioned ballot or return it to the Rules Committee for another evaluation. The ballots were brought from New Hampshire to Washington, where they were kept under guard, and the review continued from February through April. The carefully devised process turned out to contain so many opportunities for irreconcilable partisan conflicts, however, that the committee experienced a succession of tie votes on enough contested ballots to affect the outcome of the election. When the frustrated committee members realized in mid-May that they would be unable to agree upon which person to seat, they decided simply to go ahead and file a report. An accompanying resolution placed before the full Senate the questions the committee was unable to resolve, as well as the disputed ballots on which the committee held tie votes.

Having spent "over 200 hours" on the case, the Rules and Administration Committee had already established a new record for the time devoted to deliberating on a single subject. Then, beginning on June 11, the full Senate proceeded to discuss the case for more than six weeks, with Wyman and Durkin and their attorneys again observing in the back of the chamber. As a few southern Democrats joined with the minority Republicans to ensure that the Democrats would not achieve the 60 votes needed to end debate, the Senate over a period of several weeks in June and early July took an unprecedented six cloture votes on the subject, none of which succeeded. Durkin continued to hold out for a Senate solution, even amid Republican taunts that he dared not face a second election, and his party colleagues supported him. With each passing day, however, senators devoted less and less time to the New Hampshire dispute, turning their attention to other topics, as members of both parties recognized they were incapable of reaching a solution. By July 28, the Senate had actually resolved only one of the thirty-five disputed points referred to it by the Rules Committee, yet neither faction appeared willing to compromise.

As the August recess approached, the Senate remained hopelessly deadlocked. On July 28, the *Washington Post* ran an editorial charging that it would be "incredible" if the Senate were to "go on vacation for a month without settling the New Hampshire Senate election case." The newspaper suggested that Wyman and Durkin should try to reach some agreement to settle the matter. Following up on the suggestion, Louis Wyman wrote to Durkin that day, urging him to support a new election. Durkin initially refused but then, on July 29, reversed his earlier position and announced to a New Hampshire television audience his intention to agree to a new election. The next morning, July 30, he reported this change to the Democratic leadership, thus relieving the Senate from further deliberations on the topic. Later that same day, the Senate voted 71 to 21 to declare the seat vacant as of August 8. New Hampshire then arranged to hold a special election on September 16, 1975.

Conclusion

In a record-breaking turnout for a special election, New Hampshire voters gave Democrat John Durkin a convincing victory by a margin of more than 27,000 votes. As it happened, Norris Cotton, the innocent initiator of the events, administered the oath of office to Durkin. Once the Senate had declared the seat vacant, the New Hampshire governor had appointed Cotton to fill the vacancy, and he served from August 8 to September 18, 1975. In December 1975 the Senate agreed to reimburse Durkin and Wyman for a combined total of $227,000 in legal fees and to pay each of them $150 a day for the period from January to August 1975.

The New Hampshire contest, the closest election in Senate history, had captured the attention of the national press. Citizens of New Hampshire were embarrassed by the flood of publicity, some of it very unfavorable. Weary of a dispute marred by vicious personal slurs and disturbed that the state had been left with only one senator for more than seven months, they wanted an end to the controversy. In fact, on July 30 the governor and council of New Hampshire adopted a resolution that was immediately transmitted to Washington, threatening that, if the Senate went on vacation without resolving the matter, the state attorney general should go to court to have senators' salaries withheld.

As had been the case with so many of the contested elections handled by the Senate, the body was unable to avoid partisanship in its review and deliberations. Once the dispute reached the Senate floor, Republicans, fearing the Democrats planned to use their overwhelming numbers to declare Durkin the winner, managed to hold solidly together on vote after vote. They were joined on cloture votes by enough southern Democrats to prevent the Senate from acting. The strategy did succeed in blocking action, but, when combined with the Democrats' equally staunch support of Durkin, it led to a seven-month process that left the Senate appearing partisan, confused, and ineffectual to the American public.

Sources

U.S. Congress. Senate. *Congressional Record.* 94th Cong., 1st sess. (See pp. 9–11, 13–15, 199, 200, 434–55, 596–97, 894–95, 1067–69, 1133, 1146, 1471–95, 18617, 1887–906, 18993–97, 19004–22, 19315, 19319–49, 19470, 19477, 19511–13, 19725–43, 19746–52, 20082, 20083, 20101–29, 20154–55, 20192–214, 20363–404, 20507–37, 20705, 20715–32, 20735–47, 20774, 21041–44, 21047–50, 21166, 21184–87, 21406, 21407, 21417–18, 21424–25, 21590, 21807–22, 22177, 22274–77, 22303–9, 22539–47, 22827, 22830–46, 22856, 23012–20, 23084, 23089, 23561, 23727, 23597, 23794–95, 25308–10, 25316, 25463, 25939–42, 25954–62.)

———. Senate Report No. 94–156. Parts 1 and 2. 94th Cong., 1st sess., 1975.

Cotton, Norris. *In the Senate: Amidst the Conflict and the Turmoil.* New York, 1978.

Riddick, Floyd M.: Senate Parliamentarian. Oral History Interviews, June 26, 1978, to February 15, 1979, for the Senate Historical Office. Washington, D. C. (See pp. 488–531.)

Tibbetts, Donn. *The Closest U. S. Senate Race in History: Durkin v. Wyman.* Manchester, NH, 1976.

Case 138

Edmond A. Edmondson v. Henry L. Bellmon

(1919–) (1921–)

Oklahoma

Election Case
January 9, 1975 to March 4, 1976

Issues
Campaign irregularities

Result: Bellmon retained seat

Chronology:
Petition filed: Jan. 9, 1975
Referred to committee: Jan. 14, 1975
Committee report: Jan. 27, 1976
Senate vote: Mar. 4, 1976

Background

Former Oklahoma Governor Henry L. Bellmon (R) first won election to the United States Senate in 1968. When Bellmon ran for reelection six years later, he was challenged by Democrat Edmond A. Edmondson, who had served for twenty years in the House of Representatives.

On November 5, 1974, incumbent Henry Bellmon defeated Ed Edmondson by 3,835 votes. Edmondson challenged the results on the ground that there had been improprieties in regard to the voting machines in Tulsa County. The Oklahoma supreme court ruled 9 to 0 on December 19, 1974, that, although the irregularities occurred, Edmondson had not demonstrated that they had had an impact on the outcome of the election. Once the court challenge was decided, the state went ahead and issued a certificate of election to Bellmon.

Statement of the Case

Unwilling to drop his challenge, Ed Edmondson filed a petition with the U.S. Senate on January 9, 1975. He charged violations of the laws of the state of Oklahoma and asked the Senate to accept jurisdiction over the contest. Four days later, on January 13, Henry Bellmon filed a response to the Edmondson petition together with a motion to dismiss. That same day, the Committee on Rules and Administration considered the petition, the motion and the answer and unanimously recommended to the Senate that Henry Bellmon be seated without prejudice to Edmondson's contest of the election. When the Ninety-fourth Congress convened on January 14, 1975, the Senate seated Bellmon without prejudice and referred the matter to the Committee on Rules and Administration.

Edmondson's petition and complaint challenged the voting results in Tulsa County and alleged that the following violations occurred:

1) The United States Senate contest was listed on the ballot after the state races, rather than before them as state law required.

2) The voting machines lacked devices for straight-party voting, again, contrary to law.

3) Five hundred forty-five of the 640 machines used in Tulsa County prominently displayed erroneous and misleading instructions as to straight-party voting, even though it was not possible on those machines.

Edmondson contended that, where the master Democratic party lever was missing from a voting machine, many voters had pulled the lever for the Democratic candidate for the U.S. House of Representatives, thinking it was the lever for all Democratic candidates. He pointed out that in Tulsa County Bellmon had won by 22,000 votes, while in the remaining counties Edmondson had led by 18,000 votes.

Response of the Senate

The Subcommittee on Privileges and Elections discussed the case on June 3 and then postponed further consideration until after it resolved the John Durkin-Louis Wyman election contest. It completed that matter in the summer of 1975 by declaring the New Hampshire seat vacant and calling for a new election (See Case 137). Following a staff investigation in Oklahoma in August and October 1975, the committee held hearings on the Edmondson-Bellmon case in November and December, obtaining new evidence that had not been presented to the Oklahoma supreme court. After reviewing this additional data, expert witnesses testifying on Edmondson's behalf asserted that, "but for the violations of the law, there was a high probability that Mr. Edmondson would have received sufficient votes in Tulsa County to win in the statewide election."

On December 15, 1975, the Rules and Administration Committee members voted 5 to 3, along party lines with Democrats in the majority, that they were unable to identify a winner in the disputed election. The committee therefore referred the final determination to the Senate, which could, if necessary, declare a vacancy and call a special election. Republican members of the committee complained about the party-line nature of the vote, and Bellmon's Oklahoma colleague, Dewey F. Bartlett (R) contrasted the Senate's action with the case of Dennis Chavez and Patrick Hurley in 1954 (See Case 132). In that instance, he declared, the Senate, then under Republican control, refused to disfranchise New Mexico voters simply because of the failings of election officials.

On January 27, 1976, the Rules and Administration Committee presented its report on the case to the Senate. The majority report found that irregularities and violations of Oklahoma law had occurred that could have affected the outcome of the election, because "the statutes violated were substantive in nature, affecting the franchise." The form of the irregularities made it impossible for the committee to "determine who would have won the election had the violations of law not occurred." A minority report agreed with the Oklahoma supreme court ruling that Henry Bellmon had won the election. The three Republican senators rejected Edmondson's contention that many Tulsa County voters failed to vote in the U.S. Senate race due to confusion over the misleading instructions. They pointed out that in fact 97 percent of those who voted in that county did vote in the Senate race—a higher percentage than in any other county. Charging that the majority report was "a partisan document," the minority recommended that Edmondson's challenge to the election be dismissed, because Bellmon had been duly elected by the voters of Oklahoma.

When the Senate began considering the resolution submitted by the majority on March 1, it granted Edmondson the privilege of the floor for the occasion and permitted attorneys for both parties to sit at tables in the rear of the chamber. The body also allowed the use of visual aids in the case, and two voting machines from Tulsa were brought to the floor for a demonstration, one with and one without the misleading instructions for straight-party voting. During the debate, Bellmon spoke once, asserting that the Senate would set a bad precedent if it declared the seat vacant, since there were no charges of misconduct against either candidate and Edmondson had not requested a recount. It was simply a close election, he contended, and throwing out the results could lead the losers of all close elections to appeal to the Senate.

The debate continued until March 4, when the Senate finally voted 47 to 46 to table the majority's resolution. Nine Democrats joined all Senate Republicans in voting to end the challenge against Bellmon, who had energetically lobbied his colleagues for their support. By voice vote, the Senate then agreed that Henry Bellmon should retain his seat.

Conclusion

Henry Bellmon remained in the Senate until 1981. In 1986 he was once again elected governor of Oklahoma. Ed Edmondson tried for the Senate again in 1978 but failed to win nomination.

Sources

U.S. Congress. Senate. *Congressional Record.* 94th Cong., 1st sess. (See pp. 8, 35092–93, 40871–72, 41014–20, 41104–19, 41567.) 2d sess. (See pp. 4782, 4929–56, 5144–59, 5465–69, 5472–79.)

———. Senate Report No. 94–597. 94th Cong., 2d sess., 1976.

Bellmon, Henry. *The Life and Times of Henry Bellmon.* Tulsa, OK, 1992. (See pp. 283–87.)

Case 139

Herman E. Talmadge

(1913–)

Georgia

Censure Case
May 24, 1978 to October 11, 1979

Issues
Financial misconduct

Result: Censured ("Denounced")

Chronology:
Request for investigation: May 24, 1978
Committee report: Oct. 3, 1979
Senate vote: Oct. 11, 1979

Background

In 1978, Herman E. Talmadge (D-GA) was an influential and respected senator. Initially elected to the Senate in 1956 as a proponent of states' rights, he had gained national recognition and esteem through his work on the Watergate investigation. Yet, despite Talmadge's political stature, the 1970s were a decade of personal suffering for him. His son had drowned in 1975 and his wife Betty had divorced him two years later. During the litigation over the divorce property settlement, newspaper accounts of the trial revealed a number of financial irregularities by Talmadge. When it became apparent that in five years he had written only $600.00 in checks for cash, the senator explained that he received most of his pocket money in small amounts of cash from constituents. Betty Talmadge had testified in court that her husband kept large amounts of cash in an overcoat at their home to pay for all household expenses. She also described a large stock transaction that had never been disclosed as required by law.

The Senate had changed considerably as an institution during Herman Talmadge's tenure. When he arrived in 1957, there were few laws or rules regulating senatorial conduct. But since the Thomas Dodd censure case in 1967 (See Case 135), the pace of reform had quickened. During the 1970s Congress passed more government reform legislation than at any other time in history. Responding to the Dodd case, the Senate in 1968 adopted standards of conduct and limited financial disclosure requirements for members and some Senate employees. This action was followed by passage of the 1971 Federal Election Campaign Act, which required reports on campaign contributions and expenditures and set monetary limits on media advertising.

In 1977, the Senate changed the name of the Select Committee on Standards and Conduct to the Select Committee on Ethics and formalized the mechanism for managing serious complaints. The new Ethics Committee then published its rules of procedure for responding to complaints. The multi-stage process consisted of a preliminary inquiry, initial review, and investigation with trial-type hearings. The committee also created procedures for considering specific subjects, such as sensitive materials or whether there should be media coverage of hearings. If the committee determined that a case warranted the use of outside counsel, it had the authority to hire one. The committee would then report its conclusions and recommendations to the Senate. The Talmadge case was the first conducted by the committee under these procedures.

The allegations against Herman Talmadge were the most serious made against a senator since Thomas Dodd's censure by the Senate in 1967. In fact, many of the regulations Talmadge was charged with violating had not existed at the time of the Dodd censure and had been established in response to that case.

Statement of the Case

Soon after the Select Committee on Ethics learned of the newspaper reports regarding Herman Talmadge, it determined that a preliminary inquiry was needed, in light of additional press accounts that the senator had accepted excessive reimbursement from the Senate. Then, on May 24, 1978, the senator asked the committee to review his practice of accepting small cash gifts. The committee appointed a special counsel and unanimously agreed that there was sufficient evidence to justify moving to the next stage with an initial review. In response to the newspaper articles alleging that the senator had submitted incorrect vouchers and received overpayments, both Talmadge and the committee conducted audits of his office accounts. Based on the results of the audits, Talmadge repaid the Senate $37,125.90 for excess reimbursements he had received between 1972 and 1978. On December 18, 1978, after studying the special counsel's intial report, the committee voted to conduct a full investigation of five allegations, the third stage of the process.

Prior to the hearings, Talmadge filed a number of legal motions. The most significant related to an issue that had not been resolved during the Dodd inquiry, the standard of proof applicable to evidence. Talmadge urged adopting the standard used in criminal cases, that a charge must be proven "beyond a reasonable doubt," but the committee determined that it would require only "clear and convincing evidence," the same standard used in civil cases. The senator also sought to exclude documents that had been stolen from his office by his former employee Daniel Minchew, but the committee denied this motion.

Public hearings into the charges against Herman Talmadge began on April 30, 1979, and concluded on July 12. Daniel Minchew, the senator's former administrative assistant who was the subject of a related criminal investigation, became a key committee witness. Although the committee had serious problems with Minchew's credibility, the members believed his testimony could not be totally discounted. Minchew testified that, following the senator's instructions, he had opened a secret account at Riggs Bank in which he had deposited reimbursement checks and campaign contributions. These campaign contributions were not reported as required by law. According to Minchew, proceeds from the account went to Herman Talmadge, his wife, and his son. Minchew himself had received $18,000 from the account, which he claimed was repayment for expenditures he had made on the senator's behalf. The committee members, however, believed that he had taken the money for his personal use. Both Betty Talmadge and Minchew testified that the senator habitually carried $100 bills, but Talmadge could not remember the names of any of the contributors who he claimed provided the small cash donations he used as spending money.

Because the committee had determined that the senator's testimony was essential, Talmadge agreed to appear at the hearings and also called his own witnesses. In defending his actions, Herman Talmadge stated that his office had given financial matters a "low priority," that he was unaware of the over-reimbursements, and that he had learned of the Riggs account only in 1978. He attacked the veracity of his wife and the former employee.

Response of the Senate

The committee filed its report with the Senate on October 4, 1979, finding violations or failures of administrative oversight in four areas, although the report's carefully worded conclusion failed to specify who committed the offenses. Other sections of the report, however, went considerably further in attributing to Talmadge direct knowledge or participation in the misconduct. The committee found evidence of the following wrongdoing: (1) between 1973 and 1978, the senator had submitted vouchers for and received $43,435.00 in excess reimbursements (since the vouchers were signed either by autopen or by staff members, the committee concluded that the senator had failed properly to supervise their preparation); (2) Talmadge's required financial disclosure reports were inaccurate for the years 1972 to 1977; (3) campaign finance reports mandated by the Federal Election Campaign Act were filed late for 1973, and inaccurate reports were filed in 1974; and (4) more than $10,000 in campaign funds were not reported, were deposited by the senator's campaign chairman in a bank account, and were used for non-campaign purposes, in violation of both campaign laws and a Senate rule.

Based on these findings, the committee submitted a resolution stating that the senator "knew, or should have known," about these acts and was therefore responsible for them through "the gross neglect of his duty" to oversee the administration of his office. Because this conduct tended "to bring the Senate into dishonor and disrepute," the committee voted unanimously to recommend that Talmadge be "denounced" and required to reimburse the Senate for any outstanding overpayment.

Resolutions addressing misconduct in previous cases had recommended that the Senate "censure" or "condemn" a colleague, but Herman Talmadge pressed the committee to use the term "reprimand." While not accepting this alternative, the committee explained that it had specifically avoided using the words "censure" and "condemn" because the members believed Talmadge's transgressions were substantially different from those in earlier cases. They, therefore, chose words that specifically did not depend on "analogy to dissimilar historical circumstance for interpretation." The vice chairman of the committee, Harrison Schmitt (R-NM), had urged the use of the word "censure." Although his motion was defeated, he added his separate views to the report. The Capitol Hill newspaper, *Roll Call,* reported that the Senate parliamentarian was confused about the precise meaning of the term "denounce," stating, "It's not censure and it's not reprimand.... Where it falls [between the two] I sure don't know."

In addition to proposing its resolution, the committee referred a number of possible violations of criminal law to the U.S. attorney general, but the Department of Justice issued no indictments against Herman Talmadge. The committee further recommended reforms in Senate accounting procedures, including bookkeeping, voucher procedures, use of autopens to sign vouchers, and internal audits for suspected abuse. The report also suggested that rules be adopted to define "official" and "reimbursable" expenses.

When the Senate considered the committee's proposed resolution on October 11, 1979, Talmadge was permitted to have his attorney present. After the committee chairman, Adlai E. Stevenson III (D-IL), reported on the investigation, Harrison Schmitt reviewed the evidence and reiterated his arguments that censure was the appropriate term to use in this case of serious misconduct. In all but two previous cases, the Senate had used the word censure. The two exceptions, Hiram Bingham (Case 112) and Joseph McCarthy (Case 133), were "condemned" by the Senate, but that word, Schmitt noted, "seems to have been treated by historians as tantamount to censure." Still, if the Senate adopted the committee's term, "denounced," he declared, "the strongest possible meaning" should be placed on the punishment. In response to senators' questions, Chairman Stevenson stressed that the resolution did not attribute knowledge of the wrongdoing to Talmadge but rather that "he knew or should have known."

The Senate debate demonstrated that some members still had misgivings about the Ethics Committee's process. Thomas Eagleton (D-MO), for example, commented that, while the new procedures constituted an improvement, they were very time consuming and forced committee members to serve as both judge and jury at trial-type hearings. He recommended appointing an independent outsider to conduct the hearings.

No amendments were proposed to the resolution, which the Senate debated for only one afternoon and then adopted by a vote of 81 to 15. Herman Talmadge had not contested the resolution, but after it passed, he rose and spoke. Acknowledging that he had been negligent in overseeing his office and campaign finances, he emphasized that neither the committee nor the Senate had found that he had engaged in intentional wrongdoing and that censure had not been sought. While rededicating himself to his fellow senators and to the people of Georgia, Talmadge also stated his intention to continue to serve in the Senate for a "number of years to come." When he finished, other senators expressed their friendship and support for him.

Conclusion

A traditional explanation by scholars and senators for the institutional reluctance to discipline individual members has been that the voters provide the final judgment. Herman Talmadge believed this and during the investigation declared that the charges would not affect his reelection. "The ultimate ethics committee," he maintained, "are the people of Georgia." When Talmadge sought reelection in 1980, however, he faced significant opposition in the state's Democratic primary for the first time in twenty-four years. Receiving less than 50 percent of the vote, he succeeded in winning a runoff against the state's lieutenant governor. After a fall campaign in which Talmadge's ethical conduct was a significant issue, he was defeated by the Republican candidate, Mack Mattingly. Later, in his memoir, Talmadge wrote that he regretted not having fought for full exoneration on the Senate floor.

The Talmadge case exemplifies the evolution of reforms initiated immediately before and after the Dodd case. Thomas Dodd's legal challenges had resolved key issues, establishing the committee's jurisdiction and affirming the general process. In the decade between the Dodd and Talmadge cases, the Ethics Committee was created and a code of conduct adopted, making it possible for the first time to evaluate senators' behavior against clear standards. Perhaps these changes explain the relatively brief Senate floor debate over Talmadge.

In the Talmadge case the committee resolved two other important issues. It established the standard of evidence for its work as comparable to that used in civil rather than criminal cases and set the precedent that, with or without direct knowledge, senators have ultimate responsibility for any wrongdoing related to their public office.

Sources

U.S. Congress. Senate. *Congressional Record.* 96th Cong., 1st sess. (See pp. 27766–94.)

———. Senate Report No. 96–337. 96th Cong., 1st sess., 1979.

Sherrill, Robert. "Herman Talmadge: How a Demagogue Adapts." In *Gothic Politics in the Deep South: Stars of the New Confederacy*. New York, 1968.

Talmadge, Herman E. and Mark Royden Winchell. *Talmadge: A Political Legacy, A Politician's Life*. Atlanta, 1987.

Case 140

Harrison A. Williams, Jr.

(1919–)

New Jersey

Expulsion Case
May 5, 1981 to March 11, 1982

Issues
Convicted of corruption

Result: Resigned before Senate could act

Chronology:
Inquiry begun: May 5, 1981
Committee report: Sept. 3, 1981
No Senate action

Background

In February 1980, press reports linked Harrison A. Williams, Jr. (D-NJ) to the FBI's ABSCAM sting operation and investigation of business crime and political corruption. Williams, serving in his fourth term and chairman of the Senate Committee on Labor and Human Resources, was indicted on October 30, 1980, on nine counts, including bribery, receipt of an unlawful gratuity, conflict of interest, and conspiracy to defraud the United States. At the trial in United States District Court in Brooklyn, New York, the FBI produced videotapes of Williams promising to use his influence to aid a supposed Arab sheik (impersonated by an FBI agent) in return for a multi-million dollar loan to a titanium-mining corporation in which the senator had a secret financial interest. On May 1, 1981, the jury found Williams guilty on all counts. (In other ABSCAM cases, six members of the House of Representatives were also found guilty; one, Michael "Ozzie" Myers, was expelled; two resigned; and the others were defeated for reelection.)

Statement of the Case

The Senate Select Committee on Ethics commenced a preliminary inquiry of Harrison Williams' ABSCAM involvement after the initial press reports appeared in early 1980. The committee deferred further action, however, so as not to jeopardize either the Department of Justice case or Williams' right to a fair trial, free of prejudicial publicity. Once the jury returned a guilty verdict, these reasons for deference were removed, although Williams, who steadfastly insisted that he was innocent, continued to press upon the trial judge his post-trial motions to set aside the jury verdict on grounds of procedural due process. On May 5, the committee adopted a resolution authorizing an investigation of the senator, the final, most active, stage in its multi-stage procedure. It also engaged Robert S. Bennett as special counsel. On July 14, 15, and 28, 1981, the Ethics Committee held hearings at which Williams was represented by counsel and was permitted to call and examine witnesses. "While I may have crossed over the line which divides appropriate service to constituents from excessive boasting and posturing," Williams said, "I never engaged in any illegal conduct; I never corrupted my office and I never intended to do anything that would bring dishonor to the Senate."

Despite Williams' claims, on August 24 the Ethics Committee unanimously found his conduct "ethically repugnant" and recommended his expulsion. In its report issued on September 3, the committee concluded, among other things, that he had offered to use his influence to win a government contract and that he intended to conceal his interest in the mining venture. The report declared that these and Williams' other actions tended "to bring the Senate into dishonor and disrepute, and only the most severe sanction is appropriate for such an abuse of the public trust."

In September Ethics Committee Chairman Malcolm Wallop (R-WY) announced to the Senate that debate on the resolution would begin in November. In the meantime, he had arranged for key portions of the video- and audiotapes that had been used as evidence in Williams' trial to be played in a Senate office building on several occasions, so that senators could view the evidence for themselves before voting. Stressing the gravity of the issue, Wallop repeatedly took the floor through the rest of the month and again in November to remind senators of their duty to take the time to review the tapes.

The committee report had originally recommended that the full Senate postpone action on the case until after the District Court judge ruled on the pending due process motions filed by Williams. On the other hand, the committee members believed it was bad for both the Senate and Williams himself to have Senate action delayed too long. For this reason, debate was first set for November, even though the judge had not yet ruled, then postponed until December 3. Meanwhile, on November 23, after Senate leaders rejected Williams' request to be represented by private legal counsel on the Senate floor, he filed suit against the Senate in federal court. Williams charged that the Ethics Committee acted unlawfully as investigator, judge, and jury and that the full Senate threatened to violate his constitutional right to counsel. Although District Judge Gerhard Gesell refused to issue a temporary restraining order against the Senate expulsion debate, Senate leaders did decide to postpone considering the issue so that Daniel Inouye (D-HI), who had agreed to serve as Williams' chief advocate on the floor, would have time to prepare his case. The debate was therefore rescheduled for January 1982.

On December 21, 1981, Federal District Judge George C. Pratt denied Williams' due process motions to dismiss his indictment, for judgment of acquittal (setting aside the jury verdict), and for a new trial, and on February 17, 1982, Williams was sentenced to three years in prison and fined $50,000.

Response of the Senate

After several further delays, the Senate on March 3 finally began debating whether to expel Harrison Williams. Majority Leader Howard Baker (R-TN) explained that the body would follow procedures similar to those used in the past, with committees not allowed to meet for more than two hours after the Senate convened, no other business to be transacted, and a quorum of senators actually present in the chamber.

Malcolm Wallop (R-WY) and Howell Heflin (D-AL) spoke for the Ethics Committee and Daniel Inouye served as advocate for Williams. Heflin emphasized that the committee had operated in an entirely bipartisan manner and had reached a unanimous conclusion. He contended that information presented by newspaper columnist Jack Anderson in recent weeks, alleging wrongdoing by the FBI in the case, also should not affect the Senate's action. Regardless of what the FBI had done, Williams had clearly offered to use his influence as a senator and had conspired to keep his share in the venture secret.

Harrison Williams also addressed the Senate, at great length, in his own behalf. Before he started, he offered to be placed under oath and to waive his immunity under the "Speech and Debate" clause of the Constitution (Article I, section 6), but Senate leaders objected that there was no precedent for such action, this was not an evidentiary proceeding, and such a precedent could place pressure on senators in future cases to take similar oaths. Eventually, it was agreed that Williams would simply assure the Senate that he would not use immunity as a defense if he were ever charged with perjury for statements he made in his defense on the Senate floor. Declaring his complete innocence, Williams called the recommendation for expulsion "preposterous." After describing at length how he became involved in the questionable venture, he focused on what he called the entrapment and misconduct by the government in the case.

Inouye argued that in the past expulsion from the Senate had been reserved for cases of treason, but committee member Thomas Eagleton (D-MO) retorted, "If nontreasonous behavior be the sole benchmark of fitness to serve in this body, then one must ask how fit is this body in which we serve?" Several senators, chief among them Alan Cranston (D-CA), suggested censure as a more appropriate sanction. While recognizing that Williams had acted in a "manner unbecoming a senator," Cranston explained that censure, not being irrevocable like expulsion, was more appropriate while Williams was still pursuing his appeals. Later, if all the appeals were denied, the Senate could still decide to expel him. Wallop responded, pointing out that Williams had continued his involvement in the questionable enterprise over a period of many months and that the performance of the FBI was not the question but rather Williams' conduct. Eagleton then noted that, just because Williams had not had the grace to withdraw from the Senate, "we should not perpetrate our own disgrace by asking him to stay." When it became apparent that the censure movement lacked support and that the Senate would most likely vote for expulsion, Harrison Williams resigned from the Senate on March 11, 1982.

Conclusion

Harrison Williams served twenty-one months of his three-year prison sentence and was released on January 31, 1986.

The Senate was careful to take no action against Williams until the legal process had run its course, in order not to prejudice the case. Once he had been convicted and sentenced, however, the body was prepared to move against him. Committee members made clear during the debate that, even if Williams had not been convicted, the Senate would have had every right to conduct its own review of his behavior to determine whether he had violated any Senate rules.

While Daniel Inouye was correct that the Senate had previously only expelled members for disloyalty, several senators involved in corruption cases either had resigned like Williams, or had died before the Senate could vote on expulsion.

Sources

U.S. Congress. Senate. *Congressional Record.* 97th Cong., 1st sess. (See pp. 19774, 20414, 20556–57, 21301, 21502, 21622–23, 21881, 22018–19, 27098–99, 27478, 27885, 29219–20.) 2d sess. (See pp. 3–4, 1164, 2599, 2770, 2888, 2972–3081, 3294–343, 3463–86, 3624–46, 3797–829, 3973–4006.)

———. Senate Report No. 97–187. 97th Cong., 1st sess., 1981.

———. Senate Ethics Committee, *Trial Proceedings (Trial Transcript Excerpts and Tape Recording Transcripts in the Case of The United States of America v. Harrison A. Williams, Jr.* Committee Print. 97th Cong., 1st sess. 1981, 6 vols.

Case 141

David F. Durenberger

(1934–)

Minnesota

Censure Case
September 27, 1988 to July 25, 1990

Issues
Financial misconduct

Result: Censured ("Denounced")

Chronology:
Complaint received: Sept. 27, 1988
Committee report: July 20, 1990
Senate vote: July 25, 1990

Background

On September 27, 1988, the Select Committee on Ethics received a complaint from thirty-nine members of the Minnesota Bar charging financial improprieties by David F. Durenberger (R-MN). At the time, the senator was in the midst of his third senatorial campaign.

Statement of the Case

The complaint alleged that a financial agreement between David Durenberger and Piranha Press, which had published his books *Neither Madmen Nor Messiahs* and *Prescription for Change,* violated laws and rules within the committee's jurisdiction. In fairness to Durenberger, the committee waited until after the election to look into the charges. Then, based on the initial evidence and a response it received from Durenberger, the committee voted unanimously on March 1, 1989, to proceed with a preliminary inquiry, the first stage of the Ethics Committee's three-stage process. The results of that inquiry led the committee on August 3 to move to the second stage, an initial review, and to retain as special counsel Robert S. Bennett, who had served in that capacity during the 1981 Harrison Williams investigation (See Case 140). In December 1989, during the course of the Piranha Press inquiry, Minnesota newspapers printed a number of allegations about David Durenberger's ownership and use of a Minneapolis condominium, which became the subject of a second inquiry. By May 1990, the committee had found sufficient evidence of misconduct in both instances to proceed to the third stage, a full investigation with trial-like public hearings.

The committee held hearings on June 12 and 13, 1990. In his opening statement, Durenberger spoke movingly of his personal history and problems. Then, at the close of the opening statements, the senator waived his due process rights provided by the committee, including the rights to cross-examine witnesses, call and question his own witnesses, and testify on his own behalf. Instead, he asked the committee to rely on the written record in reaching its decision. This action terminated hearings that had been expected to receive extensive media coverage. In the written record, the senator had defended himself by arguing that he had made mistakes but that he had acted in good faith with no intention of violating any rules. The committee, however, rejected this defense, based on the evidence collected by the special counsel.

The committee unanimously agreed on July 18, 1990, that David Durenberger had "abused his United States Senate office and misused United States Senate funds." In its report issued two days later, the committee found that the senator's relationship with Piranha Press had been carefully structured to circumvent the limits on the amount of honoraria income a senator could receive. In 1985, David Durenberger had signed an agreement with the Press to speak to more than one hundred organizations to promote his books. Each group paid a fee to Piranha Press, which then paid Durenberger quarterly stipends for his efforts. At that time, ethics laws contained no limits on income from stipends while there was a limit on the amount of honoraria that could be received from speaking engagements. During a two-year period, the senator received $100,000 in stipend payments for these supposedly promotional appearances. The committee concluded that the purpose of the arrangement was not to sell the books but rather to allow Durenberger to deliver speeches to organizations that invited him because of his position as senator, not as author of the books, and to collect more payment than the law permitted.

Regarding the second part of the inquiry, the report found that, from 1984 to 1989, Durenberger had devised a complex series of transactions to obscure his ownership of the Minneapolis condominium he used on his visits there. The arrangement allowed him improperly to claim government reimbursement for rent paid. He charged the government a sufficiently high rate per day for the one hundred days a year that he used the unit for business that the reimbursements covered all his annual costs for the condominium. According to the committee report, such financial practices violated both Senate rules and governmental ethics. Other violations included: failing to report on his financial disclosure forms reimbursement from forty-three organizations for travel costs for Piranha Press and trips to Boston for personal business; converting a $5,000 campaign contribution to personal use through a transfer to Piranha Press; and accepting free limousine services in Boston, thus breaking the Senate rule regulating acceptance of gifts from anyone with a direct interest in legislation before Congress.

The committee did note that, at the time of these actions, Durenberger had been under severe personal stress that had impaired his judgment, but that this fact did not excuse his conduct.

The committee submitted to the Senate a resolution stating that Durenberger's conduct "has been reprehensible" and "in violation of statutes, rules and Senate standards and acceptable norms of ethical conduct." It recommended that he be "denounced" and that he be required to reimburse the Senate for the per diem funds and to donate the excess honoraria income to charity. Before the final report was released, David Durenberger wrote to the committee asking that he be "reprimanded" rather than denounced by the full Senate. In support of his request, he cited his lack of malicious intent and the many measures he had taken to comply with ethics legislation and rules. This plea was denied, based on Special Counsel Robert Bennett's recommendation in his report to the committee. In the 1981 case of Harrison Williams, Bennett declared, he had supported expulsion because the New Jersey senator had acted with "criminal intent." Durenberger, he believed, had not. On the other hand, he contended that a reprimand or other sanction not requiring action by the full Senate would be insufficient, because Durenberger had behaved unethically by "knowingly and willfully" violating laws, rules, and Senate standards.

The report also recommended that the investigation's results be referred to the Federal Election Commission and the Department of Justice.

Response of the Senate

On July 25, 1990, the full Senate considered the committee's resolution. Because David Durenberger unexpectedly informed his colleagues at the beginning of the session that he would not contest the resolution of censure, much of the debate addressed concerns about the disciplinary process and the role of the special counsel. Howell Heflin (D-AL), chairman of the Ethics Committee, emphasized the bipartisan nature of the committee's deliberations and outlined the reasons for the panel's recommendations. He did express concern about the committee's role as prosecutor, judge, and jury. For future investigations, he suggested that the Senate might adopt a procedure similar to one that had been recently enacted by the House of Representatives, which divided the investigative and adjudicative functions into two separate subcommittees. One panel could then function as a grand jury and the other as a trial jury.

While agreeing that the committee's work had not been partisan, Trent Lott (R-MS), a committee member, urged that the investigative process be improved. The multiplicity of stages caused a case to drag on, in this instance for almost two years. Meanwhile, the accused individual remained under a cloud. Lott recommended streamlining the procedure by eliminating some of the stages. Committee Chairman Heflin, however, explained that the multistage process was actually designed to protect the individual being investigated. Under the committee's rules the two early portions of an inquiry were carried out in closed session, and only the third stage—the formal investigation and hearing—was conducted in public. In fact, on a number of occasions, he declared, the confidentiality of the procedure had protected senators against whom unjust charges had been brought with the committee. Heflin also defended the special counsel's work as following the rules established by the committee.

The debate also reflected continuing uncertainty over the terms used in disciplining members. Trent Lott addressed the choice of "denouncement" rather than "censure." Past cases, he said, showed different levels of punishment. Thus, there could be "denouncement, condemnation, censure, and expulsion by the full Senate." He indicated that the committee had chosen denouncement in order to distinguish Durenberger's from previous cases because of the mitigating circumstances and lack of venal intent. When Howell Heflin was questioned about the term, however, he responded that it fell within the parameters of censure. The differences in terminology could be subject to individual interpretation, he explained, but the point was that the Senate as a whole "acts to show its displeasure . . . its disapproval in strong language."

A number of senators praised David Durenberger's hard work and legislative accomplishments and reaffirmed their friendship and sympathy for him, while accepting the committee's decision. At the conclusion of the debate, the Senate passed the resolution denouncing Durenberger by a vote of 96 to 0. After the vote, David Durenberger addressed the Senate, stating, "For past mistakes, I ask your forgiveness. For future challenges, I need your friendship."

Conclusion

The Senate action to denounce David Durenberger did not end his difficulties. On April 20, 1993, the senator was indicted and pleaded not guilty to two felony charges related to filing false claims for reimbursement. A federal judge dismissed the indictment in December 1993, basing his ruling on the "speech and debate" clause of the Constitution (Article I, section 6) that protects senators from prosecution for actions taken in their official capacities. The Senate had submitted a brief to the court in support of Durenberger's argument that the courts could not use affidavits from third parties that he had submitted to the Ethics Committee. The judge, however, observed that the case could probably be made without using the inadmissable evidence, and a grand jury reindicted the senator on the same charges on February 25, 1994.[1] In the midst of these legal problems, Durenberger announced on September 16, 1993, that he would not seek reelection in 1994.

In 1991, as part of further changes in ethics provisions, Congress banned the acceptance of honoraria, as well as of stipends related to official position or duties. The debate in this case reflected the Senate's continuing discomfort

[1] In February 1995 the U.S. Circuit Court of Appeals for the District of Columbia ruled that Durenberger could not use the constitutional protection because he was charged with lying about his condominium on his disclosure form.

with a process that is part investigatory and part adjudicatory, as well as with the expanded role of the special counsel.

The Durenberger case also identifies some emerging issues in misconduct cases. Legal costs for both the committee and senators being investigated have increased substantially. These costs were apparently an important factor in Durenberger's decision to waive his due process rights in the committee hearing. As the number of statutes regulating congressional behavior has increased, so has the role of executive branch agencies, such as the Justice Department, in providing oversight and prosecution of members. If this trend continues, senators charged with misconduct may increasingly face indictments after the Senate completes its internal disciplinary action.

Sources

U.S. Congress. Senate. *Congressional Record.* July 25, 1990. (See pp. S10557–75 (daily edition).)

———. *Congressional Record.* August 6, 1993. (See pp. S10832–33 (daily edition).)

———. Select Committee on Ethics and the Special Counsel, Report of. Investigation of Senator David F. Durenberger. 1990) Senate Report No. 101–382, 101st Cong., 2d sess., 1990.

APPENDICES

APPENDIX A

Table of Cases by Name

APPENDIX B

Table of Election Cases by State

State	Case No.
Alabama	56, 62, 68, 98, 114
Arkansas	16, 44, 50
California	134
Connecticut	6, 12, 19
Delaware	2, 84
Florida	24, 51, 55, 80
Georgia	52, 57
Idaho	79
Illinois	21, 28, 95, 110
Indiana	30, 76, 122, 136
Iowa	29, 105
Kansas	35, 61, 72, 83
Kentucky	11, 25, 38, 42
Louisiana	45, 63, 117
Maryland	8, 49, 94, 99, 127, 130
Massachusetts	23
Michigan	102, 129
Minnesota	32, 33, 106, 116
Mississippi	53, 54, 67, 126
Missouri	65
Montana	78, 82, 89
New Hampshire	27, 71, 74, 137
New Jersey	13, 47
New Mexico	107, 118, 132
New York	73
North Carolina	59, 115
North Dakota	108, 123
Ohio	9, 75, 86
Oklahoma	138
Oregon	69, 85
Pennsylvania	1, 31, 88, 109, 113
Rhode Island	14
South Carolina	66
Tennessee	4, 48, 120, 121, 125
Texas	58, 81, 103
Utah	91
Vermont	26
Virginia	37, 46
Washington	82
West Virginia	37, 77, 87, 97, 100, 119, 124, 128
Wisconsin	96
Wyoming	82

APPENDIX C

Topical Arrangement of Cases

Election Cases (A indicates appointment case; Q indicates qualification case)

1. Albert Gallatin (PA) (1793–1794) Q
2. Kensey Johns (DE) (1794) A
4. William Blount and William Cocke (TN) (1796) Q
6. Uriah Tracy (CT) (1801) A
8. Samuel Smith (MD) (1809) A
9. Stanley Griswold (OH) (1809) Q
11. Jesse Bledsoe (KY) (1815)
12. James Lanman (CT) (1825) A
13. Ephraim Bateman (NJ) (1827–1828)
14. Elisha R. Potter v. Asher Robbins (RI) (1833–1834)
16. Ambrose H. Sevier (AR) (1837) A
19. John M. Niles (CT) (1844) Q
21. James Shields (IL) (1849) Q
23. Robert C. Winthrop (MA) (1851) A
24. David L. Yulee v. Stephen R. Mallory (FL) (1851–1852)
25. Archibald Dixon (KY) (1852) A
26. Samuel S. Phelps (VT) (1854) A
27. Jared W. Williams (NH) (1854) A
28. Lyman Trumbull (IL) (1855–1856) Q
29. James Harlan (IA) (1855–1857)
30. Henry S. Lane v. Jesse D. Bright;
    William M. McCarty v. Graham N. Fitch (IN) (1857–1859)
31. Simon Cameron (PA) (1857)
32. James Shields (MN) (1858)
33. Henry Mower Rice (MN) (1858) Q
35. Frederick P. Stanton v. James H. Lane (KS) (1861–1862) Q
37. Waitman T. Willey and John S. Carlile (VA) (1861) Q
44. William M. Fishback; Elisha Baxter; William D. Snow (AR) (1864–1866)
45. R. King Cutler; Charles Smith; Michael Hahn (LA) (1864–1865)
46. Joseph E. Segar and John C. Underwood (VA) (1865)
47. John P. Stockton (NJ) (1865–1866)
48. David T. Patterson (TN) (1866) Q
49. Phillip F. Thomas (MD) (1867–1868) Q
50. John T. Jones and Augustus H. Garland; Alexander McDonald and
    Benjamin F. Rice (AR) (1868)
51. William Marvin v. Thomas W. Osborn (FL) (1868)
52. Richard H. Whiteley and Henry P. Farrow v. Joshua Hill and H.V.M.
    Miller (GA) (1868–1871) Q
53. Adelbert Ames (MS) (1870) Q
54. Hiram Revels (MS) (1870) Q
55. Ossian B. Hart v. Abijah Gilbert (FL) (1870)
56. George Goldthwaite (AL) (1871–1872)

57. Thomas M. Norwood v. Foster Blodgett, Jr. (GA) (1871) Q
58. Joseph J. Reynolds v. Morgan C. Hamilton (TX) (1871)
59. Joseph C. Abbott v. Zebulon B. Vance and
    Matt W. Ransom (NC) (1871–1872) Q
61. Samuel C. Pomeroy and Alexander Caldwell (KS) (1872–1873)
62. Francis W. Sykes v. George E. Spencer (AL) (1872–1876)
63. Louisiana Cases: John Ray v. William L. McMillen;
    William L. McMillen, James B. Eustis, and Robert H. Marr v.
    P.B.S. Pinchback; Henry M. Spofford and Thomas C. Manning v.
    William P. Kellogg (LA) (1873–1880)
65. Lewis V. Bogy (MO) (1873)
66. David T. Corbin v. Matthew C. Butler (SC) (1877–1879)
67. L.Q.C. Lamar (MS) (1877)
68. John T. Morgan (AL) (1877)
69. La Fayette Grover (OR) (1877–1878)
71. Charles H. Bell (NH) (1879) A
72. John J. Ingalls (KS) (1879–1882)
73. Elbridge G. Lapham and Warner Miller (NY) (1881)
74. Henry W. Blair (NH) (1885) A
75. Henry B. Payne (OH) (1886)
76. David Turpie (IN) (1887–1888)
77. Daniel B. Lucas v. Charles J. Faulkner (WV) (1887) Q
78. William A. Clark v. Wilbur F. Sanders;
    Martin Maginnis v. Thomas C. Power (MT) (1890)
79. George L. Shoup, William J. McConnell, and William H. Clagett v.
    Fred T. Dubois (ID) (1890–1892)
80. Robert H.M. Davidson v. Wilkinson Call (FL) (1891–1892)
81. Horace Chilton (TX) (1891–1892) A
82. John B. Allen (WA); Asahel C. Beckwith (WY);
    Lee Mantle (MT) (1893) A
83. Joseph V. Ady v. John Martin (KS) (1893–1895)
84. Henry A. du Pont (DE) (1895–1897)
85. Henry W. Corbett (OR) (1897–1898) A
86. Marcus A. Hanna (OH) (1898–1899)
87. John T. McGraw v. Nathan B. Scott (WV) (1899–1900) Q
88. Matthew Quay (PA) (1899–1900) A
89. William A. Clark (MT) (1899–1900)
91. Reed Smoot (UT) (1903–1907) Q
94. John W. Smith (MD) (1908)
95. William Lorimer (IL) (1910–1912)
96. Isaac Stephenson (WI) (1911–1912)
97. Clarence W. Watson and William E. Chilton (WV) (1912–1913)
98. Henry D. Clayton and Franklin P. Glass (AL) (1913–1914) A
99. William Purnell Jackson v. Blair Lee (MD) (1913–1914) A
100. William E. Chilton v. Howard Sutherland (WV) (1917–1918)
102. Henry Ford v. Truman H. Newberry (MI) (1918–1922)
103. George E.B. Peddy v. Earle B. Mayfield (TX) (1923–1925)

105. Daniel F. Steck v. Smith W. Brookhart (IA) (1925–1926)
106. Magnus Johnson v. Thomas D. Schall (MN) (1925–1926)
107. Holm O. Bursum v. Sam G. Bratton (NM) (1925–1926)
108. Gerald P. Nye (ND) (1925–1926) A
109. William B. Wilson v. William S. Vare (PA) (1926–1929)
110. Frank L. Smith (IL) (1926–1928)
113. Joseph R. Grundy (PA) (1929–1930)
114. J. Thomas Heflin v. John H. Bankhead II (AL) (1931–1932)
115. George M. Pritchard v. Josiah W. Bailey (NC) (1931–1933)
116. Einar Hoidale v. Thomas D. Schall (MN) (1932–1933)
117. Huey P. Long and John H. Overton (LA) (1932–1934)
118. Dennis Chavez v. Bronson M. Cutting (NM) (1935)
119. Henry D. Hatfield v. Rush D. Holt (WV) (1935) Q
120. George L. Berry (TN) (1937) A
121. John R. Neal v. A.T. (Tom) Stewart (TN) (1939)
122. Raymond E. Willis v. Frederick Van Nuys (IN) (1939)
123. William Langer (ND) (1941–1942) Q
124. Clarence E. Martin v. Joseph Rosier (WV) (1941) A
125. John R. Neal v. A.T. (Tom) Stewart (TN) (1943)
126. Theodore G. Bilbo (MS) (1946–1947)
127. D. John Markey v. Herbert R. O'Conor (MD) (1946–1948)
128. Tom Sweeney v. Harley M. Kilgore (WV) (1947–1949)
129. Frank E. Hook v. Homer Ferguson (MI) (1949)
130. Millard Tydings v. John Marshall Butler (MD) (1950–1951)
132. Patrick J. Hurley v. Dennis Chavez (NM) (1952–1954)
134. Pierre E.G. Salinger (CA) (1964) Q
136. Richard L. Roudebush v. R. Vance Hartke (IN) (1970–1972)
137. John A. Durkin v. Louis C. Wyman (NH) (1974–1975)
138. Edmond A. Edmondson v. Henry L. Bellmon (OK) (1975–1976)

Expulsion Cases

5. William Blount (TN) (1797)
7. John Smith (OH) (1807–1808)
34. Clement C. Clay, Jr. (AL); Robert A. Toombs (GA); Jefferson Davis and Albert G. Brown (MS); Stephen R. Mallory (FL); Judah P. Benjamin (LA) (1861)
36. James M. Mason and Robert M.T. Hunter (VA); Thomas L. Clingman and Thomas Bragg (NC); James Chesnut, Jr. (SC); A.O.P. Nicholson (TN); William K. Sebastian and Charles B. Mitchel (AR); John Hemphill and Louis T. Wigfall (TX) (1861)
38. John C. Breckinridge (KY) (1861)
39. Waldo P. Johnson and Trusten Polk (MO) (1861–1862)
40. Jesse D. Bright (IN) (1861–1862)
41. Benjamin Stark (OR) (1862)
42. Lazarus W. Powell (KY) (1862)
43. James F. Simmons (RI) (1862)

64. Crédit Mobilier Scandal: James W. Patterson (NH); William B. Allison (IA); James A. Bayard, Jr. (DE); George S. Boutwell (MA); Vice President Schuyler Colfax (IN); James Harlan (IA); John A. Logan (IL); Roscoe Conkling (NY); Henry Wilson (MA) (1873)
92. Joseph R. Burton (KS) (1904–1906)
101. Robert M. La Follette (WI) (1917–1919)
131. Joseph R. McCarthy (WI) and William Benton (CT) (1951–1953)
140. Harrison A. Williams, Jr. (NJ) (1981–1982)

Censure Cases

3. Humphrey Marshall (KY) (1796)
10. Timothy Pickering (MA) (1810–1811)
15. George Poindexter (MS) (1835)
17. John Ruggles (ME) (1838)
18. Benjamin Tappan (OH) (1844)
20. John M. Clayton (DE); Spencer Jarnagin (TN); Walter T. Colquitt (GA) (1846)
22. Thomas Hart Benton (MO) and Henry S. Foote (MS) (1850)
60. Powell Clayton (AR) (1872–1873)
70. Stanley Matthews (OH) (1878–1879)
90. John L. McLaurin and Benjamin R. Tillman (SC) (1902)
93. Charles H. Dietrich (SD) (1904)
104. Burton K. Wheeler (MT) (1924)
111. Arthur R. Gould (ME) (1926–1928)
112. Hiram Bingham (CT) (1929)
133. Joseph R. McCarthy (WI) (1954)
135. Thomas J. Dodd (CT) (1966–1967)
139. Herman E. Talmadge (GA) (1978–1979)
141. David F. Durenberger (MN) (1988–1990)

APPENDIX D

Cross Reference of Case Numbers from 1972 Edition and Current Numbers

(Cases in brackets are those dropped from the present volume)

Current Numbers		1972 Numbers
1.	Albert Gallatin (PA) (1793–1794)	1
2.	Kensey Johns (DE) (1794)	2
3.	Humphrey Marshall (KY) (1796)	3
4.	William Blount and William Cocke (TN) (1796)	4
5.	William Blount (TN) (1797)	5
6.	Uriah Tracy (CT) (1801)	6
7.	John Smith (OH) (1807–1808)	7
8.	Samuel Smith (MD) (1809)	9
9.	Stanley Griswold (OH) (1809)	8
10.	Timothy Pickering (MA) (1810–1811)	10
11.	Jesse Bledsoe (KY) (1815)	11
12.	James Lanman (CT) (1825)	12
13.	Ephraim Bateman (NJ) (1827–1828)	13
[—	George Poindexter and Daniel Webster (1833) [Dropped—No Senate action; not referred to committee]	14]
14.	Elisha R. Potter v. Asher Robbins (RI) (1833–1834)	15
15.	George Poindexter (MS) (1835)	16
16.	Ambrose H. Sevier (AR) (1837)	17
17.	John Ruggles (ME) (1838)	18
18.	Benjamin Tappan (OH) (1844)	20
19.	John M. Niles (CT) (1844)	19
20.	John M. Clayton (DE); Spencer Jarnagin (TN); Walter T. Colquitt (GA) (1846)	21
21.	James Shields (IL) (1849)	22
22.	Thomas Hart Benton (MO) and Henry S. Foote (MS) (1850)	23
23.	Robert C. Winthrop (MA) (1851)	24
24.	David L. Yulee v. Stephen R. Mallory (FL) (1851–1852)	25
25.	Archibald Dixon (KY) (1852)	26
26.	Samuel S. Phelps (VT) (1854)	27
27.	Jared W. Williams (NH) (1854)	28
[—	John J. Crittenden (1855) [Dropped—No Senate action; not referred to committee]	29]
28.	Lyman Trumbull (IL) (1855–1856)	30
29.	James Harlan (IA) (1855–1857)	31
30.	Henry S. Lane v. Jesse D. Bright; William M. McCarty v. Graham N. Fitch (IN) (1857–1859)	32
31.	Simon Cameron (PA) (1857)	33
32.	James Shields (MN) (1858)	35

Current Numbers		1972 Numbers
33.	Henry Mower Rice (MN) (1858)	34
[—	Louis T. Wigfall (1861) TX [Now combined with Case 36]	36]
34.	Clement C. Clay, Jr. (AL); Robert A. Toombs (GA); Jefferson Davis and Albert G. Brown (MS); Stephen R. Mallory (FL); Judah P. Benjamin (LA) (1861)	37
35.	Frederick P. Stanton v. James H. Lane (KS) (1861–1862)	46
36.	James M. Mason and Robert M.T. Hunter (VA); Thomas L. Clingman and Thomas Bragg (NC); James Chesnut, Jr. (SC); A.O.P. Nicholson (TN); William K. Sebastian and Charles B. Mitchel (AR); John Hemphill and Louis T. Wigfall (TX) (1861)	38
37.	Waitman T. Willey and John S. Carlile (VA) (1861)	39
38.	John C. Breckinridge (KY) (1861)	40
39.	Waldo P. Johnson and Trusten Polk (MO) (1861–1862)	42 and 43
40.	Jesse D. Bright (IN) (1861–1862)	41
41.	Benjamin Stark (OR) (1862)	47
42.	Lazarus W. Powell (KY) (1862)	44
43.	James F. Simmons (RI) (1862)	45
44.	William M. Fishback; Elisha Baxter; William D. Snow (AR) (1864–1866)	48
45.	R. King Cutler and Charles Smith; Michael Hahn (LA) (1864–1865)	49
46.	Joseph E. Segar and John C. Underwood (VA) (1865)	50
47.	John P. Stockton (NJ) (1865–1866)	51
48.	David T. Patterson (TN) (1866)	52
49.	Phillip F. Thomas (MD) (1867–1868)	53
50.	John T. Jones and Augustus H. Garland v. Alexander McDonald and Benjamin F. Rice (AR) (1868)	54
51.	William Marvin v. Thomas W. Osborn (FL) (1868)	55
52.	Richard H. Whiteley and Henry P. Farrow v. Joshua Hill and H.V.M. Miller (GA) (1868–1871)	56
53.	Adelbert Ames (MS) (1870)	57
54.	Hiram Revels (MS) (1870)	59
55.	Ossian B. Hart v. Abijah Gilbert (FL) (1870)	58
56.	George Goldthwaite (AL) (1871–1872)	62
57.	Thomas M. Norwood v. Foster Blodgett, Jr. (GA) (1871)	60
58.	Joseph J. Reynolds v. Morgan C. Hamilton (TX) (1871)	61
59.	Joseph C. Abbott v. Zebulon B. Vance and Matt W. Ransom (NC) (1871–1872)	63
60.	Powell Clayton (AR) (1872–1873)	64
61.	Samuel C. Pomeroy and Alexander Caldwell (KS) (1872–1873)	65
[—	William L. McMillen (1873) [Dropped—no separate referral to committee; No Senate action]	75]
62.	Francis W. Sykes v. George E. Spencer (AL) (1872–1876)	76
63.	Louisiana Cases: John Ray v. William L. McMillen; William L. McMillen, James B. Eustis, and Robert H. Marr v. P.B.S. Pinchback; Henry M. Spofford and Thomas C. Manning v. William P. Kellogg (LA) (1873–1880)	77

APPENDIX E
Committees to Which Cases Referred

Year	Name and Number	Committee
1793	Gallatin (1)	Committee of Elections
1794	Gallatin (1) cont.	Committee of Elections
	Johns (2)	Committee of Elections
1796	Marshall (3)	specially appointed
	Blount / Cocke (4)	no committee
1797	Blount (5)	specially appointed
1801	Tracy (6)	no committee
1807–1808	J. Smith (7)	specially appointed
1809	S. Smith (8)	no committee
	Griswold (9)	specially appointed
1810–1811	Pickering (10)	no committee
1815	Bledsoe (11)	no committee
1825	Lanman (12)	specially appointed
1827–1828	Bateman (13)	specially appointed
1833–1834	Potter / Robbins (14)	specially appointed
1835	Poindexter (15)	specially appointed
1837	Sevier (16)	Judiciary
1838	Ruggles (17)	specially appointed
1844	Tappan (18)	specially appointed
	Niles (19)	specially appointed
1846	Clayton / Jarnagin / Colquitt (20)	specially appointed
1849	Shields (21)	specially appointed
1850	Foote / Benton (22)	specially appointed
1851	Winthrop (23)	Judiciary
	Yulee / Mallory (24)	specially appointed

Year	Name and Number	Committee
1852	Yulee / Mallory (24) cont.	specially appointed
	Dixon (25)	no committee
1854	Phelps (26)	Judiciary
	Williams (27)	Judiciary
1855	Trumbull (28)	Judiciary
	Harlan (29)	Judiciary
1856	Trumbull (28) cont.	Judiciary
	Harlan (29) cont.	Judiciary
1857	Harlan (29) cont.	Judiciary
	H.S. Lane / Bright / McCarty / Fitch (30)	Judiciary
	Cameron (31)	Judiciary
1858	H.S. Lane / Bright et al. (30) cont.	Judiciary
	Shields (32)	Judiciary
	Rice (33)	Military Affairs and Militia
1859	H.S. Lane / Bright et al. (30) cont.	Judiciary
1861	Clay / Toombs / Davis / Brown / Mallory / Benjamin (34)	no committee
	Stanton / J.H. Lane (35)	Judiciary
	Mason / Hunter / Clingman / Bragg / Chesnut / Nicholson / Sebastian / Hemphill / Wigfall (36)	no committee
	Willey / Carlile (37)	no committee
	Breckinridge (38)	no committee
	Johnson / Polk (39)	Judiciary
	Bright (40)	Judiciary
1862	Stanton / J.H. Lane (35) cont.	Judiciary
	Johnson / Polk (39) cont.	Judiciary
	Bright (40) cont.	Judiciary
	Stark (41)	Judiciary and specially appointed
	Powell (42)	Judiciary
	Simmons (43)	Judiciary
1864	Fishback / Baxter / Snow (44)	Judiciary
	Cutler / C. Smith / Hahn (45)	Judiciary
1865	Fishback / Baxter / Snow (44) cont.	Judiciary
	Cutler / C. Smith / Hahn (45) cont.	Judiciary
	Segar / Underwood (46)	no committee
	Stockton (47)	Judiciary

Year	Name and Number	Committee
1866	Fishback / Baxter / Snow (44) cont.	Judiciary
	Stockton (47) cont.	Judiciary
	D. Patterson (48)	Judiciary
1867	Thomas (49)	Judiciary
1868	Thomas (49) cont.	Judiciary
	Jones / Garland / McDonald / Rice (50)	no committee
	Marvin / Osborn (51)	no committee
	Whiteley / Farrow / Hill / Miller (52)	Judiciary
1869	Whiteley / Farrow / Hill / Miller (52) cont.	Judiciary
1870	Whiteley / Farrow / Hill / Miller (52) cont.	Judiciary
	Ames (53)	Judiciary
	Revels (54)	no committee
	Hart / Gilbert (55)	Judiciary
1871	Whiteley / Farrow / Hill / Miller (52) cont.	Judiciary
	Goldthwaite (56)	Privileges and Elections
	Norwood / Blodgett (57)	Privileges and Elections
	Reynolds / Hamilton (58)	Privileges and Elections
	Abbott / Vance / Ransom (59)	Privileges and Elections
1872	Goldthwaite (56) cont.	Privileges and Elections
	Abbott / Vance / Ransom (59) cont.	Privileges and Elections
	P. Clayton (60)	specially appointed
	Pomeroy / Caldwell (61)	Privileges and Elections and specially appointed
	Sykes / Spencer (62)	Privileges and Elections
1873	P. Clayton (60) cont.	specially appointed
	Pomeroy / Caldwell (61) cont.	Privileges and Elections and specially appointed
	Sykes / Spencer (62) cont.	Privileges and Elections
	Louisiana Cases (63)	Privileges and Elections
	Crédit Mobilier (64)	specially appointed
	Bogy (65)	Privileges and Elections
1874–1876	Sykes / Spencer (62) cont.	Privileges and Elections
	Louisiana Cases (63) cont.	Privileges and Elections
1877	Louisiana Cases (63) cont.	Privileges and Elections
	Corbin / Butler (66)	Privileges and Elections
	Lamar (67)	no committee
	Morgan (68)	no committee
	Grover (69)	Privileges and Elections

Year	Name and Number	Committee
1878	Louisiana Cases (63) cont.	Privileges and Elections
	Corbin / Butler (66) cont.	Privileges and Elections
	Grover (69) cont.	Privileges and Elections
	Mathews (70)	specially appointed
1879	Louisiana Cases (63) cont.	Privileges and Elections
	Corbin / Butler (66) cont.	Privileges and Elections
	Mathews (70) cont.	specially appointed
	Bell (71)	Privileges and Elections
	Ingalls (72)	Privileges and Elections
1880	Louisiana Cases (63) cont.	Privileges and Elections
	Ingalls (72) cont.	Privileges and Elections
1881	Lapham / Miller (73)	Privileges and Elections
1885	Blair (74)	no committee
1886	Payne (75)	Privileges and Elections
1887	Turpie (76)	Privileges and Elections
	Lucas / Faulkner (77)	Privileges and Elections
1888	Turpie (76) cont.	Privileges and Elections
1890	Clark / Sanders / McGinnis / Power (78)	Privileges and Elections
	Shoup / McConnell / Clagett / Dubois (79)	Privileges and Elections
1891	Shoup et al. (79) cont.	Privileges and Elections
	Davidson / Call (80)	Privileges and Elections
	H. Chilton (81)	Privileges and Elections
1892	Shoup et al. (79) cont.	Privileges and Elections
	Davidson / Call (80) cont.	Privileges and Elections
	H. Chilton (81) cont.	Privileges and Elections
1893	Allen / Beckwith / Mantle (82)	Privileges and Elections
	Ady / Martin (83)	Privileges and Elections
1894	Ady / Martin (83) cont.	Privileges and Elections
1895	Ady / Martin (83) cont.	Privileges and Elections
	du Pont (84)	Privileges and Elections
1896	du Pont (84) cont.	Privileges and Elections
1897	du Pont (84) cont.	Privileges and Elections
	Corbett (85)	Privileges and Elections

Year	Name and Number	Committee
1898	Corbett (85) cont.	Privileges and Elections
	Hanna (86)	Privileges and Elections
1899	Hanna (86) cont.	Privileges and Elections
	McGraw / Scott (87)	Privileges and Elections
	Quay (88)	Privileges and Elections
	Clark (89)	Privileges and Elections
1900	McGraw / Scott (87) cont.	Privileges and Elections
	Quay (88) cont.	Privileges and Elections
	Clark (89) cont.	Privileges and Elections
1902	McLaurin / Tillman (90)	Privileges and Elections
1903	Smoot (91)	Privileges and Elections
1904	Smoot (91) cont.	Privileges and Elections
	Burton (92)	Privileges and Elections
	Dietrich (93)	specially appointed
1905–1906	Smoot (91) cont.	Privileges and Elections
	Burton (92) cont.	Privileges and Elections
1907	Smoot (91) cont.	Privileges and Elections
1908	J.W. Smith (94)	no committee
1910	Lorimer (95)	Privileges and Elections and specially appointed
1911	Lorimer (95) cont.	Privileges and Elections and specially appointed
	Stephenson (96)	Privileges and Elections
1912	Lorimer (95) cont.	Privileges and Elections and specially appointed
	Stephenson (96) cont.	Privileges and Elections
	Watson / W.E. Chilton (97)	Privileges and Elections
1913	Watson / W.E. Chilton (97) cont.	Privileges and Elections
	H.D. Clayton / Glass (98)	Privileges and Elections
	Jackson / Lee (99)	Privileges and Elections
1914	H.D. Clayton / Glass (98) cont.	Privileges and Elections
	Jackson / Lee (99) cont.	Privileges and Elections
1917	W.E. Chilton / Sutherland (100)	Privileges and Elections
	La Follette (101)	Privileges and Elections

Year	Name and Number	Committee
1918	W.E. Chilton / Sutherland (100) cont.	Privileges and Elections
	La Follette (101) cont.	Privileges and Elections
	Ford / Newberry (102)	Privileges and Elections
1919	La Follette (101) cont.	Privileges and Elections
	Ford / Newberry (102) cont.	Privileges and Elections
1920–1922	Ford / Newberry (102) cont.	Privileges and Elections
1923	Peddy / Mayfield (103)	Privileges and Elections
1924	Peddy / Mayfield (103) cont.	Privileges and Elections
	Wheeler (104)	specially appointed
1925	Peddy / Mayfield (103) cont.	Privileges and Elections
	Steck / Brookhart (105)	Privileges and Elections
	Johnson / Schall (106)	Privileges and Elections
	Bursom / Bratton (107)	Privileges and Elections
	Nye (108)	Privileges and Elections
1926	Steck / Brookhart (105) cont.	Privileges and Elections
	Johnson / Schall (106) cont.	Privileges and Elections
	Bursum / Bratton (107) cont.	Privileges and Elections
	Nye (108) cont.	Privileges and Elections
	Wilson / Vare (109)	Privileges and Elections and specially appointed
	F.L. Smith (110)	Privileges and Elections and specially appointed
	Gould (111)	Privileges and Elections
1927	Wilson / Vare (109) cont.	Privileges and Elections and specially appointed
	F.L. Smith (110) cont.	Privileges and Elections and specially appointed
	Gould (111) cont.	Privileges and Elections
1928	Wilson / Vare (109) cont.	Privileges and Elections and specially appointed
	F.L. Smith (110) cont.	Privileges and Elections and specially appointed
1929	Wilson / Vare (109) cont.	Privileges and Elections and specially appointed
	Bingham (112)	Judiciary
	Grundy (113)	Privileges and Elections

Year	Name and Number	Committee
1930	Grundy (113) cont.	Privileges and Elections
1931	Heflin / Bankhead (114)	Privileges and Elections
	Pritchard / Bailey (115)	Privileges and Elections
1932	Heflin / Bankhead (114) cont.	Privileges and Elections
	Pritchard / Bailey (115) cont.	Privileges and Elections
	Hoidale / Schall (116)	Privileges and Elections
	Long / Overton (117)	Privileges and Elections and Judiciary
1933	Pritchard / Bailey (115) cont.	Privileges and Elections
	Hoidale / Schall (116) cont.	Privileges and Elections
	Long / Overton (117) cont.	Privileges and Elections and Judiciary
1934	Long / Overton (117) cont.	Privileges and Elections and Judiciary
1935	Chavez / Cutting (118)	Privileges and Elections
	Hatfield / Holt (119)	Privileges and Elections
1937	Berry (120)	Privileges and Elections
1939	Neal / Stewart (121)	Privileges and Elections
	Willis / Van Nuys (122)	Privileges and Elections
1941	Langer (123)	Privileges and Elections
	Martin / Rosier (124)	Privileges and Elections
1942	Langer (123) cont.	Privileges and Elections
1943	Neal / Stewart (125)	Privileges and Elections
1946	Bilbo (126)	Special Nat. Defense and Spec. Campaign
	Markey / O'Conor (127)	Rules and Administration
1947	Bilbo (126) cont.	Spec. Nat. Defense and Spec. Campaign
	Markey / O'Conor (127) cont.	Rules and Administration
	Sweeney / Kilgore (128)	Rules and Administration
1948	Markey / O'Conor (127) cont.	Rules and Administration
	Sweeney / Kilgore (128) cont.	Rules and Administration
1949	Sweeney / Kilgore (128) cont.	Rules and Administration
	Hook / Ferguson (129)	Rules and Administration

Year	Name and Number	Committee
1950	Tydings / Butler (130)	Rules and Administration
1951	Tydings / Butler (130) cont.	Rules and Administration
	McCarthy / Benton (131)	Rules and Administration
1952	McCarthy / Benton (131) cont.	Rules and Administration
	Hurley / Chavez (132)	Rules and Administration
1953	McCarthy / Benton (131) cont.	Rules and Administration
	Hurley / Chavez (132) cont.	Rules and Administration
1954	Hurley / Chavez (132) cont.	Rules and Administration
	McCarthy (133)	specially appointed
1964	Salinger (134)	Rules and Administration
1966–1967	Dodd (135)	Standards and Conduct
1970–1972	Roudebush / Hartke (136)	no committee
1974	Durkin / Wyman (137)	Rules and Administration
1975	Durkin / Wyman (137) cont.	Rules and Administration
	Edmondson / Bellmon (138)	Rules and Administration
1976	Edmondson / Bellmon (138) cont.	Rules and Administration
1978–1979	Talmadge (139)	Ethics
1981–1982	Williams (140)	Ethics
1988–1990	Durenberger (141)	Ethics

APPENDIX F
State Abbreviations

AL	Alabama	MT	Montana
AK	Alaska	NE	Nebraska
AZ	Arizona	NV	Nevada
AR	Arkansas	NH	New Hampshire
CA	California	NJ	New Jersey
CO	Colorado	NM	New Mexico
CT	Connecticut	NY	New York
DE	Delaware	NC	North Carolina
FL	Florida	ND	North Dakota
GA	Georgia	OH	Ohio
HI	Hawaii	OK	Oklahoma
ID	Idaho	OR	Oregon
IL	Illinois	PA	Pennsylvania
IN	Indiana	RI	Rhode Island
IA	Iowa	SC	South Carolina
KS	Kansas	SD	South Dakota
KY	Kentucky	TN	Tennessee
LA	Louisiana	TX	Texas
ME	Maine	UT	Utah
MD	Maryland	VT	Vermont
MA	Massachusetts	VA	Virginia
MI	Michigan	WA	Washington
MN	Minnesota	WV	West Virginia
MS	Mississippi	WI	Wisconsin
MO	Missouri	WY	Wyoming

APPENDIX G
Political Party Abbreviations

Adams	Adams
Adams-Clay F	Adams-Clay Federalist
Adams-Clay R	Adams-Clay Republican
AJ	Anti-Jackson
Am	American (Know-Nothing)
Anti-Admin	Anti-Administration
C	Conservative
CRR	Crawford Republican
D	Democrat
F	Federalist
FL	Farmer-Labor
FS	Free Soil
I	Independent
ID	Independent Democrat
IR	Independent Republican
J	Jacksonian
JR	Jacksonian Republican
L	Liberty
LO	Law and Order
LR	Liberal Republican
N	Nullifier
NR	National Republican
OP	Opposition
PO	Populist
PR	Progressive
Pro-Admin	Pro-Administration
R	Republican [1]
RA	Readjuster
S	Silver
SR	Silver Republican
U	Unionist
UU	Unconditional Unionist
W	Whig

[1] Refers to two different parties widely separated in time: Jeffersonian Republicans of the late eighteenth and early nineteenth centuries, and the present Republican party, which was founded in the 1850s. The dates of the case in question should make clear which of the two parties is intended.

Index[1]

(Arabic numerals refer to case numbers; small roman numerals are page numbers in Introduction.)

Case No.

[1] In general, only the names of principals in cases are included. Other individuals, such as presidents of the United States, carry explanatory phrases; for example, senators who took a lead in debate on a case are indicated with "remarks by."